2004
YEAR BOOK OF
VASCULAR SURGERY®

The 2004 Year Book Series

Year Book of Allergy, Asthma, and Clinical Immunology™: Drs Rosenwasser, Boguniewicz, Milgrom, Routes, and Spahn

Year Book of Anesthesiology and Pain Management™: Drs Chestnut, Abram, Black, Lang, Roizen, Trankina, and Wood

Year Book of Cardiology®: Drs Gersh, Cheitlin, Graham, Kaplan, Sundt, and Waldo

Year Book of Critical Care Medicine®: Drs Dellinger, Parrillo, Balk, Bekes, Dries, and Roberts

Year Book of Dentistry®: Drs Zakariasen, Boghosian, Burgess, Hatcher, Horswell, McIntyre, and Zakariasen

Year Book of Dermatology and Dermatologic Surgery™: Drs Thiers and Lang

Year Book of Diagnostic Radiology®: Drs Osborn, Birdwell, Dalinka, Gardiner, Groskin, Levy, Maynard, and Oestreich

Year Book of Emergency Medicine®: Drs Burdick, Cone, Cydulka, Hamilton, Handly, and Quintana

Year Book of Endocrinology®: Drs Mazzaferri, Becker, Kannan, Kennedy, Kreisberg, Meikle, Molitch, Osei, Poehlman, and Rogol

Year Book of Family Practice®: Drs Bowman, Apgar, Dexter, Miser, Neill, and Scherger

Year Book of Gastroenterology™: Drs Lichtenstein, Dempsey, Ginsberg, Katzka, Kochman, Morris, Nunes, Reddy, Rosato, and Stein

Year Book of Hand Surgery®: Drs Berger and Ladd

Year Book of Medicine®: Drs Barkin, Frishman, Klahr, Loehrer, Mazzaferri, Phillips, Pillinger, and Snydman

Year Book of Neonatal and Perinatal Medicine®: Drs Fanaroff, Maisels, and Stevenson

Year Book of Neurology and Neurosurgery®: Drs Gibbs and Verma

Year Book of Nuclear Medicine®: Drs Coleman, Blaufox, Royal, Strauss, and Zubal

Year Book of Obstetrics, Gynecology, and Women's Health®: Drs Mishell, Kirschbaum, and Miller

Year Book of Oncology®: Drs Loehrer, Arceci, Glatstein, Gordon, Morrow, Schiller, and Thigpen

Year Book of Ophthalmology®: Drs Rapuano, Cohen, Eagle, Grossman, Myers, Nelson, Penne, Regillo, Sergott, Shields, and Tipperman

Year Book of Orthopedics®: Drs Morrey, Beauchamp, Peterson, Swiontkowski, Trigg, and Yaszemski

Year Book of Otolaryngology-Head and Neck Surgery®: Drs Paparella, Keefe, and Otto

Year Book of Pathology and Laboratory Medicine®: Drs Raab, Grzybicki, Bejarano, Bissell, and Stanley

Year Book of Pediatrics®: Dr Stockman

Year Book of Plastic and Aesthetic Surgery™: Drs Miller, Bartlett, Garner, McKinney, Ruberg, Salisbury, and Smith

Year Book of Psychiatry and Applied Mental Health®: Drs Talbott, Ballenger, Frances, Jensen, Markowitz, Meltzer, and Simpson

Year Book of Pulmonary Disease®: Drs Phillips, Barker, Blanchard, Dunlap, Lewis, and Maurer

Year Book of Rheumatology, Arthritis, and Musculoskeletal Disease™: Drs Panush, Hadler, Hellmann, Hochberg, Lahita, and Seibold

Year Book of Sports Medicine®: Drs Shephard, Alexander, Cantu, Nieman, Sanborn, and Shrier

Year Book of Surgery®: Drs Copeland, Bland, Cerfolio, Daly, Eberlein, Howard, Luce, Mozingo, and Seeger

Year Book of Urology®: Drs Andriole and Coplen

Year Book of Vascular Surgery®: Dr Moneta

2004

The Year Book of VASCULAR SURGERY®

Editor-in-Chief
Gregory L. Moneta, MD
Professor of Surgery, Chief of Vascular Surgery, Oregon Health & Science University, Oregon Health & Science University Hospital, Portland VA Medical Center, Portland, Oregon

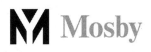 Mosby

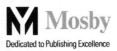

Dedicated to Publishing Excellence

Vice President, Continuity Publishing: Timothy M. Griswold
Developmental Editor: Beth Martz
Senior Manager, Continuity Production: Idelle L. Winer
Senior Issue Manager: Pat Costigan
Composition Specialist: Betty Dockins
Illustrations and Permissions Coordinator: Kimberly E. Hulett

2004 EDITION

Printed in the United States of America
Composition by Thomas Technology Solutions, Inc.
Printing/binding by Sheridan Books, Inc

Editorial Office:
Elsevier
300 East
170 South Independence Mall West
Philadelphia, PA 19106-3399

International Standard Serial Number: 0749-4041
International Standard Book Number: 0-323-02067-4

Contributors

Daniel G. Clair, MD

Assistant Professor of Surgery, Columbia and Cornell Universities, Columbia Campus Site Chief, New York Presbyterian Division of Vascular Surgery, New York, New York

Roy M. Fujitani, MD

Associate Professor of Surgery and Chief, Division of Vascular Surgery, University of California Irvine Medical Center, Orange, California

Randolph L. Geary, MD

Department of General Surgery, Wake Forest University School of Medicine, Winston-Salem, North Carolina

Larry W. Kraiss, MD

Associate Professor of Surgery and Interim Chief, Division of Vascular Surgery, University of Utah School of Medicine, Salt Lake City, Utah

Timothy K. Liem, MD

Clinical Assistant Professor of Surgery, Oregon Health & Science University; Attending Surgeon, Legacy Emanuel Hospital/Oregon Health & Science University, Portland, Oregon

Frank B. Pomposelli, Jr, MD

Clinical Chief of Vascular Surgery, Beth Israel Deaconess Medical Center, Boston, Massachusetts

Michael T. Watkins, MD

Associate Professor of Surgery, Harvard Medical School; Director, Vascular Surgery Research Laboratories, Massachusetts General Hospital, Boston, Massachusetts

Table of Contents

Journals Represented

Mosby and its editors survey approximately 500 journals for its abstract and commentary publications. From these journals, the editors select the articles to be abstracted. Journals represented in this YEAR BOOK are listed below.

Acta Neurologica Scandinavica
American Journal of Cardiology
American Journal of Epidemiology
American Journal of Human Genetics
American Journal of Hypertension
American Journal of Kidney Diseases
American Journal of Medicine
American Journal of Neuroradiology
American Journal of Physiology
American Journal of Roentgenology
American Journal of Surgery
American Surgeon
Annals of Internal Medicine
Annals of Surgery
Annals of Thoracic Surgery
Annals of Vascular Surgery
Archives of Neurology
Archives of Surgery
Arthroscopy
British Journal of Surgery
British Journal of Urology International
Cardiovascular Surgery
Chest
Circulation
Clinical Infectious Diseases
Clinical Radiology
Contraception
Diabetes
Diabetic Medicine
European Journal of Radiology
European Journal of Surgery
European Journal of Vascular and Endovascular Surgery
Journal of Applied Physiology
Journal of Internal Medicine
Journal of Neurosurgery
Journal of Surgical Research
Journal of Thoracic and Cardiovascular Surgery
Journal of Urology
Journal of Vascular Surgery
Journal of the American Geriatrics Society
Journal of the American Medical Association
Kidney International
Lancet
Mayo Clinic Proceedings
Medicine and Science in Sports and Exercise
Nephrology, Dialysis, Transplantation
Neurosurgery

New England Journal of Medicine
Pain
Pharmacotherapy
Plastic and Reconstructive Surgery
Radiology
Spine
Stroke
Surgery
Surgical Neurology
Thrombosis Research
Vascular Medicine
Vascular and Endovascular Surgery
World Journal of Surgery

STANDARD ABBREVIATIONS

The following terms are abbreviated in this edition: acquired immunodeficiency syndrome (AIDS), cardiopulmonary resuscitation (CPR), central nervous system (CNS), cerebrospinal fluid (CSF), computed tomography (CT), deoxyribonucleic acid (DNA), electrocardiography (ECG), health maintenance organization (HMO), human immunodeficiency virus (HIV), intensive care unit (ICU), intramuscular (IM), intravenous (IV), magnetic resonance (MR) imaging (MRI), ribonucleic acid (RNA), and ultrasound (US).

NOTE

The YEAR BOOK OF VASCULAR SURGERY® is a literature survey service providing abstracts of articles published in the professional literature. Every effort is made to assure the accuracy of the information presented in these pages. Neither the editors nor the publisher of the YEAR BOOK OF VASCULAR SURGERY® can be responsible for errors in the original materials. The editors' comments are their own opinions. Mention of specific products within this publication does not constitute endorsement.

To facilitate the use of the YEAR BOOK OF VASCULAR SURGERY® as a reference tool, all illustrations and tables included in this publication are now identified as they appear in the original article. This change is meant to help the reader recognize that any illustration or table appearing in the YEAR BOOK OF VASCULAR SURGERY® may be only one of many in the original article. For this reason, figure and table numbers will often appear to be out of sequence within the YEAR BOOK OF VASCULAR SURGERY®.

Introduction

The 2004 YEAR BOOK OF VASCULAR SURGERY contains abstracts and commentary of 288 scientific articles. Some are more "scientific" than others and, of course, not all are pivotal works. Some, however, are of obvious importance, some may seem to be important but will prove to be worthless, and others that are truly important have been "ignored" by the editor (me). I am not always as insightful as I would like to think. If you feel your article has been slighted by the fact that it was not in this year's YEAR BOOK, you should not feel alone. I review many thousands of articles for possible inclusion in the YEAR BOOK OF VASCULAR SURGERY. Selections reflect some editorial bias. In fact, selections reflect a good deal of editorial bias. While some authors may have an exaggerated perception of the importance of their work, it is clearly also possible that I am insufficiently informed to make a perfect decision on all possible articles. If a particular article is not included, it is not because I disagree with the author, or don't like the author. It is simply because choices and decisions have to be made, and not all choices and decisions prove to be correct in the long run. I will say, however, while clearly not every article in this year's YEAR BOOK will stand the test of time as to its importance, all are interesting given the current status of knowledge of vascular disease and its therapies.

I continue to be impressed with the diversity and overall high quality of publications related to vascular surgery and vascular disease. While some credit must be given to the editors and editorial boards of the journals, the majority of the credit goes to the authors. It is my guess that much of the research and many of the manuscripts involve a large component of "after 6" and "weekend" effort on the part of the primary authors. This type of extraordinary effort is often not sufficiently acknowledged or appreciated. It usually does not pay the bills and always cuts into time for family and recreation. It is, however, a mark of a professional to endeavor to contribute to their field simply because it is the right thing to do. Physicians are successful people. With success inevitably comes responsibility. Taking care of patients is important, but all physicians also have a responsibility to take care of medicine.

I continue to be interested in the science of vascular disease. As I have previously acknowledged, I myself am not a scientist. Perhaps for that reason I greatly admire those who are scientists. Science and laboratory work will provide the foundation for progress that will ultimately benefit patients. Those who substantially contribute to the understanding of the genetics and molecular biology of vascular disease will ultimately benefit far more patients than most of us ever will by operating 3 or 4 days a week.

There are clearly some trends in the basic research of vascular disease. The availability of genetic microarrays is resulting in many studies examining the relative expression of various genes in different types of vascular disease. The role of infectious agents and serum markers in the genesis and prognosis of atherosclerotic disease, as well as the basic biology of atherosclerosis, continue to be of interest. The field of therapeutic angiogenesis, however, at least for the time being, has been a disappointment. Clinical applications of enhanced angiogenesis as a treatment for critical ischemia have been promised for years but thus far have not appeared. It appears that inhibition of angiogenesis as a treatment for cancer, rather than promotion of angiogenesis as a treatment for arterial disease, is more likely to be clinically useful in the foreseeable future.

Over 25,000 people a year in the United States die a potentially preventable death from aortic disease. An encouraging trend is that in the last year or 2, aortic disease seems to be gradually gaining a greater level of public awareness. A *Wall Street Journal* front page article in the fall of 2003 focused on problems with diagnosis and treatment of thoracic and abdominal aortic disease. At Frank Veith's November 2003 New York symposium, former senator Bob Dole gave a speech emphasizing the need for physician education regarding aortic disease. It is therefore appropriate that endovascular therapy of the aorta has remained a hot topic and be featured prominently in the 2004 YEAR BOOK OF VASCULAR SURGERY.

We are continuing to learn more about the complications and details of aortic endografting. Articles in this year's YEAR BOOK highlight the importance of preserving pelvic flow in patients with aortic endografts, the possibility of limiting radiation exposure during implantation of these grafts, and the complications of migration, kinking, and other conformational changes of the graft and the native aorta over time. One of the first reports of the Lifeline Registry for aortic endografts is included in this year's YEAR BOOK. I am, however, waiting for convincing evidence that aortic stent grafts are effective in community practice. We need to know what the patients are like that are actually getting these grafts in community practice. Certainly, there are high-volume community practices of aortic endografting. These practices must provide us the technical and long-term results of their procedures. Aortic endografts are heavily promoted by industry, and industry targets community practice. After all, that is where most of the money will be made. I hope in future editions of the YEAR BOOK the results of widespread application of aortic endografting can be highlighted through the inclusion of high-quality peer-reviewed reports from community practice. It is irresponsible for high volume community practices not to objectively report their results with this new procedure.

Old-fashioned, but reliable and effective, operative therapy for infrarenal aortic aneurysm continues to be of interest. Pesky, but not always appreciated, complications of bowel and cognitive dysfunction after open aortic surgery are highlighted this year. We continue to see papers documenting both excellent, and less than excellent, results with open abdominal aortic aneurysm repair. The spectrum of aneurysm repair with open surgery is changing with an increasing predominance of more complicated open procedures. How this will effect the overall results of open aneurysm repair will be determined over the next few years.

The thoracic aorta is appropriately gaining an increased number of publications. There is improved understanding of the thoracic aorta as a source of distal embolization and also better understanding of the natural history of intramural hematomas and their relationship to subsequent aortic dissection. New procedures, principally catheter based, are being developed for treatment of thoracic aortic disease. These procedures may allow effective and low-morbidity treatment of thoracic aneurysms and thoracoabdominal aneurysms outside of a few very high-volume specialized centers.

Many articles on peripheral arterial occlusive disease this year were selected from the "medical" literature. Clearly, internists have discovered peripheral arterial disease. Articles from internal medicine sources are included to provide perspective on how these patients are viewed by our "nonprocedural" colleagues.

Of course, there continue to be reports of the results of arterial grafting for lower extremity ischemia. I must confess, however, I have grown somewhat weary of repetitive series from a single institution documenting overall results with infrainguinal bypass grafts, including, I must admit, those from our own institution. How we deal with operations is obviously important. However, authors who can communicate how they achieved successful surgery are more interesting than those who can merely document their success. I have pretty well figured out just how well we as surgeons do with operations. As I continue to mature as a surgeon, I am becoming more interested in how my patients deal with operations.

Research and intervention for cerebrovascular disease is a bit betwixt and between. Carotid endarterectomy is well established as effective therapy, at least for patients with high-grade internal carotid artery stenosis associated with hemispheric symptoms. Thrombolytic therapy for acute cerebral ischemia has proven to be a bit of a bust and clearly has not lived up to the hopes of several years ago. Angioplasty and stenting of the internal carotid artery is an area of current intense interest. All of a sudden, there are thousands of "high-risk" carotid patients, many of whom are asymptomatic and who are being treated with carotid angioplasty. I wonder where these patients came from and how anyone can justify treating in any way a high-risk patient with asymptomatic cerebrovascular disease? We are literally being flooded with hype but not much in the way of real data. I recently received a flyer for a continuing medical education course suggesting US Food and Drug Administration (FDA) approval for carotid angioplasty and stenting is "expected in 2004." What baloney. It is now obvious to all that carotid angioplasty and stenting can be done. The current status of the field is somewhat akin to that of carotid endarterectomy prior to the result of the publication of the ECST, NASCET, and the ACAS trial. Things will eventually sort out. At this point, however, we all need to be interested but wary of those with an agenda. Loss of objectivity is dangerous.

A few years ago, I was on the membership committee for The American Association for Vascular Surgery. As part of a potential member's application, a case list was required. From analysis of those case lists, it is clear many of our colleagues devote a large component of their practice to vascular access. This year's YEAR BOOK therefore has nearly 20 articles concerning vascular access. Vascular access is a field that has rapidly responded to criticism and the Dialysis Outcome and Quality Imitative (DOQI) guidelines. Endovascular technology and techniques are assuming a greater role in the care of dialysis patients. The results of technology and DOQI have not, however, been uniformly favorable. Establishing and maintaining reliable dialysis access needs to be the focus of even more intensive research efforts. Details of some recent efforts are provided in chapter 11 of the YEAR BOOK.

In the field of venous disease, interest continues to grow in the evaluation of D-dimer testing to potentially limit the need for venous US to rule out the presence of deep venous thrombosis. The assays for D-dimer are getting better, quicker, and more widely available. I believe as soon as we can educate physicians and administrators as to the appropriate patient groups to target with D-dimer testing, and which of the many available assays to use, that this technology will go a long way in improving the efficiency and decreasing the expense of assessing for the presence of acute deep venous thrombosis. Vena caval filters have been developed that are removable. I suspect these filters will become the standard, especially for those patients where the filter has been placed basically for short-term prophylaxis.

I wish to express my thanks to my contributing editors. It is important that perspectives other than those of the editor be included in the YEAR BOOK. I put the contributing editors in a difficult position by asking them to review articles that I choose for them. The fact they do their jobs so well greatly enhances the overall quality of the YEAR BOOK. Finally, I express my appreciation to the YEAR BOOK staff at Elsevier and give special thanks to Jenna Bowker for her invaluable assistance in organizing the enormous amount of material required for production of the YEAR BOOK OF VASCULAR SURGERY. Projects like this do not get done without the skills and dedication of people like Jenna.

Gregory L. Moneta, MD
Editor-in-Chief

1   Basic Considerations

Circulating Endothelial Progenitor Cells, Vascular Function, and Cardio-vascular Risk

Hill JM, Zalos G, Halcox JPJ, et al (NIH, Bethesda, Md; Emory Univ, Atlanta, Ga)

N Engl J Med 348:593-600, 2003   1–1

Objective.—Endothelial progenitor cells express various endothelial-specific cell-surface markers and have many different endothelial actions. Previous studies have suggested that circulating endothelial progenitor cells might play a role in ongoing endothelial repair processes. The effects of circulating endothelial progenitor cells on endothelial dysfunction and on progression of cardiovascular disease were investigated.

Methods.—Peripheral blood samples were obtained from 45 men (mean age, 50 years). Some of the men had conventional cardiovascular risk factors, but all were free of cardiovascular disease. Circulating endothelial progenitor cells were measured in colony-forming units. The results were compared with the subjects' cardiovascular risk and endothelium-independent function, measured by high-resolution brachial artery US.

Results.—Circulating endothelial progenitor cell number was strongly correlated with cardiovascular risk, based on combined Framingham risk

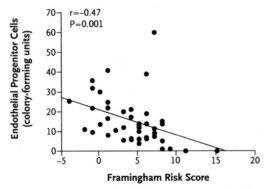

FIGURE 2.—Association between cardiovascular risk factors and endothelial-progenitor-cell colony counts. The number of colony-forming units was strongly correlated with the subjects' Framingham risk scores. Levels of endothelial progenitor cells were expressed as the mean number of colonies per well in at least 4 separate determinations for each subject. Higher Framingham risk scores indicate greater cardiovascular risk. (Reprinted by permission of *The New England Journal of Medicine* from Hill JM, Zalos G, Halcox JP, et al: Circulating endothelial progenitor cells, vascular function, and cardiovascular risk. *N Engl J Med* 348:593-600. Copyright 2003, Massachusetts Medical Society. All rights reserved.)

score: $r = -0.47$ (Fig 2). The progenitor cell number was also significantly correlated with flow-mediated reactivity within the brachial artery; this association was even stronger than that between conventional risk factors and vascular reactivity. In vitro studies demonstrated endothelial progenitor cells from subjects with higher cardiovascular disease risk factors showed higher cellular senescence scores than cells from subjects at low risk.

Discussion.—Circulating endothelial progenitor cell level may be a useful indicator of vascular functioning and overall cardiovascular risk. Ongoing injury caused by cardiovascular risk factors may result in depletion of endothelial progenitor cells over time. Further research will be needed to test this hypothesized "risk factor-induced exhaustion" of progenitor cells, as well as the relationship between progenitor cells and cardiovascular event risk.

▶ The article implies there is ongoing injury and repair of the endothelium. When the balance favors injury, one result is atherosclerosis. Little is known about endothelial repair that may prevent atherosclerosis. This article is of major importance because it is among the first to focus on the endothelial repair side of the equation.

G. L. Moneta, MD

Increased Risk of Atherosclerosis Is Confined to CagA-Positive *Helicobacter pylori* Strains: Prospective Results From the Bruneck Study
Mayr M, Kiechl S, Mendall MA, et al (Austrian Academy of Sciences, Innsbruck, Austria; Univ Clinic, Innsbruck, Austria; Mayday Univ Hosp, London)
Stroke 34:610-615, 2003   1–2

Background.—*Helicobacter pylori* seropositivity has been postulated to be a risk factor in cardiovascular and cerebrovascular disease, but the pathogenetic role of *H pylori* in coronary artery disease is unclear, with a recent meta-analysis showing only limited support for a positive association. This study investigated whether cytotoxin-associated gene A (CagA), found in the most virulent *H pylori* strains, is related to intima-media thickness (IMT)—and early plaque development in carotid arteries.

Methods.—Six hundred eighty-four cases were evaluated prospectively. Seropositivity to *H pylori* and to CagA was assessed, as well as IMT and atherosclerosis of the carotid arteries.

Results.—Only elevated levels of immune reactions to mycobacterial heat shock protein 65 showed a relationship with seropositivity for *H pylori*; none of the other cardiovascular risk factors or markers of systemic inflammation were linked. The highest levels of seropositivity were noted in patients who harbored virulent *H pylori* strains. Patients who were seropositive to CagA had significantly enhanced common carotid IMT. Those infected with CagA-negative *H pylori* strains did not show this association. There was a dose-response relationship between anti-CagA antibodies and both IMT and atherosclerosis risk. An increased risk of atherosclerosis with CagA seropositivity occurred in the presence of elevated C-reactive protein levels. The relationship of CagA antibody levels and atherosclerosis was more pronounced among younger persons.

Conclusions.—The contribution of *H pylori* to the pathogenesis of atherosclerosis appears to involve virulent CagA-positive strains only. The immune inflammatory reactions may be aggravated by the presence of the virulent *H pylori*, with a significant increase in the risk of carotid atherosclerosis.

▶ Not all *H pylori* are created equal. Those with the CagA gene associated with *H pylori* that produce a specific toxin (VacA toxin) seem to cause an immune inflammatory response that may increase atherosclerosis. The association of chronic infection with atherosclerosis may have little to do with infection per se and everything to do with immune response to infection.

G. L. Moneta, MD

Localization of a Gene for Peripheral Arterial Occlusive Disease to Chromosome 1p31
Gudmundsson G, Matthiasson SE, Arason H, et al (Natl Univ Hosp, Reykjavik, Iceland; Genetic Research Service Ctr, Reykjavik, Iceland; Icelandic Heart Assoc, Reykjavik, Iceland; et al)
Am J Hum Genet 70:586-592, 2002   1–3

Background.—Atherosclerosis underlies several of the most lethal diseases in humans, including stroke and myocardial infarction. However, peripheral arterial occlusive disease (PAOD) represents atherosclerosis of the large and medium arteries of the limbs, particularly of the lower extremities, and includes the aorta and iliac arteries. Data on the mapping of a locus for PAOD and the first example of linkage to a specific chromosomal location were presented.

Methods.—Cross-matching a population-based list of Icelandic patients with PAOD who had undergone angiography or revascularization with the use of a genealogy database of Iceland as a whole yielded 116 extended families containing 272 patients. All patients had undergone angiography, and 85% had angioplasty or vascular surgery.

Results.—A genome-wide scan with microsatellite markers revealed significant linkage of PAOD with chromosome 1p31, with an allele-sharing LOD score of 3.93. This locus has been designated as PAOD1. The subtraction from this analysis of 35 patients with a history of stroke increased the LOD score to 4.93.

Conclusion.—PAOD has recognized risk factors, but there may also be genetic factors that are specific to this particular subtype of atherosclerotic occlusive disease.

▶ We have all seen patients who have severe peripheral arterial disease with minimal risk factors and, conversely, patients with extensive risk but minimal disease. Intuitively, we know that there must be something else in these patients that determines susceptibility. This study supports this notion and suggests that susceptibility to vascular disease may have a genetic component that can be described independent of standard vascular risk factors. It will be especially interesting to learn what protein the newly identified gene *PAOD1* encodes.

L. W. Kraiss, MD

Toll-Like Receptor 4 Polymorphisms and Atherogenesis
Kiechl S, Lorenz E, Reindl M, et al (Univ Clinic, Innsbruck, Austria; Wake Forest Univ, Winston-Salem, NC; Bruneck Hosp, Italy; et al)
N Engl J Med 347:185-192, 2002   1–4

Background.—Intravascular inflammation has proatherogenic effects. Thus, an efficient immune defense against microorganisms may provide an early advantage against bacterial pathogens at the expense of chronic vascular damage in later years.

Methods.—Eight hundred ten persons were monitored for 5 years and screened for the TLR4 polymorphisms Asp299Gly and Thr399IIe. The Asp299Gly TLR4 polymorphism attenuates receptor signaling and reduces the inflammatory response to gram-negative pathogens. High-resolution duplex US was used to determine the extent and progression of carotid atherosclerosis.

Findings.—Compared with persons with wild-type TLR4, 55 persons with the Asp299Gly TLR4 allele had lower concentrations of some proinflammtory cytokines, acute-phase reactants, and soluble adhesion molecules, including interleukin-6 and fibrinogen. These persons were more susceptible to severe bacterial infections but had a decreased risk of carotid atherosclerosis, with an odds ratio of 0.54. In addition, this group had a smaller intima-media thickness in the common carotid artery.

Conclusion.—The Asp299Gly TLR4 polymorphism appears to be associated with a reduced risk of atherosclerosis. These findings suggest that the immune response plays a role in atherogenesis.

▶ With the explosion of information from the human genome and from DNA sequencing in defined human populations, we are about to be deluged with reports linking specific genes and their polymorphisms (slight differences in a gene's DNA sequence that may affect activity of the gene product) with various disease processes. In this study, adults were screened for polymorphisms in TLR4, a receptor that activates immune responses to bacteria, among other things. Individuals carrying TLR4 polymorphisms demonstrated less carotid artery atherosclerosis (intima-media thickness and plaque) than persons with the normal TLR4 gene. These data fit nicely with a growing body of data linking systemic inflammation with atherosclerosis progression. In fact, statins are now felt to work in part through anti-inflammatory effects independent of lipid-lowering. A cautionary note, however: the authors do not prove cause and effect, and in an animal model of atherosclerosis (ApoE-/- mouse) complete deletion of the TLR4 gene did not reduce atherosclerosis. So continue taking your statin for now.

R. L. Geary, MD

C-Reactive Protein Predicts Progression of Atherosclerosis Measured at Various Sites in the Arterial Tree: The Rotterdam Study
van der Meer IM, de Maat MPM, Hak AE, et al (Erasmus Med Ctr, Rotterdam, The Netherlands; Gaubius Lab, TNO-PG, Leiden, The Netherlands; Numico Research, Wageningen, The Netherlands)
Stroke 33:2750-2755, 2002   1–5

Background.—It has been proposed that the measurement of C-reactive protein (CRP), in addition to traditional risk factors, may improve the prediction of cardiovascular disease. However, the role of CRP as a predictor of the progression of subclinical atherosclerosis is not known. Whether CRP is predictive of progression of atherosclerosis measured at various sites in the arterial tree was determined.

Methods.—The study group comprised 773 patients aged 55 years or older who were participating in the Rotterdam Study. CRP levels were assessed in these patients, and subclinical atherosclerosis was assessed at various sites at 2 time points, with a mean duration of 6.5 years between measurements.

Results.—After adjustment for age, sex, and smoking habits, the odds ratios (ORs) associated with CRP levels in the highest compared with the lowest quartile were increased for progression of carotid, aortic, iliac, and lower extremity atherosclerosis. The OR for generalized progression of atherosclerosis as indicated by a composite progression score was 4.5 (95% confidence interval, 2.3-8.5). With the exception of aortic atherosclerosis, there was

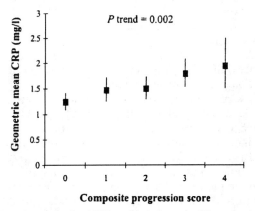

FIGURE 2.—Geometric mean level and 95% confidence intervals of C-reactive protein (*CRP*) for each value of the composite progression score. Means are adjusted for baseline levels of traditional cardiovascular risk factors. (Courtesy of van der Meer IM, de Maat MPM, Hak AE, et al: C-reactive protein predicts progression of atherosclerosis measured at various sites in the arterial tree: The Rotterdam Study. *Stroke* 33:2750-2755, 2002.)

little change in these estimates after additional adjustment for multiple car-diovascular risk factors. The ORs for progression of atherosclerosis associ-ated with high CRP levels were as high as the ORs associated with the tradi-tional cardiovascular risk factors (high cholesterol, hypertension, and smoking). Geometric mean levels of CRP increased with the number of sites showing progression of atherosclerosis (Fig 2).

Conclusions.—CRP is predictive of progression of atherosclerosis mea-sured at various sites in the arterial tree.

▶ Building on the fact elevation of CRP is associated with myocardial infarc-tion and stroke, the authors also found an association with progression of in-dicators of peripheral arterial disease as well. The results should not be sur-prising as atherosclerosis is clearly a systemic disorder, with various risk factors assuming greater or lessor importance depending on what site in the arterial tree is scrutinized.

G. L. Moneta, MD

Influence of C3 Deficiency on Atherosclerosis

Buono C, Come CE, Witztum JL, et al (Harvard Med School, Boston; Univ of California, San Diego, La Jolla; St Michael's Hosp, Toronto)
Circulation 105:3025-3031, 2002   1–6

Background.—Individuals with atherosclerotic disease produce antibod-ies specific to atheroma antigens, such as oxidized low-density lipoproteins (LDLs) and heat shock protein 60/65. Antibody responses to oxidation-spe-cific epitopes of oxidized LDL may modulate atherosclerotic disease, but the mechanisms by which these antibodies influence atherogenesis are unclear. Several studies have suggested that complement activation is involved in atherogenesis. Components of the terminal complement pathway are often found in human atheromas. Studies have also found C3 and C4 deposition in arterial lesions. The effects of C3 deficiency on the extent and phenotype of atherosclerosis were investigated.

Methods.—Aortic atherosclerosis was analyzed in LDL receptor (ldlr)/C3-deficient mice (ldlr$^{-/-}$C3$^{-/-}$) and ldlr$^{-/-}$C3$^{+/-}$ littermate control mice after 15 weeks on a 1.25% (wt/wt) cholesterol diet.

Results.—No significant differences were found between the 2 groups in serum lipoprotein profiles and immunoglobulin levels. The lipid-positive en face lesional area in the thoracic and abdominal aorta was greater in the C3-deficient mice than in the control mice (3.9% vs 2.1%); likewise, the C3-de-ficient mice had a greater lipid-positive area in aortic arch sections compared with the control mice (0.04 mm^2 vs 0.02 mm^2). Analysis of aortic arch sec-tions showed greater lesional macrophage content and less collagen content in C3-deficient mice versus control mice.

Conclusions.—This study showed that the progression of atheromas from foam cell–rich and lipid-rich lesions to lesions with prominent smooth mus-cle cells and collagens depends, in part, on the presence of an intact complement system. Complement activation should be a consideration in the evaluation of the mechanisms and prognostic significance of inflammatory variables associated with atherosclerosis.

▶ The concept that atheromas at least begin as a chronic inflammatory lesion of the arterial wall seems reasonably well accepted. Up to this point, whether or not the various inflammatory mediators postulated to induce the inflammation leading to atherosclerosis have a common pathway has not been determined. The article suggests the complement system may serve as that pathway. Ultimately, atherosclerosis may be an immune modulated disease.

G. L. Moneta, MD

Association Between Enhanced Soluble CD40L and Prothrombotic State in Hypercholesterolemia: Effects of Statin Therapy
Cipollone F, Mezzetti A, Porreca E, et al (Univ of Chieti, Italy)
Circulation 106:399-402, 2002   1–7

Background.—The high incidence of thrombotic complications reported in association with hypercholesterolemia may be related to an enhanced thrombotic risk. Previous studies have documented persistent platelet activation and increased thrombin generation in patients with hypercholesterolemia and the capability of simvastatin to reverse these abnormalities. The CD40 ligand (CD40L) is expressed on CD4+ T cells and activated platelets. It is hypothesized that inhibition of CD40 signaling would prevent the initiation and progression of atherosclerosis. In addition, soluble CD40L (sCD40L) has been implicated in acute coronary syndromes, and elevated sCD40L is predictive of an increased risk of future cardiovascular events in healthy individuals. The in vivo expression of sCD40L was investigated in hypercholesterolemia and was characterized and correlated with the extent of the prothrombotic state and whether it could be modified by statins.

Methods.—Eighty patients with hypercholesterolemia and 80 matched healthy control subjects participated in the study. Serum, plasma, and urine samples were obtained for biochemical analysis and enzyme immunoassay after participants fasted for 12 hours. Serum sCD40L and plasma P-selectin, sIL2-R, prothrombin fragment 1 + 2 (F1 + 2), and factor VIIa (FVIIa) were determined by enzyme-linked immunosorbent assay. Immunoreactive 11-dehydro-thromboxane B_2 was extracted and measured by radioimmunoassay.

Results.—Patients with hypercholesterolemia had enhanced levels of sCD40L, FVIIa and F1 + 2 compared with healthy participants. sCD40L correlated with total cholesterol and low density lipoprotein cholesterol, and sCD40L was positively associated with in vivo platelet activation. The inhibition of cholesterol biosynthesis by pravastatin or cerivastatin was associated with comparable, significant reductions in sCD40L, FVIIa, and F1 + 2.

Conclusions.—These findings suggest that sCD40L may represent the molecular link between hypercholesterolemia and the prothrombotic state.

It seems that statin therapy may significantly reduce sCD40L and the pro-thrombotic state.

▶ The expression of CD40L on T cells and activated platelets is upregulated in hypercholesterolemia. CD40L interacts with cells in the arterial wall to induce inflammatory and prothrombotic responses. Statins appear to disrupt this pathway. This study identifies another thrombophilic disorder that is important in arterial disease and one that may be treatable with statins.

G. L. Moneta, MD

Folic Acid Improves Endothelial Function in Coronary Artery Disease via Mechanisms Largely Independent of Homocysteine Lowering
Doshi SN, McDowell IFW, Moat SJ, et al (Univ of Wales, Cardiff)
Circulation 105:22-26, 2002   1–8

Introduction.—Elevated total plasma homocysteine (tHcy) levels are known to be an independent and potentially modifiable risk factor for coronary artery disease (CAD). Folic acid supplementation can reduce total plasma tHcy levels by 25% and can improve endothelial functioning in patients with CAD, but it is not known whether this improvement results from a reduction in tHcy level or from some other effect of folic acid. The relationship between changes in tHcy and endothelial functioning was examined in a double-blind study of patients with significant CAD.

Methods.—Thirty-three patients were randomly assigned to receive either 5 mg of folic acid daily or placebo for 6 weeks. Those eligible for the study were not actively smoking or had recently quit smoking and were not taking antioxidant vitamins, folic acid, or fish oils. Other exclusion criteria included a recent acute coronary event, diabetes mellitus, uncontrolled hypertension, and impaired renal functioning. Endothelial function was assessed by flow-mediated dilatation (FMD) at 2 and 4 hours after the first dose of folic acid and after 6 weeks of treatment.

Results.—The folic acid and placebo groups were similar in baseline clinical and biochemical variables. Both groups had impaired FMD at baseline. The treated group had marked FMD improvement at 2 and 4 hours after the first folic acid dose. After 6 weeks of treatment a small additional improvement was seen. In both groups, tHcy levels fell in the early phase, and at 6 weeks, tHcy levels were significantly reduced by folic acid. No correlation was found between improvement in FMD and reductions in either tHcy or free (non–protein-bound) homocysteine levels at any time.

Conclusion.—Findings confirm the benefits of high-dose folic acid treatment in patients with CAD. However, a reduction in homocysteine levels is unlikely to account for the early and possibly long-term improvement in endothelial function observed with folic acid treatment.

▶ In my opinion, this article does little to clarify a mechanism of benefit of folic acid therapy. In this study, patients were given acutely very high doses of folic acid, amounts not possible through dietary supplementation alone, and endo-thelial function improved without changes in homocysteine levels. However, this observation does not exclude the possibility of long-term improvement of endothelial function mediated by lower levels of folic acid that eventually lower homocysteine levels over the long term.

G. L. Moneta, MD

Blood Levels of Long-Chain n–3 Fatty Acids and the Risk of Sudden Death
Albert CM, Campos H, Stampfer MJ, et al (Brigham and Women's Hosp, Boston; Massachusetts Gen Hosp, Boston; Harvard School of Public Health, Boston)
N Engl J Med 346:1113-1118, 2002   1–9

Background.—The Physicians' Health Study (PHS) has reported an association between fish consumption and a reduced risk of sudden cardiac death. This association is believed to be caused by the presence of long-chain n–3 polyunsaturated fatty acids (PUFAs) found in fish. A prospective, nested case–control analysis of the fatty acid composition of whole blood from men without a history of cardiovascular disease who were participants in the PHS was performed so that the relationship between long chain n–3 fatty acids and sudden cardiac death could be examined.

Study Design.—The PHS monitored more than 22,000 male physicians with no history of cardiovascular disease. A blood sample was obtained at baseline. Dietary information was obtained at 12 months. Cardiovascular event information was updated annually. Over the 17 years of follow-up, 94 sudden cardiac deaths occurred, and baseline blood samples were available for these cases. Each of these participants was age-, and smoking status–matched with 2 healthy control subjects from the PHS sample. The link between long-chain n–3 fatty acids and sudden cardiac death was examined by evaluation of whole blood from both case and control subjects for fatty acid content by gas–liquid chromatography.

Findings.—Baseline whole blood levels of long-chain n–3 fatty acids were inversely related to the risk of sudden cardiac death, even after adjustment for potential confounding variables.

Conclusions.—This prospective case–control study of healthy male physicians demonstrated that baseline whole blood levels of long-chain n–3 fatty acids were inversely associated with the subsequent risk of sudden cardiac death. Increasing the intake of long-chain n–3 fatty acids by dietary change or supplementation is a low-cost and low-risk intervention that could be applied to this population.

▶ The long-chain omega-3 PUFAs found in fish, including eicosapentaenoic acid and docosahexaenoic acid, are thought to have antiarrhythmic and antiplatelet properties. These properties may account for the benefits derived from regular fish consumption. The limitations of this study include the fact the analysis is based on a single baseline measurement and therefore may not accurately reflect levels of long-chain omega-3 PUFAs over sustained periods. We should not translate this to mean that we should start routinely to screen for levels of long-chain omega-3 fatty acid blood levels in our patients. It will be prudent to follow closely the refinement of prophylactic risk-factor management in reducing sudden death from cardiovascular disease. Like the proverb says, "If you give a man a fish, he will eat for a day, but if you teach him how to fish, he eats for the rest of his life" (and avoids sudden death). (See also Abstract 12–5.)

R. M. Fujitani, MD

Height in Young Adulthood and Risk of Death From Cardiorespiratory Disease: A Prospective Study of Male Former Students of Glasgow University, Scotland

McCarron P, Okasha M, McEwen J, et al (Natl Cancer Inst, Bethesda, Md; Univ of Bristol, England; Univ of Glasgow, Scotland)
Am J Epidemiol 155:683-687, 2002   1–10

Objective.—Some studies have found an inverse relationship between adult height and cardiovascular disease. This association may involve various early life factors and socioeconomic circumstances. Prospective data on a large, socially homogeneous group were used to examine the effects of height on cardiovascular mortality.

Methods.—The analysis used data on 8361 men undergoing medical examinations as students at Glasgow University between 1948 and 1968. National registry data were used to assess cause-specific mortality through 1998. Associations between adult height and cardiovascular and other causes of disease were assessed.

Results.—A total of 863 men died during a median follow-up of 41.3 years. A Cox proportional hazards model found no relationship between height and all-cause mortality. However, an inverse relationship was found between height and all cardiovascular disease mortality: the age-adjusted hazard ratio was 0.79 per 10 cm increase in height (95% CI, 0.66-0.93). A similar association was noted for coronary heart disease mortality (adjusted hazard ratio, 0.76; 95% CI, 0.62-0.93). The data also suggested inverse associations with stroke and respiratory disease mortality, but these were nonsignificant. No associations were noted for death from cancer or noncardiorespiratory causes.

Conclusions.—Findings in a relatively socially homogeneous population of men support the inverse association between adult height and cardiovascular mortality. Early life factors affecting final adult height also seem to influence the risk of cardiorespiratory disease. Study of the mechanisms of this association may lend useful insights for primary prevention.

▶ It is generally known in the epidemiology world that height is a reasonable surrogate for the overall nutritional status and social economic status of a population. It seems unlikely increased height itself is what leads to less cardiovascular mortality. Factors influencing height are more likely important. In this study, however, many potential confounding variables were controlled. Perhaps the answer is simply bigger people have bigger vessels, and therefore everything else being equal, proportionally more luminal narrowing is required to lead to a coronary event.

G. L. Moneta, MD

Presence of Increased Stiffness of the Common Carotid Artery and Endothelial Dysfunction in Severely Obese Children: A Prospective Study
Tounian P, Aggoun Y, Dubern B, et al (Armand-Trousseau Teaching Hosp, Paris; Necker Enfants-Malades Teaching Hosp, Paris; Hôtel-Dieu Teaching Hosp, Paris)
Lancet 358:1400-1404, 2001   1–11

Background.—There is a strong association between obesity in adults and cardiovascular disease, primarily through an increased risk of insulin resistance, dyslipidemia, and high blood pressure. There is now a substantial amount of evidence indicating that obesity in childhood provides the metabolic foundation for adult cardiovascular disease. Epidemiologic studies also suggest obesity-induced atherosclerosis may begin in childhood, but this process has never been demonstrated. Arterial changes in obese children and the association between these changes and cardiovascular risk factors were examined.

Methods.—The study included 48 severely obese normotensive children and 27 control children. Noninvasive US measurements were obtained in both groups to investigate arterial mechanics and endothelial function. Plasma lipid concentrations, indexes of insulin resistance, and body composition were assessed in the obese children.

Results.—The obese children had significantly lower arterial compliance than the healthy control children (median, 0.132 vs 0.143 mm²/mm Hg) as well as lower distensibility (0.60 vs 0.70 mm Hg¹·10⁻². Conversely, the obese children had higher values than the control children for wall stress (3.36 vs 2.65 mm Hg·10²) and incremental elastic modulus (1.68 vs 0.96).

The obese children also had lower values for endothelium-dependent and independent function compared with the control children. Endothelial dysfunction was correlated with low plasma apolipoprotein A-I and with insulin resistance indexes. An android fat distribution was positively correlated with indexes of insulin resistance and plasma triglyceride concentrations and was negatively correlated with plasma high-density lipoprotein cholesterol concentration and arterial compliance.

Conclusion.—This study identified an association between severe obesity in children and endothelial dysfunction. Low levels of plasma apolipoprotein A-I, insulin resistance, and android fat distribution may be the main risk factors for these arterial changes that are possible early events in the genesis of atheroma.

▶ While it is easy to be critical of obese people, the proper emotion is pity. These people are heading down a path of misery and premature disability and death. I watched my former partner slowly die for years. He knew what was happening but could do nothing about it. I don't know the explanation for this sort of denial. However, I am quite sure that neither Lane Bryant nor bariatric surgery is the answer to this increasingly important social problem.

G. L. Moneta, MD

Obesity Accelerates the Progression of Coronary Atherosclerosis in Young Men

McGill HC Jr, for the Pathobiological Determinants of Atherosclerosis in Youth (PDAY) Research Group (Univ of Texas, San Antonio; Southwest Found for Biomedical Research, San Antonio, Texas; Ohio State Univ, Columbus; et al)
Circulation 105:2712-2718, 2002   1–12

Background.—Obesity is a risk factor for adult coronary heart disease (CHD) and is increasing in prevalence among the young. The Pathobiological Determinants of Atherosclerosis in Youth (PDAY) study was organized in 1985 to examine the effects of CHD risk factors in 2133 men and in 688 women autopsied between the ages of 15 and 34 years.

Study Design.—The PDAY study involved 15 centers. Research subjects included those aged 15 to 34 years who died of external causes within 72 hours of injury and were autopsied within 48 hours of death. Gross atherosclerotic lesions in the right coronary artery, American Heart Association lesion grade in the left anterior descending coronary artery, serum lipid concentrations, serum thiocyanate concentrations (smoking), intimal thickness of renal arteries (hypertension), glycohemoglobin concentrations (hyperglycemia), body mass index (BMI), and thickness of panniculus adiposus were evaluated.

Findings.—BMI was associated with both fatty streaks and raised lesions in the right coronary artery and with American Heart Association grade and stenosis in the left anterior descending coronary artery in young men. These effects of obesity were even greater in young men with a thick panniculus adiposus. Obesity was associated with non–high-density lipoprotein cholesterol levels and inversely with high-density lipoprotein cholesterol levels. Obesity was inversely associated with smoking. Obesity was also associated with hypertension and an increased glycohemoglobin concentration. BMI was not significantly associated with atherosclerosis in young women.

Conclusions.—Autopsy results demonstrate that obesity is associated with the extent and severity of early atherosclerotic lesions in adolescent and young men. Because obesity is a modifiable contributor to CHD, efforts to control childhood obesity are justified.

▶ The seeds of death are planted early.

G. L. Moneta, MD

Cardiac Benefits of Fish Consumption May Depend on the Type of Fish Meal Consumed: The Cardiovascular Health Study
Mozaffarian D, Lemaitre RN, Kuller LH, et al (Univ of Washington, Seattle; Univ of Pittsburgh, Pa; Wake Forest Univ, Winston-Salem, NC; et al)
Circulation 107:1372-1377, 2003   1–13

Background.—There is an inverse relationship between fish consumption and fatal ischemic heart disease (IHD) and arrhythmic death. The prevention of fatal arrhythmias is attributed to the antiarrhythmic effects of long-chain n-3 polyunsaturated fatty acids (PUFAs) in fish, but the n-3 PUFA content varies with different types of fish. Few data are available concerning the various types of fish and IHD risk. It was postulated that (1) eating fish with higher n-3 PUFA content would show an inverse relationship with IHD death but not with nonfatal myocardial infarction (MI) rates, since n-3 PUFAs do not influence atherogenesis or plaque stability, and (2) eating fish lower in n-3 PUFA content would show no relationship with IHD death or nonfatal MI rates.

Methods.—Baseline usual fish consumption was determined for 3910 adults age 65 years or older who had no known cardiovascular disease. The number of deaths and nonfatal MIs were documented over a mean follow-up of 9.3 years.

Results.—The weekly mean fried fish or fish sandwich consumption was 0.7 serving and that for tuna or other broiled or baked fish was 2.2 servings. Two hundred forty-seven IHD deaths and 363 incident nonfatal MIs occurred. Persons who had greater tuna/other fish intake evidenced a lower risk of total IHD death and arrhythmic IHD death but no decline in the number of nonfatal MIs. Compared to consumption once a month or less, when consumption of tuna/other fish was 3 or more times a week, the total IHD death risk was 49% lower and the risk of arrhythmic IHD death was 58% lower. No lower risk was linked to greater fried fish/fish sandwich intake in any of the cardiovascular areas, but instead, there was a trend toward an association with higher risk of total IHD death, arrhythmic IHD death, and nonfatal MI.

Conclusions.—Persons who ate more tuna or other baked or broiled fish had a lower risk of IHD death, especially arrhythmic IHD death. The strongest relationships were between fish intake and arrhythmic IHD death and the weakest were between fish intake and nonfatal MI. Because fried fish/fish sandwich consumption was not associated with a decline in risk, the cardiac benefits of a fish meal can vary with the n-3 PUFA content or the preparation method.

▶ How fish meals may lower risk of cardiac death is unknown. Plasma phospholipid long-chain n-3 fatty acids are present in broiled or baked fish but apparently not fried fish. These fatty acids have an antiarrhythmic effect and, indeed, reductions in cardiac death due to arrhythmia were correlated with baked or broiled fish meals but not fried fish meals. In simple terms, it appears you are fooling yourself getting a fish sandwich rather than a Big Mac.

G. L. Moneta, MD

Meta-Analysis of Wine and Beer Consumption in Relation to Vascular Risk

Di Castelnuovo A, Rotondo S, Iacoviello L, et al (Consorzio Mario Negri Sud, Santa Maria Imbaro, Italy; Catholic Univ, Campobasso, Italy)
Circulation 105:2836-2844, 2002   1–14

Background.—Many epidemiologic studies have shown an inverse association between moderate alcohol consumption and vascular risk. The all-cause mortality rate as a function of alcohol has been described as a *J*-shaped curve, which reflects a lower risk of coronary heart disease (CHD) with moderate consumption and an increased risk of certain cancers and cirrhosis at higher amounts. Many studies have addressed the question of whether different alcoholic beverages are equal in their protective effect against CHD or whether a specific beverage might offer greater protection; however, findings are inconclusive. The American Heart Association recently stated that the usual standards to recommend alcohol consumption as a preventive measure against CHD are not met and that wine is indistinguishable from other alcoholic beverages in this regard. However, these conclusions have been challenged in other studies. A meta-analysis of the relationship between wine or beer consumption and vascular risk is presented.

Methods.—A PUBMED search identified 26 studies for inclusion in this review. A general variance-based method and fitting models were applied to pooled data from these studies to determine a quantitative estimation of the vascular risk associated with consumption of either wine or beer.

Results.—From 13 studies involving 209,418 individuals, the relative risk associated with wine intake was 0.68 relative to nondrinkers. Strong evidence from 10 studies involving 176,042 participants supported a *J*-shaped association between different amounts of wine intake and vascular risk. This inverse association was statistically significant up to a daily intake of 150 mL of wine. In 15 studies involving 208,036 individuals, the overall relative risk of moderate beer consumption was 0.78. However, a meta-analysis of 7 studies involving 136,382 individuals found no significant relationship between different amounts of beer intake and vascular risk.

Conclusions.—It would seem that a significant inverse association exists between light to moderate consumption of wine and vascular risk and that a similar though smaller association exists between beer consumption and vascular risk. However, the association with beer consumption is difficult to interpret because no relationship was established between different amounts of beer intake and vascular risk.

▶ I wonder as I sit on the deck drinking a beer and reviewing this article if I should switch to wine. I decide not to. It is 85 degrees in Portland, the sun is shining. Beer seems better.

G. L. Moneta, MD

Very Late Survival After Vascular Surgery
Kazmers A, Kohler TR (Wayne State Univ, Detroit; Dept of Veterans Affairs, Ann Arbor, Mich; Seattle Veterans Affairs Med Ctr)
J Surg Res 105:109-114, 2002   1–15

Background.—Today, radionuclide ventriculography (RNVG) is seldom performed for cardiac assessment. RNVG was performed routinely from 1984 through 1988, before major elective vascular surgery to help stratify operative risk. The very late survival data obtained from veterans having RNVG before their vascular surgery was assessed.

Methods.—The 310 patients (mean age, 65 years; range, 44-92 years) having preoperative RNVG were followed up by direct contact, Veterans Administration databases, and the Social Security Death Index for a mean of 6.64 years (range, 0-16.2 years). The RNVG was performed to define left ventricular ejection fraction (EF) and to determine the presence of ventricular wall motion abnormalities before these patients underwent major elective vascular surgery.

Results.—RNVG found that the mean EF was 53%. The 30-day postoperative mortality rate was 2.6%. The current survival rate is 10% after carotid surgery, 12% after aortic aneurysm repair, 15% after extremity reconstruction, and 0% after visceral artery reconstruction; no significant difference in survival was noted at 30 days or at 1, 5, or 10 years. Carotid surgery patients survived for a mean of 6.42 years, aneurysm repair patients for a mean of 7.11 years, extremity reconstruction patients for a mean of 6.81 years, and visceral artery reconstruction patients for a mean of 6.29 years.

Age, diabetes, smoking, and an abnormally low EF (50% or less) were independently related to mortality during follow-up. On analysis of variance, only an abnormal EF was significantly associated with number of days of survival. Patients with a normal EF had a mean survival of 7.99 years; those with a low EF had a mean survival of 4.78 years. None of the patients who had severe left ventricular dysfunction or postoperative cardiac complications were alive at the last evaluation.

Patients whose EF was 35% or less survived for a mean of 2.72 years, while those whose EF was over 35% had a mean survival of 7.37 years. Those with postoperative cardiac complications survived for a mean of 4.28 years, while those with no postoperative cardiac complications had a mean survival of 7.14 years.

Conclusion.—The presence of diabetes, active smoking at the time of surgery, left ventricular dysfunction, and postoperative cardiac complications led to reduced survival for these patients evaluated with RNVG before undergoing vascular surgery. The overall mortality rate was not related to the presence of angina or previous myocardial infarction. Aggressive coronary evaluation methods may not alter very late survival.

▶ The article brings into focus the fact that patients with arterial disease requiring surgery are approaching the end of life. The patients analyzed in this article encompass the time of my vascular surgical residency at the University of Washington. Fifteen years later, less than 10% of these patients survive. I doubt such sobering statistics exist for any other field of surgery.

G. L. Moneta, MD

Differential Gene Expression in Human Abdominal Aorta: Aneurysmal Versus Occlusive Disease
Armstrong PJ, Johanning JM, Calton WC Jr, et al (Geisinger Med Ctr, Danville, Pa)
J Vasc Surg 35:346-355, 2002   1–16

Objective.—Abdominal aortic aneurysms (AAA) and arterial occlusive disease (AOD) are both associated with inflammation and atherosclerosis. Little is known about the genetic mechanisms underlying these disease processes. Gene array techniques were used to compare gene expression in specimens of AAA and AOD versus normal aorta.

Methods.—Complementary DNA probes were generated with the use of RNA from 7 aortic specimens of human AAA, from 5 specimens of AOD, and from 5 specimens from healthy control subjects. Differences in expression of a human cell interaction array of 265 genes were compared among the groups.

Findings.—Eleven genes showed differences in expression between pathologic and normal aorta. Genes for collagen V α1, glycoprotein IIIA, and α2-macroglobulin were significantly downregulated in the AAA specimens, and genes for laminin α4 and insulin-like growth factor 2 receptor were significantly upregulated in AOD. Both aortic pathologic states were associated with upregulation of matrix metalloproteinase (MMP)-9, intercellular adhesion molecule-1, and tumor necrosis factor-β receptor. Finally, both AAA and AOD specimens showed downregulation of integrin α5, ephrin A5, and rho/rac guanine nucleotide exchange factor.

Evaluation of 16 MMPs found that MMP-9 was the only one to be upregulated in both aortic disease states. Tissue inhibitor of metalloproteinase-1 tended to be upregulated in AAA. Across groups, 8 of the 15 most highly expressed genes were either extracellular matrix or secreted proteins. Collagen VI α1 was the only one of these to show a significant change; however, biglycan tended to be downregulated in AAA.

Conclusions.—This gene expression study notes differential expression of several genes in both AAA and AOD compared with healthy aorta. Other genes differ in expression between the 2 aortic pathologic states. These 2 aortic diseases may be characterized by similarities of genetic expression, but altered expression of certain genes plays some role in the differentiation between AAA and AOD.

▶ This study is a proof-of-concept experiment. It is not surprising that there are differences in gene expression between aorta exhibiting stenotic versus aneurysmal disease. It is axiomatic that important differences in biological structure must result from differences in protein expression that in turn reflect differential gene expression. The results are consistent with the prevailing paradigm that alterations in extracellular matrix metabolism are important in vascular disease. The specific applicability of these results is very limited since only about 1% (265) of the 20,000 to 30,000 genes of the human genome were analyzed. In addition, gene expression studies are most informative when they also demonstrate that the relevant proteins are also present in the proportions suggested by the genetic analysis. Nevertheless, this study indicates that a genome-wide screen of aneurysmal versus occlusive disease patients would be interesting.

L. W. Kraiss, MD

The Association Between Venous Structural Alterations and Biomechanical Weakness in Patients With Abdominal Aortic Aneurysms
Goodall S, Crowther M, Bell PR, et al (Univ of Leicester, England)
J Vasc Surg 35:937-942, 2002   1–17

Background.—Patients with abdominal aortic aneurysm (AAA) may have additional aneurysms at sites remote from the abdominal aorta. There is considerable evidence indicating a systemic nature of this degenerative disease. There have, however, been no in vitro studies to investigate the tensile properties of venous tissue in patients with aneurysms. An effort was made to determine whether features associated with vessel wall weakness observed in patients with AAAs are present in venous tissue of these patients.

Methods.—Eleven patients who underwent aneurysm repair and 11 patients who underwent colectomy for diverticulosis were included in the study. A segment of inferior mesenteric vein was harvested from patients in both groups for evaluation. Matrix composition of the vessel was determined with stereology, and the vessel dimensions were measured with a computerized image analysis system. Stress-strain measurements were obtained with elongation of inferior mesenteric vein tissue with a tensile-testing machine.

Results.—Histologic evaluation demonstrated fragmentation of elastin fibers within the medial layer of venous tissue obtained from patients with AAAs. The medial elastin content in tissue from these patients was 19.4%, compared with 26.8% in venous tissue from patients in the control group. Results of mechanical testing showed a significant reduction in the tensile strength, from 2.885 MPa in the control group to 1.405 MPa in the AAA group. This reduction corresponded with a reduction of 59% in vessel stiffness; the mean Young's modulus of elasticity was 2.72 MPa in the AAA group compared with 5.361 MPa in the control group.

Conclusions.—Reductions were found in tensile strength and stiffness in venous tissue from patients with AAAs and were associated with disruption and decreased elastin content of the vein wall. These changes are analogous to alterations in the arterial aneurysmal wall and provide confirmation of the systemic nature of AAA.

▶ This is another in a series of studies that have suggested a generalized tissue defect of some sort in patients with AAAs. Previously, others have shown that patients with AAAs have more incisional and groin hernias than patients with aortoiliac occlusive disease. Most vascular surgeons also recognize that aneurysm patients as a rule tend to have larger saphenous veins than patients with occlusive disease alone. This line of inquiry of trying to identify a generalized tissue problem in patients with aneurysm disease makes sense. We already know that there are genetic diseases, such as Ehlers-Danlos and Marfan syndromes, that weaken arterial walls. I suspect that aneurysm disease is merely part of a spectrum of diseases that act through genetically induced alterations of the vessel wall. Some of these genetic defects will require interactions with risk factors, such as tobacco, to become phenotypically manifest, whereas others, such as those associated with Ehlers-Danlos or Marfan syndrome, will be able to produce clinically important changes without a so-called second hit.

G. L. Moneta, MD

Impaired Vasoreactivity Despite an Increase in Plasma Nitrite in Patients With Abdominal Aortic Aneurysms

Knipp BS, Peterson DA, Rajagopalan S, et al (Univ of Michigan, Ann Arbor)
J Vasc Surg 35:363-367, 2002   1–18

Introduction.—Autogenous bypass grafts tend to dilate over time, unlike vein grafts for occlusive disease, which do not dilate over time. Patients with abdominal aortic aneurysms (AAAs) were compared with patients with peripheral arterial occlusive disease (PAOD) and with control subjects without known vascular disease to determine whether there were any between-group differences in vasoreactivity.

Methods.—Brachial artery vasoreactivity was examined in blinded fashion, after endothelium-dependent (ED) and endothelium-independent (EI) flow-mediated vasodilation, in age-matched men with AAAs or PAOD and control subjects (11, 9, and 10 patients, respectively). There were no significant differences in pretrial systolic or diastolic blood pressure, body mass index, or antilipidemic medications among the groups. Exclusion criteria were diabetes and tobacco use within 3 months.

All participants underwent quantitative US scan measurements of brachial artery diameters at rest and after either forearm ischemia (ED) or administration of 0.4 mg sublingual nitroglycerin (EI). Plasma nitric oxide

$(NO_x = NO_2 + NO_3)$ was ascertained by the Saville assay. Asymmetric dimethylarginine, an endogenous inhibitor of NO_x synthase, was determined by liquid chromatography.

Results.—The mean initial brachial artery diameters did not vary significantly (4.85 mm, AAA group; 4.82 mm, PAOD group; 4.68 mm, control subjects). Vasodilation in the presence of ED or EI was significantly lower ($P = .02$ and $P = .03$, respectively) for the AAA group (-1.17 and 8.33, respectively), compared with control subjects (2.96 and 13.88, respectively). Plasma NO_x was significantly increased ($P = .01$) in the AAA group (7.86 µmol/L), compared with both control subjects (5.13 µmol/L) and the PAOD group (4.85 µmol/L) (Fig 1). Asymmetric dimethylarginine levels were reduced in the AAA group (0.34 µmol/L) versus the PAOD group (0.46 µmol/

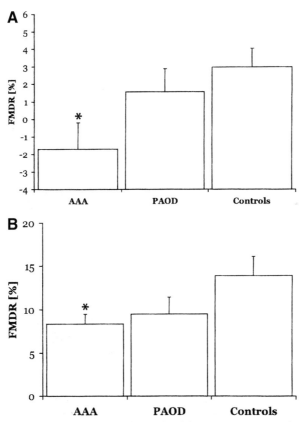

FIGURE 1.—**A**, After reactive hyperemia, flow mediated diameter ratio (*FMDR*) of patients with abdominal aortic aneurysms (*AAAs*) was significantly less ($P = .02$) than that of healthy control subjects. FMDR of patients with peripheral arterial occlusive disease (*PAOD*) was less than that of healthy control subjects, but difference was not significant ($P = .41$). **B**, after administration of nitroglycerine, the FMDR of patients with AAAs was significantly less ($P = .03$) than that of healthy control subjects. The FMDR of patients with PAOD was less than that of healthy control subjects, but the difference was not statistically significant ($P = .15$). (Reprinted from Knipp BS, Peterson DA, Rajagopalan S, et al: Impaired vasoreactivity despite an increase in plasma nitrite in patients with abdominal aortic aneurysms. *J Vasc Surg* 35:363-367, 2002. Copyright 2002 by Elsevier.)

L). There was no correlation between aneurysm size and ED or EI vasodilation or plasma NO_x.

Conclusion.—A divergence between ED and EI vasoreactivity and systemic NO metabolites were documented for the first time in patients with AAAs. It may be that a dysfunctional vessel wall response, rather than a lack of NO, is important in the pathogenesis of AAAs.

▶ This is a very intriguing and provocative study that raises many additional questions to pursue. The study was carefully done and strongly suggests that vasomotor reactivity in patients with aneurysms is especially impaired while the ability to generate vasodilator substances is not. Establishing a compelling pathophysiological link between impaired responsiveness to vasodilators and aneurysm formation is now the challenge.

L. W. Kraiss, MD

Doxycycline in Patients With Abdominal Aortic Aneurysms and in Mice: Comparison of Serum Levels and Effect on Aneurysm Growth in Mice
Prall AK, Longo GM, Mayhan WG, et al (Univ of Nebraska, Omaha; Methodist Hosp, Omaha, Neb; Washington Univ, St Louis)
J Vasc Surg 35:923-929, 2002   1–19

Background.—The rate of abdominal aortic aneurysm (AAA) growth and the risk of rupture are both related to aneurysm size. Doxycycline has been shown to inhibit aneurysm formation in a rodent model of AAA and may slow aneurysm expression in humans. However, the dose necessary to obtain the murine inhibitory effect is 6 mg/kg, much higher than the standard antibiotic doses used in humans (1 to 1.5 mg/kg).

Side effects of doxycycline are dose related, so it is unclear whether patients would tolerate doses that are 4 to 6 times higher than normal. It is also not known whether the serum levels obtained in animal models can be safely attained in patients. The goals of this study were to determine the serum concentrations needed to inhibit aneurysm formation in a murine model of AAA and to compare these findings with the plasma concentrations in patients with AAA with those obtained with a standard dose of doxycycline.

Methods.—Doxycycline was administered to 4 groups of 10 C57BL/6 mice at doses of 0, 10, 50, and 100 mg/kg beginning at 7 weeks of age. AAA was induced at 8 weeks of age. Blood samples were obtained 10 weeks after surgery to assess the levels of doxycycline. Aortic size was measured at AAA induction and at death. For comparison with humans, 14 patients with AAA were given 100 mg of doxycycline twice a day for at least 3 months. Blood samples were taken from these patients at 3 or 6 months to determine the plasma levels of the drug. The circulating levels of doxycycline for mice and humans were assessed with high-performance liquid chromatography.

Results.—Doses of 10, 50, and 100 mg/kg accounted for a 33%, 44%, and 66% reduction, respectively, of the aneurysmal growth in the mice (Fig

Aortic Diameter vs. Doxycycline Serum Level

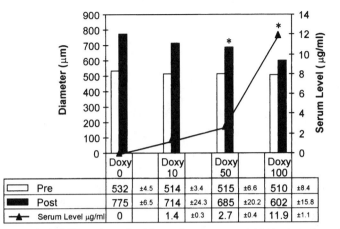

	Doxy 0		Doxy 10		Doxy 50		Doxy 100	
Pre	532	±4.5	514	±3.4	515	±6.6	510	±8.4
Post	775	±6.5	714	±24.3	685	±20.2	602	±15.8
Serum Level µg/ml	0		1.4	±0.3	2.7	±0.4	11.9	±1.1

FIGURE 2.—Effects of different doses of oral doxycycline on aneurysm inhibition in murine model. (aortic diameter on *left axis*) and relationship to serum doxycycline levels (*right axis*). Treatment groups of 50 mg/kg and 100 mg/kg showed statistically significant attenuation in aortic growth when compared with control group (0 mg/kg). *Asterisk* indicates $P < .05$. (Reprinted from Prall AK, Longo GM, Mayhan WG, et al: Doxycycline in patients with abdominal aortic aneurysms and in mice: Comparison of serum levels and effect on aneurysm growth in mice. *J Vasc Surg* 35:923-929, 2002. Copyright 2002 by Elsevier.)

2). The circulating doxycycline levels in the patients ranged from 1.8 to 9.42 (g/mL, similar to the values obtained in mice.

Conclusion.—The circulating levels of doxycycline in the patients were comparable to those obtained in mice. Doxycycline inhibits murine aortic expansion by 33% to 66%. These findings suggest that standard doxycycline doses could inhibit the growth of AAAs in humans.

▶ The authors recognize that one of the problems of pharmacologic research is that giving huge doses of drugs to animals does not necessarily mimic drug levels that can be achieved in humans. This article is therefore an important preliminary step toward an eventual clinical trial seeking to evaluate whether the growth of AAAs can be slowed pharmacologically. Beta-blockers didn't work out; maybe doxycycline will.

G. L. Moneta, MD

Early-Onset Carotid Atherosclerosis Is Associated With Increased Intima-Media Thickness and Elevated Serum Levels of Inflammatory Markers
Magyar MT, Szikszai Z, Balla J, et al (Univ of Debrecen, Hungary)
Stroke 34:58-63, 2003   1–20

Background.—Prospective studies have found that increased common carotid artery intima-media thickness (IMT) is a powerful predictor of coronary and cerebrovascular complications. Most studies on carotid artery disease focus on elderly patients. However, because age is the primary risk factor for carotid artery disease, examination of an elderly patient group may mask the effects of risk factors for early atherosclerosis. Thus, the role of several potential risk factors of early atherosclerosis in persons younger than 55 years were evaluated.

Methods.—The study group included 45 patients with greater than 30% stenosis of the internal carotid artery, 20 patients with carotid occlusion, and 35 control participants. Plasma lipids, oxidative resistance of low-density lipoprotein, homocysteine, inflammatory markers, plasma viscosity, and red blood cell deformability were measured in fasting blood samples from the study participants, and stenosis and IMT of the common carotid artery were evaluated by duplex US.

Results.—Compared with control participants, the patients had significantly higher white blood cell (WBC) counts, plasma fibrinogen, C-reactive protein (CRP), and lipoprotein(a) levels. Patients also had increased IMT. There was a tendency for higher homocysteine levels in patients. Patients who smoked had higher WBC counts, fibrinogen, and CRP levels than nonsmoking patients. After controlling for the effect of smoking, WBC counts, and natural logarithmic transform of homocysteine, IMT remained significantly higher in patients than in control participants. WBC, fibrinogen, and CRP levels were highest in patients in the highest IMT quartile.

Conclusions.—Inflammatory markers and homocysteine have a more important role than lipid factors in the development of early onset carotid atherosclerosis.

▶ All of us who take care of patients with atherosclerosis recognize there is no uniform pattern of risk factors or biochemical abnormalities that apply to every patient. The idea that different risk factors may have different levels of importance, in varying arterial beds, depending on age, I believe fits clinical observation. Of course, why there is this differential effect of risk factors is the important question. My guess is that it will relate to the interactions of gene expression and risk factor exposure. I predict within a few years atherosclerotic research will move from the analysis of risk factors and inflammatory markers to primarily a field of genetic analysis.

G. L. Moneta, MD

Active and Passive Smoking, Chronic Infections, and the Risk of Carotid Atherosclerosis: Prospective Results From the Bruneck Study
Kiechl S, Werner P, Egger G, et al (Innsbruck Univ Hosp, Austria; Bruneck Hosp, Italy; St George's Hosp Med School, London)
Stroke 33:2170-2176, 2002   1–21

Background.—There is substantial variation in the susceptibility of the vasculature to the deleterious effects of smoking. Some smokers have severe premature atherosclerosis develop, whereas others remain free of advanced atheroma until their elderly years. This study was conducted to estimate the contribution of chronic infections to the variability of atherosclerosis severity among smokers.

Methods.—Researchers performing the community-based Bruneck Study used high-resolution US to assess 5-year changes in carotid atherosclerosis. *Early atherogenesis* was defined as the development of nonstenotic plaques and *advanced atherogenesis* as the development/progression of vessel stenosis by more than 40%.

Results.—The risk of early atherogenesis was strongly dependent on lifetime smoking exposure and continued to be elevated long after the cessation of smoking. A surprising finding was that current and ex-smokers faced an increased risk of atherosclerosis only in the presence of chronic infections, whereas current, past, and nonsmokers without infections did not differ significantly from one another in their estimated risk burden (Fig 3). Similar to those with first-hand smoking exposures, persons exposed to environmental tobacco smoke were found to be vulnerable to the manifestation of chronic infection, and only infected persons experienced a high risk of atherosclerosis. The risk of advanced atherogenesis was related in a dose-dependent manner to the number of daily cigarettes, returned to normal shortly after the cessation of smoking, and emerged independent of infectious illness.

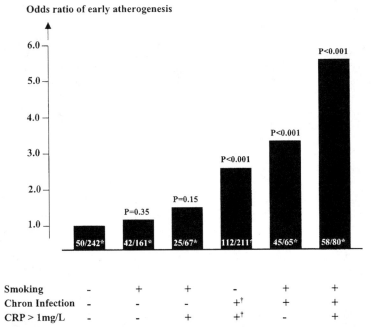

FIGURE 3.—Adjusted odds ratios [95% CIs] of early atherogenesis in the carotid arteries according to smoking, infection status, and levels of C-reactive protein (CRP). Analysis was conducted in the entire population sample. Adjustment is as described in Figure 2. *Number of subjects with early atherogenesis per number of subjects at risk; †chronic infection or CRP >1 mg/L or both. *Abbreviation: Chron*, Chronic. (Kiechl S, Werner P, Egger G, et al: Active and passive smoking, chronic infections, and the risk of carotid atherosclerosis: prospective results from the Bruneck Study. *Stroke* 33:2170-2176, 2002.)

Conclusions.—This study provides the first epidemiologic evidence that the proatherogenic effects of cigarette smoking are partially mediated by the chronic infections often found in smokers.

▶ The article demonstrates an association between smoking and chronic infection in patients with carotid atherosclerosis. It does not clarify if smoking and chronic infection combined to lead to atherosclerosis or if smoking and atherosclerosis combined to lead to conditions favoring chronic infection. The old chicken and egg problem revisited once again.

G. L. Moneta, MD

Prospective, Randomized, Double-blind Trial Investigating the Effect of Doxycycline on Matrix Metalloproteinase Expression Within Atherosclerotic Carotid Plaques
Axisa B, Loftus IM, Naylor AR, et al (Univ of Leicester, England)
Stroke 33:2858-2865, 2002   1–22

Purpose.—Previous reports have linked high levels of matrix metalloproteinases (MMPs), especially MMP-1 and MMP-9, to an increased risk of plaque rupture. The effects of MMP inhibition with doxycycline on MMP levels in carotid atheromas were assessed.

Methods.—The prospective randomized study included 100 patients undergoing carotid endarterectomy. For 2 to 8 weeks preoperatively, patients were treated with doxycycline, 200 mg/day, or placebo. Surgical specimens of carotid plaques were tested for concentrations of MMPs and doxycycline.

Results.—In the treated group, mean doxycycline concentration in the surgical specimens was 6.0 (g/g wet weight). Carotid plaque concentration of MMP-1 was reduced from 14.8 ng/100 g wet weight in the placebo group to 10.3 ng/100 g wet weight in the doxycycline group. This effect was ascribed to a reduction in MMP-1 transcript. Concentrations of other MMPs, including MMP-9, and of tissue inhibitors of MMP-1 and MMP-2, were unaffected by doxycycline.

Conclusions.—The nonspecific MMP inhibitor doxycycline is concentrated in carotid artery plaques, producing a significant reduction in MMP-1 concentration. The effects of MMP inhibition on clinical event rates in patients with atherosclerosis remain to be determined.

▶ MMPs are zinc-dependent endopeptidases that have been established as being the major physiologic regulators of the extracellular matrix. The localized increase in expression of several MMPs within the shoulder and fibrous cap of atherosclerotic plaques (notably MMP-1 and MMP-9), coupled with an increased proteolytic activity, have been implicated in increasing the risk for plaque rupture. Doxycycline is known to be a direct MMP antagonist. This interesting report speculates that doxycycline may modulate adverse clinical events through its role of MMP inhibition. One wonders what adjunctive role the antimicrobial effect of doxycycline has on possible *Chlamydia pneumoniae* colonization of the carotid atheroma in affecting clinical events? Carefully conducted prospective clinical trials may help us answer this provocative question.

R. M. Fujitani, MD

Increased Expression of HDJ-2 (hsp40) in Carotid Artery Atherosclerosis: A Novel Heat Shock Protein Associated With Luminal Stenosis and Plaque Ulceration

Nguyen TQ, Jaramillo A, Thompson RW, et al (Washington Univ, St Louis)

J Vasc Surg 33:1065-1071, 2001   1–23

Introduction.—There is evidence that both humoral and cellular autoimmune processes directed toward heat shock proteins (hsp) augment the pathogenesis of atherosclerosis. A novel 46-kDa hsp, HDJ-2, has been cloned and characterized from human tissue. There is evidence that the hsps, including hsp60 and hsp70, are involved in the autoimmune response linked with atherosclerosis. The role of HDJ-2 in the pathogenesis of atherosclerosis was examined.

Methods.—The level of HDJ-2 messenger RNA (mRNA) expression was compared with the level of hsp60 and hsp70 mRNA expression in 26 carotid endarterectomy specimens and 17 normal specimens. The level of expression of HDJ-2 mRNA was correlated with the presence of plaque ulceration and the extent of luminal stenosis.

Results.—Expression of HDJ-2 and hsp70 was significantly higher in carotid artery plaques than in normal arteries: HDJ-2, 6.7 versus 0.1 ($P = .001$); hsp70, 9.5 versus 3.7 ($P = .002$). The difference in hsp60 expression between carotid artery plaques and normal arteries was not significantly different. Increased HDJ-2 expression in carotid artery plaques was observed and was independent of hsp70 (Pearson correlation, $r = 0.11$; Bartlett analysis, χ^2, $P = .71$). Within the ulcerated plaque group, there was an association between the extent of stenosis and high HDJ-2 mRNA expression ($r = 0.896$; $P = .016$). There was no association between the extent of stenosis and high HDJ-2 mRNA expression within the nonulcerated plaque group ($r = 0.530$; $P = .076$) or within the entire cohort ($r = 0.0085$; $P = .97$).

Conclusion.—Expression of HDJ-2 is significantly increased in atherosclerotic carotid artery plaques, compared to hsp60 and hsp70. It is associated with luminal stenosis in ulcerated atherosclerotic carotid artery plaques.

▶ This study bolsters a not-so-new idea that atherosclerosis exhibits many features of autoimmunity. The increased expression of HDJ-2 is convincingly correlated with atherosclerotic disease in the carotid artery, and even more intriguing, with plaque ulceration. The long-term significance of this study is unknown since it only shows that HDJ-2 expression correlates with carotid artery disease without demonstrating cause and effect or informing us of the particular function of HDJ-2 in carotid atherogenesis. The article will prove to be a seminal observation when and if additional studies exploring the obvious questions raised by these findings are published. For instance, is there any relationship between a patient's viral serologic status and the expression of HDJ-2 in the carotid specimen? Is increased HDJ-2 the cause of or a response to plaque ulceration?

L. W. Kraiss, MD

Local Delivery of Plasmid DNA Into Rat Carotid Artery Using Ultrasound

Taniyama Y, Tachibana K, Hiraoka K, et al (Osaka Univ, Japan; Fukuoka Univ, Hakata, Japan)
Circulation 105:1233-1239, 2002   1–24

Background.—Viral vector systems are efficient in transferring foreign genes into blood vessels, but they may cause adverse events, and their safety in human beings is unproven. An alternative, nonviral method for transferring foreign genes into blood vessels that involves the use of US with microbubble material (Optison) is described.

Methods.—Human endothelial cells (ECs) and vascular smooth muscle cells (VSMCs) were cultured and transfected with luciferase plasmid DNA mixed with or without Optison. Transfection was achieved via high-frequency, low-intensity US irradiation (8 one-minute treatments at 2.5 W/cm^2 and 37°C). The activity of luciferase plasma DNA in ECs and VSMCs was examined 24 hours after transfection.

In in vivo experiments, a balloon catheter was introduced into the carotid artery of male Sprague-Dawley rats. An Optison solution containing luciferase plasmid was introduced into the balloon-injured vessel and exposed to US for 2 minutes. Luciferase activity was measured 2 days after transfection. In addition, control cDNA and an anti-oncogene (p53) plasmid cDNA were transfected via US into balloon-injured carotid arteries (with or without Optison). The intimal-to-medial area ratio was measured at 2 weeks.

Results.—Luciferase activity in vivo was greater than 7000-fold higher in ECs and VSMCs treated with US and Optison than in cells incubated with plasmid alone. Luciferase activity was also significantly higher (by >1000-fold) in balloon-injured arteries 2 days after transfection with Optison and US than after transfection with plasmid DNA alone. At 2 weeks, the intimal-to-medial area ratio was significantly lower (by half) in the arteries transfected with p53 plasma, Optison, and US than in vessels not treated by US or Optison (Fig 4). In addition, p53 plasmid DNA synthesis was significantly decreased (by about 5-fold) in the arteries transfected via US and Optison. Vessels transfected with plasmid DNA via US and Optison showed no evidence of toxic effects.

Conclusion.—The use of US plus Optison to transfect plasmid DNA into blood vessels was efficient and apparently safe. The efficacy of transfection is believed to be caused by Optison's penetration of the cell surface during therapeutic US irradiation. Transfection of p53 plasma via this method also decreased the intimal-to-medial area ratio in balloon-injured arteries. This

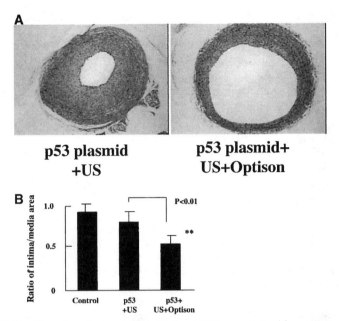

**p53 plasmid
+US**

**p53 plasmid+
US+Optison**

FIGURE 4.—Effect of transfection of naked p53 plasmid DNA on neointimal formation in rat balloon injury model at 2 weeks after transfection. A, Representative cross-sections of balloon-injured vessels transfected with p53 vector at 2 weeks after injury (hematoxylin and eosin staining). p53 plasmid + US indicates naked p53 plasma DNA by means of US alone; p53 plasmid + US + Optison indicates naked p53 plasmid DNA by means of US with Optison. B, Effect of transfection of naked p53 plasmid DNA on ratio of neointimal-to-medial area in rat balloon injury model 2 weeks after transfection. Control indicates naked control plasmid DNA; p53 + US indicates naked p53 plasmid DNA by means of US alone; and p53 + US + Optison indicates naked p53 plasmid DNA by means of US with Optison. **P < .01 versus control. Control group contains 5 animals; each HGF group contains 6 animals. (Courtesy of Taniyama Y, Tachibana K, Hiraoka H, et al: Local delivery of plasmid DNA into rat carotid artery using ultrasound. *Circulation* 105 (10):1233-1239, 2002.)

nonviral vector system may be appropriate for use during gene therapy in human beings.

▶ Practicality, efficiency and durability are the hallmark components of this fascinating article. The authors use US and microspheres to increase transfection efficiency and durability in vitro and in vivo. There is no evidence that US or the microspheres cause vascular injury in vitro or in vivo. The authors then evaluated the effect of this transfection protocol on balloon-injured arteries, finding a tremendous potential therapeutic benefit. One must wonder whether US and microspheres might provide a useful adjunct to the overall effectiveness of drug-eluting stents in preventing restenosis.

M. T. Watkins, MD

Microinjection of DNA Into the Nuclei of Human Vascular Smooth Muscle Cells

Nelson PR, Kent KC (Univ of Massachusetts, Worcester; Cornell Univ, New York)

J Surg Res 106:202-208, 2002

1–25

Introduction.—The introduction of genetic material into mammalian cells requires cellular transfection. Currently available transfection techniques are associated with a tendency to produce injury resulting in cellular function changes or cell death. The limitation of current transfection techniques led to an exploration of whether DNA might be successfully injected into human cells. A method of direct nuclear microinjection of DNA constructs was used for transfection of human vascular smooth muscle cells (SMCs).

Methods.—The nuclei of human saphenous vein SMCs, harvested by an explant technique, were microinjected with the plasmid pCMVβ containing the *lacZ* gene for β-galactosidase (β-gal). The efficiency of injection and expression were evaluated by histochemical staining for β-gal. Standard assays of viability and migration were also applied to injected SMCs.

Results.—Positive blue staining of the cells, evidence of gene expression, was found as early as 1 hour and as late as 60 hours after injection. Analysis of parameters affecting the conditions of injection were analyzed to optimize transfection efficiency. Compared with a horizontal approach, a vertical injection led to a 2-fold increase in expression of β-gal. The vertical approach was also technically easier and faster in this cell model. A maximal rate of expression of β-gal was achieved at a DNA concentration of 100 ng/μL (390 copies/injection). Maximal expression was obtained with a time of injection of 200 to 500 ms, an injection pressure of 5 to 10 psi, and a pipette size of 0.6 μm, producing an injection volume of 0.03 pL. Cytoplasmic, versus nuclear, injection yielded no gene expression. The injection process employed did not alter the ability of SMCs to migrate under videomicroscopy.

Conclusion.—A reproducible method for nuclear microinjection of DNA constructs into cultured SMCs derived from human saphenous vein has been developed. With the use of a vertical approach and optimal parameters

TABLE 1.—Optimal Parameters for Injection of Human Saphenous Vein Smooth Muscle Cells

Parameter	Optimal Setting
Approach	Vertical
DNA concentration	100 ng/μL
Pipette tip size	150 kPa
Duration of injection	500 ms
Pressure of injection	5 psi
Volume of injection	0.03 pl

(Table 1), a 60% efficiency of transfection and cell viability greater than 95% were achieved.

▶ This article provides a tremendous advance in technology associated with gene transfer. Understanding the physiologic consequences of gene transfer in vitro and in vivo is hampered by the low transfection rates (5%-15%). Even in settings of successful transfection, cellular viability is often compromised, decreasing the effective transfection rate. These authors describe a microinjection technique that maintains cellular viability at 95% and increases transfection efficiency to 65%. Furthermore, microinjection does not appear to influence human vascular SMC migration; this technique, while not widely available today may provide an effective adjunct to facilitate gene transfer studies for in vitro applications. This technique may have limited applicability to the in vivo arena.

M. T. Watkins, MD

Autoantibodies Against Oxidatively Modified Lipoproteins and Progression of Carotid Restenosis After Carotid Endarterectomy
Meraviglia MV, Maggi E, Bellomo G, et al (Ospedale San Raffaele, Milan, Italy; Ospedale Policlinico San Matteo, Pavia, Italy; Ospedale Maggiore, Novara, Italy)
Stroke 33:1139-1141, 2002   1–26

Introduction.—Oxidized low-density lipoproteins (LDLs) may be important in progression of carotid stenosis. It is not known if oxidized LDLs increase restenosis after carotid endarterectomy. This was investigated in 52 patients who underwent carotid endarterectomy.

Methods.—The study included 37 men and 15 women (ages 59-75 years; mean age, 67.3 years), who underwent carotid surgery for symptomatic stenosis of more than 75%. The presence of antibodies against oxidized LDL in the serum at the time of surgery was assessed and compared with echo Doppler flow imaging measurements of intima-media thickness 6 months after surgery.

Results.—At 6 months after surgery, a significant association was observed between the arterial wall thickness at the site of surgery and the absolute value of IgG antibodies against oxidized LDL ($P < .012$) and IgM immunocomplexes ($P < .03$).

Conclusion.—The presence of antibodies against oxidized LDL at the time of surgery predicts a greater intima-media wall thickness after surgery.

▶ This study uses intima-media thickness as a surrogate marker of carotid restenosis after carotid endarterectomy. The idea, of course, is to identify something that can be modified to prevent intimal hyperplasia associated with arterial injury. I will need a larger study with actual clinically significant levels of carotid stenosis as end points before I accept intimial medial thickening as a valuable measurement of early carotid injury that ultimately predicts potentially clinically significant carotid restenosis.

G. L. Moneta, MD

Endothelial Healing in Vein Grafts: Proliferative Burst Unimpaired by Genetic Therapy of Neointimal Disease

Ehsan A, Mann MJ, Dell' Acqua G, et al (Harvard Med School, Boston)
Circulation 105:1686-1692, 2002   1–27

Background.—Experimental evidence indicates cell cycle gene blockade therapy inhibits neointimal hyperplasia and improves endothelial cell functioning. However, little is known about endothelial healing immediately after vein grafting and how cell cycle gene blockade may affect healing of the endothelium. The effects of cell cycle gene blockade with E2F decoy oligodeoxynucleotide (ODN) on endothelial healing were examined.

Methods.—Jugular vein–carotid artery interposition grafts were performed in New Zealand white rabbits. A 2-cm vein graft was harvested and incubated for 10 minutes in either normal saline at ambient pressure or the E2F decoy ODN at 300 mm Hg. The vein graft was then placed as a carotid interpositional graft and vessels subsequently harvested at 1, 3, 7, and 14 days after surgery. At 18 and 12 hours before harvesting, bromodeoxyuridine was administered. Harvested vessels were pressure fixed and treated with silver staining. Endothelial cell density was determined by scanning electron microscopy. En face endothelial preparations were examined immunohistochemically via Häutchen preparation, and whole graft lysates were examined by Western blotting to identify proliferating cell nuclear antigen. In addition, human umbilical vein endothelial cells (HUVECs) and human umbilical artery smooth muscle cells (HUASMCs) were cultured and exposed to E2F decoy ODN, and their proliferation was examined.

Results.—In controls, on day 1, the endothelial cell density decreased significantly in the grafted vein compared with the ungrafted vein in response to acute stretching of the native vein graft wall. However, cell density increased back to baseline by day 3. The bromodeoxyuridine labeling index increased dramatically by day 2 (Fig 2, B), which indicated rapid endothelial cell proliferation. Treatment with E2F decoy ODN significantly inhibited vascular smooth muscle cell proliferation but had no effect on endothelial cell proliferation. This differential response was also seen in cultured human cells, in which E2F decoy ODN inhibited HUASMC proliferation but did not affect the proliferation of HUVECs. Furthermore, an electrophoretic mobility shift assay confirmed that E2F binding activity decreased significantly in HUASMCs but not in HUVECs.

Conclusion.—A cell cycle gene blockade with E2F decoy ODN selectively inhibits vascular smooth muscle cell activation and proliferation but does not affect endothelial cell variables. The E2F decoy ODN gene does not block the burst of endothelial cell proliferation, thus allowing normal endothelial healing.

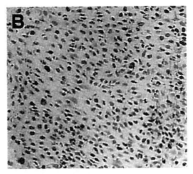

FIGURE 2B.—Bromodeoxyuridine labeling of endothelial cells. Light microscopy photomicrographs of Häutchen preparations for postoperative day 2 vein graft (magnification, ×400). (Courtesy of Ehsan A, Mann MJ, Dell' Acqua G, et al: Endothelial healing in vein grafts: Proliferative burst unimpaired by genetic therapy of neointimal disease. *Circulation* 105(14):1686-1692, 2002.)

▶ As PREVENT III rapidly approaches its target enrollment of 1400 patients, it is comforting that basic considerations in support of the E2F decoy strategy continue to trickle forth. The E2F decoy is an ODN that binds the E2F transcription factor and prevents it from promoting cell replication. It is being studied in human beings receiving vein bypass grafts where it is hoped that the initial burst of smooth muscle proliferation in bypass grafts will be blocked to improve graft durability. However, a nagging question has been whether the decoy might also block endothelial cell replication and prevent restoration of the protective monolayer at the graft lumen. In this study, the Brigham group reassures us by showing the E2F decoy selectively blocks smooth muscle cell replication but not endothelial cell replication or regeneration in a rabbit vein graft model. The result is largely academic at this point as clinical data will be available soon.

R. L. Geary, MD

Blood Monocyte Concentration Is Critical for Enhancement of Collateral Artery Growth

Heil M, Ziegelhoeffer T, Pipp F, et al (Max Planck Inst for Physiological and Clinical Research, Bad Nauheim, Germany)
Am J Physiol 283:H2411-H2419, 2002   1–28

Background.—Evidence is mounting that collateral arteries, unlike capillary growth during angiogenesis, originate from preexisting arterial anastomoses that are composed of the endothelium and the surrounding smooth muscle cell layers. The hypothesis that arteriogenesis is linked functionally to the concentration of circulating blood monocytes was tested in 2 animal models of acute femoral artery occlusion.

Methods.—Monocyte concentrations in peripheral blood of New Zealand white rabbits and mice were manipulated by single injections of the antimetabolite 5-fluorouracil (5FU). 5FU initially results in a decrease of monocytes followed by a rebound increase in monocytes in these species with the rebound occurring more rapidly in the rabbit versus the mouse. A model of acute femoral artery ligation was used to assess collateral artery growth in both species.

Results.—At day 7 of ligation, collateral conductance and the number of visible collateral arteries were increased in the rebound rabbit group. Concurrent with this increase, there was increased monocyte accumulation as demonstrated by immunohistology in the thigh 3 days after surgery. In the murine model, treatment with 5FU prompted a dramatic decrease in blood monocyte numbers, followed by a rebound effect at day 12. Blood flow in the mouse foot, as determined by laser Doppler imaging before and several times after surgery, increased from day 7 through day 21 in mice from the rebound group. In contrast, ligation during monocyte depletion caused a reduction in blood flow reconstitution, which was reversed by an injection of isolated monocytes.

Conclusions.—There is a functional link between the monocyte concentration in the peripheral blood and the enhancement of arteriogenesis.

▶ Using 2 different animal models (rabbit and mouse), these investigators provide convincing evidence to support the hypothesis that circulating monocytes rather than endothelial progenitors promote arteriogenesis during acute limb ischemia. The methods used to support this hypothesis include stimulation of monocytes utilizing rebound after 5FU administration and chronic infusion of monocyte chemoattractant protein using a mini-osmotic pump. This suggests that inflammatory processes may predominate during arteriogenesis. These authors cannot discount a role for bone marrow precursors in the development of arteriogenesis. Recent data clearly document the fact that monocyte and endothelial precursors share a common bone marrow precursor. Furthermore, clinically significant ischemia usually develops over time in a chronic fashion. It's unclear whether observations regarding arteriogenesis in acute ischemia models will be relevant to chronic ischemia.

M. T. Watkins, MD

Differential Effects of Vascular Growth Factors on Arterial and Venous Angiogenesis

Blebea J, Vu J-H, Assadnia S, et al (Pennsylvania State Univ, Hershey)
J Vasc Surg 35:532-538, 2002   1–29

Background.—Proangiogenic agents such as vascular endothelial growth factor (VEGF) and naltrexone induce new blood vessel growth. Growth factors such as the endogenous opioid growth factor (OGF) and retinoic acid inhibit angiogenesis. To date, no one has studied the differential effects of any growth factor on veins and arteries.

Methods.—In vivo angiogenesis was quantitated with the use of the chick chorioallantoic membrane (CAM) assay. Fertilized chick embryos were incubated for 3 days and explanted. A 3.2- mm methylcellulose disk containing VEGF or naltrexone or the inhibitors OGF or retinoic acid were then placed onto the surface of the CAM. An equal volume of distilled water was used as a control substance. The CAM arteries and veins were studied after 2 days of growth.

Findings.—Compared with control values, VEGF and naltrexone, the angiogenic stimulators, substantially increased the total number and length of all blood vessels. The mean length of blood vessels was reduced, suggesting that new vessel growth was induced. Also, VEGF and naltrexone proportionately increased vein and artery angiogenesis. Artery-to-vein ratios for vessel number and length were maintained. The inhibitors OGF and retinoic acid markedly reduced the total number and length of blood vessels in the CAM preparations. These agents had a disproportionately greater inhibitory effect on arterial angiogenesis, reflected in reduced artery-to-vein ratios for number and length of vessels.

Conclusion.—Naltrexone and VEGF induce vein and artery development in a proportional way. However, OGF and retinoic acid inhibited arterial angiogenesis more than venous angiogenesis. These data may be important for defining the mechanisms of action and for designing treatments.

▶ These investigators remind us how naive we may be when considering endothelial cells or smooth muscle cells as generic cell-types, irrespective of their origin. How often do we see cells cultured from veins or umbilical vessels used to model mechanisms of arterial pathology? This study shows that microvessels respond very differently depending whether they are on the arterial or venous side of the embryonic circulation. While most relevant to angiogenesis, these data are in line with a growing literature showing diversity among populations of a given cell type at different locations within the vascular tree. It should not be a shock that smooth muscle cells in an artery wall have functions unique to those in comparison to a nearby vein or that those from coronary and carotid arteries (arising from totally different embryonic populations) have different phenotypes. By focusing on these differences, we may be able to explain patterns of vascular diseases and help define what must be done to get a vein graft to optimally adapt to the arterial environment.

R. L. Geary, MD

Overexpression of von Willebrand Factor Is an Independent Risk Factor for Pathogenesis of Intimal Hyperplasia: Preliminary Studies
Qin F, Impeduglia T, Schaffer P, et al (Heart and Vascular Inst of New Jersey, Englewood)
J Vasc Surg 37:433-439, 2003   1–30

Background.—Von Willebrand factor (vWF), a multimeric glycoprotein, is expressed by endothelial cells and megakaryocytes and secreted into plasma and subendothelial space, enabling platelet adhesion at injury sites. Binding and stabilizing factor VIII is the primary function of vWF, and deficiencies produce von Willebrand disease (vWD). Because of the fact there is increased deposition in the hyperplastic intima of vascular grafts, elevated levels of vWF in patients who have cardiovascular diseases, and the finding vWF-deficient pigs show resistance to atherosclerotic progression, vWF may play a significant role in vascular remodeling processes. The role of vWF in the pathogenesis of intimal hyperplasia (IH) was evaluated.

Methods.—Mice aortic smooth muscle cells (SMC) were exposed to vWF in concentrations of 0, 5, 20, 100, 500, and 1000 ng/mL in vitro. H-thymidine incorporation indicated DNA synthesis of SMC. In an in vivo evaluation, 108 mice from inbred strains of C57BL/6J (controls) and RIIIS/J (characteristic of low plasma vWF) underwent carotid artery ligation (flow cessation model). They were divided into 3 groups: C57BL/6J, RIIIS/J, and RIIIS/J treated with desmopressin (DDAVP), 3 µg/kg/d injected intraperitoneally. Carotid arteries were harvested after 2 and 4 weeks and analyzed. Enzyme-linked immunosorbent assay determined plasma vWF levels.

Results.—In vitro, a positive dose-response curve was observed with vWF doses at 5 to 1000 ng/mL of vWF for aortic smooth muscle cells grown in fetal bovine serum–enhanced culture medium. In cells grown in culture medium without fetal bovine serum, a positive dose-response curve was observed with vWF doses between 5 and 100 ng/mL but disappeared at doses greater than 500 ng/mL. In vivo, controls exhibited graduated and prominent IH at 2 and 4 weeks. Carotid ligation did not induce IH in the RIIIS/J group, but some IH was observed in the RIIIS/J mice treated with DDAVP. There were no notable morphologic changes in the unligated arteries of the 3 groups. In carotid arteries of the control group, vWF was identified in the neointimal extracellular matrix and vasa vasora of the outer media and adventitia. RIIIS/J mice who received DDAVP had less deposition, whereas RIIIS/J mice not given DDAVP had only positive endothelial cytoplasmic staining and no intimal vWF deposits. Plasma levels of vWF were 110% in controls, 21% in RIIIS/J mice, and 45% in RIIIS/J mice treated with DDAVP. Levels drawn at 2 and 4 weeks did not differ within groups. All control mice exhibited constant baseline expression of vWF–messenger RNA (mRNA) in unligated common carotid arteries, with ligation producing significant, persistent increases in vWF-mRNA. Compared with RIIIS/J mice, vWF-mRNA was 9 times higher in the carotid arteries of C57BL/6J mice and 4 times higher in RIIIS/J mice treated with DDAVP.

Conclusions.—Smooth muscle cell proliferation in vitro was stimulated by vWF in a direct dose-response effect. IH acceleration was proportional to vWF expression without platelet activation and release of platelet-derived growth factor. Thus, controlling IH may involve modulating vWF expression.

▶ In addition to its presence in plasma, vWF is present in the subendothelial space. It accumulates in increased amounts in hyperplastic intima associated with vascular grafts. What it is doing there is anyone's guess, but it appears to be one of many "growth factors" that can stimulate smooth muscle cell proliferation.

G. L. Moneta, MD

A Chemically Modified Dextran Inhibits Smooth Muscle Cell Growth In Vitro and Intimal in Stent Hyperplasia In Vivo

Deux J-F, Prigent-Richard S, d'Angelo G, et al (X Bichat Med School, Paris; Tenon Hosp, Villetaneuse, France; CNRS-Univ Paris 13)
J Vasc Surg 35:973-981, 2002   1–31

Background.—The accumulation of neointimal smooth muscle cells (SMCs) in response to vascular injury plays a critical part in postangioplasty restenosis. Polypeptide growth factors have been identified as activators of SMC migration and proliferation, but heparin and related synthetic sulfated polysaccharides, such as β-cyclodextrin tetradecasulfate or pentosan polysulfate, are inhibitors of SMC growth. Previous studies have found the distribution of carboxymethyl, benzylamide, and sulfonate–sulfate groups along a dextran backbone allows the production of synthetic polysaccharides with antiproliferative activity for SMCs. The in vitro and in vivo SMC growth inhibitory activity of a specific nonanticoagulant chemically modified detxran, E9, was investigated in an animal model.

Methods.—SMC proliferation was followed in culture in the presence of E9 by cell counting, thymidine uptake, and cell cycle analysis in a murine model. Western blot analysis was performed on phosphorylated mitogen-activated protein kinase (MAPK) extracellular signal-regulated protein kinase 1/2 proteins, and MAPK activity on serum-stimulated SMCs was also investigated. The binding and internalization of radiolabeled and fluorescent-labeled E9 were followed with binding displacement experiments, electron microscopy, and cell fractionation. For the in vivo experiments, iliac arteries from New Zealand white rabbits were injured with balloon dilation and stent deployment. The animals were treated for 2 weeks with saline solution or E9, after which time the animals were killed and the arteries harvested for morphometric analyses (6 arteries, 18 sections).

Results.—In the in vitro experiments, nonanticoagulant E9 inhibited SMC proliferation. Tyrosine phosphorylation of MAPK 1/2 and MAPK activity were inhibited with E9 within 5 minutes of incubation. Evidence of binding and rapid cytoplasmic internalization of the synthetic compound was seen, but, in contrast to heparin, no evidence of any nuclear localization of the antiproliferative E9 was found. In the in vivo experiment, qualitative modifications of neointimal structure with a thinner fibrocellular neointima were noticed after E9 treatment. The morphometric analyses of stented arteries in the E9-treated rabbits showed an important reduction of intimal growth of 33% for intimal area and 45% for the intima/media ratio.

Conclusions.—These experiments showed that cytoplasmic internalization of the synthetic polysaccharide correlated to the SMC growth inhibition involving the MAPK pathway in an animal model. The nonanticoagulant derived dextran E9 seems to be a new candidate for potential selective treatment of SMC proliferation.

▶ Deja vu. These investigators remind us how well heparin worked to limit intimal hyperplasia after angioplasty in rats and rabbits and regurgitate the mantra that clinical trials of heparin to inhibit restenosis in human beings likely failed because too little drug was given for fear of bleeding complications. I feel compelled to remind them that very high doses of the same heparin shown by Clowes[1] to block intimal hyperplasia in rats had no effect on the response to angioplasty in primates. There are likely species differences and other factors to explain the difficulty we have had translating rodent successes into clinical successes. Using a modified nonanticoagulant dextran with antiproliferative properties similar to heparin, they reduced intimal hyperplasia after iliac artery stenting in rabbits. I wish them the best but won't hold my breath for the clinical trial.

R. L. Geary, MD

Reference

1. Clowes AW: Regulation of smooth muscle cell function by heparin. *J Vasc Surg* 15:911-913, 1992.

2 Endovascular

Endovascular Workforce for Peripheral Vascular Disease: Current and Future Needs
Wieslander CK, Huang CC, Omura MC, et al (Univ of California, Los Angeles)
J Vasc Surg 35:1218-1225, 2002   2–1

Background.—The growth of endovascular surgery is of interest to many cardiovascular specialists. Practitioners in interventional cardiology, interventional radiology, cardiovascular surgery, and peripheral vascular surgery have shown interest in performing peripheral endovascular procedures. However, the current status and future needs of peripheral endovascular utilization and training have not been well defined. The current number of patients and procedures and the numbers of treating physicians and surgeons were analyzed so that predictions and recommendations for the future could be formulated.

Methods.—Data on the number of vascular patients and procedures were obtained from the Healthcare Cost and Utilization Project Trend Query Web site. Telephone or e-mail contact with aortic endograft manufacturers was used to obtain the number of endovascular abdominal aortic aneurysm repairs. Other data gathered for this analysis included the number of different cardiovascular specialists, the number of accredited US cardiovascular fellowship programs and first year positions for 2000 to 2001, and the number of endovascular fellowship programs and first year positions (Table 5).

Results.—The numbers of vascular patients and procedures rose from 1993 to 1997, and this trend is expected to continue as the US population ages. The number of open cases has also continued to rise, despite the rapid rise of the use of endovascular procedures. However, it is expected that the number of vascular specialists will remain stable (Table 6).

TABLE 5.—Board Certification of Cardiovascular Specialists

Specialty	Total No. Certified
Cardiology[22]	19,354 (since 1941)
Cardiothoracic surgery[23]	5261 (living in 1996)
Interventional cardiology[22]	2108 (since Nov 1999)
Vascular surgery[24]	2055 (since 1982)
Interventional radiology[25]	1466 (since 1990)

(Reprinted from Wieslander CK, Huang CC, Omura MC, et al: Endovascular workforce for peripheral vascular disease: Current and future needs. *J Vasc Surg* 35:1218-1225, 2002. Copyright 2002 by Elsevier.)

TABLE 6.—Accredited Fellowship Programs in the United States

Specialty	No. of Programs	No. of First Year Positions
Interventional radiology[26]	94	240
Cardiothoracic surgery[26]	90	148
Interventional cardiology[26]	55	127
Vascular surgery[26]	89	100
Total	328	615

(Reprinted from Wieslander CK, Huang CC, Omura MC, et al: Endovascular workforce for peripheral vascular disease: Current and future needs. *J Vasc Surg* 35:1218-1225, 2002. Copyright 2002 by Elsevier.)

Conclusions.—This analysis indicates a looming critical shortage of endovascularly trained specialists. Meeting these future needs will require more surgeons to receive endovascular training.

▶ I don't think anyone really has any idea how many vascular specialists of all sorts are going to be needed in the future. I don't believe many people in the United States are denied care because of unavailability of a specialist to perform a needed procedure. Economic, social, and logistic factors seem more important.

G. L. Moneta, MD

Lifeline Registry of Endovascular Aneurysm Repair: Registry Data Report

McKinlay S, for the Lifeline Registry of Endovascular Aneurysm Repair Steering Committee (NERI, Watertown, Mass)
J Vasc Surg 35:616-620, 2002   2–2

Background.—The goal of the Lifeline Registry of Endovascular Aneurysm Repair is to collect long-term data on patients receiving endovascular grafts and open surgical reconstruction for abdominal aortic aneurysm (AAA). These data will be used to evaluate the aggregate safety and effectiveness of endovascular grafts in the treatment of aneurysmal disease. An analysis of early data collected by the Registry was presented.

Methods.—Follow-up data were collected on 1757 patients, including 1646 patients who received endovascular grafts and 111 surgical patients, who were treated for AAA.

Results.—The mean age of the graft recipients was 73.1 years, and the mean age for surgical patients was 71.1 years. The most prevalent risk factors were hypertension, myocardial infarction, and chronic obstructive pulmonary disease. Both groups had similar baseline risk factors, but the endovascular graft recipients had significantly less hypertension than patients in the surgical group. Logistic regression analysis of 1-year survival indicates that the factors most likely to decrease 1-year survival for the surgical group were renal failure and larger aneurysm size. For the patients who received an endovascular graft, the presence of renal failure, chronic obstructive pulmonary disease, congestive heart failure, larger aneurysm size, and increased age reduced the 1-year survival.

At publication, approximately 80% of endovascular recipients had been followed up for 1 year. Of these patients, 17% have experienced an endoleak, and 4.6% have experienced enlargement of the aneurysm. A total of 80 (4.9%) endovascular graft recipients were converted to surgery. The factors most frequently involved in the conversion to surgery were an increase in aneurysm diameter, aneurysm rupture, and the presence of a proximal endoleak.

Conclusion.—Early and late complications of endovascular grafting for AAA are relatively frequent. These early data demonstrate the importance of early and ongoing surveillance of endovascular graft recipients.

▶ This is the first published report of the Lifeline Registry of Endovascular Aneurysm Repair and represents the inaugural data analysis of a national endovascular registry. It offers some important insights about the demographic characteristics of the patient population treated for AAA. The early follow-up data, however, are limited to only 2 endograft devices. As with any clinical database, the accuracy of data analysis is directly correlated with the thoroughness in which the data are entered—a formidable challenge for any large-scale national registry. Yet the goal for a complete, prospectively collected database is very important since it has the potential to provide outcomes analysis that will ultimately influence the long-term care of our patients. Additional updated information about the Lifeline Registry can be found at www.lifelineregistry.org.

R. M. Fujitani, MD

Routine Use of Intravascular Ultrasound for Endovascular Aneurysm Repair: Angiography Is Not Necessary
von Segesser LK, Marty B, Ruchat P, et al (Centre Hospitalier Universitaire Vaudois, Lausanne, Switzerland; Ospedale San Giovanni, Bellinzona, Switzerland)
Eur J Vasc Endovasc Surg 23:537-542, 2002   2–3

Introduction.—The preprocedural assessment of endovascular aneurysm repair (EVAR) may change with the routine use of intravascular ultrasound (IVUS). The outcomes of endovascular abdominal aortic aneurysm (AAA) and thoracic aortic aneurysm (TAA) repair were evaluated in 80 consecutive patients with the use of preprocedural angiography versus IVUS for preoperative planning.

Methods.—The median patient age was 69 years (range, 25-90 years); 72 (80%) were men. Sixty-eight (85%) underwent AAA repair and 12 (15%) underwent TAA repair; 31 patients (39%) underwent preprocedural angiography and 49 (61%) underwent IVUS, according to surgeon preference.

Results.—Hospital mortality was 3% (1 [2%] for AAA; 1 [8%] for TAA); 7% for angiography (1/31) and 0% for IVUS (0/49) (P = NS). The median x-ray exposure time was 24 minutes (range, 9-65 minutes) for angiography versus 8 minutes (range, 0-60 minutes) for IVUS ($P < .05$). The median quantity of contrast medium was 190 mL for angiography and 0 mL for IVUS ($P < .01$). No incidence of coverage of renal or suprarenal artery orifices occurred. Conversion to open surgery was required in 5% of patients: 3% (1/31) for angiography and 6% (3/49) for IVUS. Early endoleaks occurred in 16% (13/80): 26% (8/31) for angiography and 10% (5/49) for IVUS ($P < .05$). Endoleaks resolved spontaneously in 39% (5/13); 61% (8/13) needed additional procedures.

Conclusion.—IVUS is reliable in target site identification, landing zone measurement, neck quality analysis, preprocedural quality assessment, and trouble shooting during EVAR. For most patients, preprocedural angiography is not needed for EVAR. The routine use of IVUS permits minimal use of contrast media and decreased exposure to radiation.

▶ Several issues related to this study deserve a close look. The authors report on what appears to be their initial endograft experience with the later patients not having angiography. One would assume that with increased experience alone, fluoroscopy time would diminish. As all the IVUS patients were at the latter end of the experience, differences in fluoroscopy could be explained by this alone. Additionally, the authors' experience is dominated by 2 grafts, the Talent graft and the Stenway graft, which is no longer available. No mention is made as to the relationship of the graft used to imaging technique, and it may be that the earlier graft (Stenway) may have been a more complex device to deploy, explaining the increase in fluoroscopy time. Lastly, the authors' average of 190 mL of contrast media for an elective endograft seems unusually high and is likely more than that of most experienced interventionalists. Whether this is due to stent graft design, operator experience, or imaging technique is unclear.

While this article does provide useful insight into the concept of utilizing IVUS alone as a method of intraoperative evaluation, it clearly has not proven the case for abandoning angiography. An important message is that in patients with renal impairment and favorable anatomy, IVUS can be safely used as an alternative to standard angiography to guide endograft placement.

D. G. Clair, MD

Does the Presence of an Iliac Aneurysm Affect Outcome of Endoluminal AAA Repair? An Analysis of 336 Cases
Parlani G, Zannetti S, Verzini F, et al (Policlinico Monteluce, Perugia, Italy)
Eur J Vasc Endovasc Surg 24:134-138, 2002   2–4

Introduction.—The presence of a common iliac artery (CIA) aneurysm may limit the ability of endoluminal abdominal aortic aneurysm (AAA) repair to accomplish full exclusion of the aneurysm with the stent graft. The effect of iliac aneurysms on the outcome of endovascular exclusion of AAA in terms of incidence of graft-associated endoleaks, AAA rupture, AAA growth, and the fate of the iliac aneurysmal sac was examined.

Methods.—Between April 1997 and March 2001, preoperative, operative, and follow-up data on 336 consecutive patients undergoing endovascular repair for AAAs were entered into a prospective database. The suitability for endovascular repair was evaluated via contrast-enhanced CT. A maximum CIA diameter of 20 mm or greater was considered to be an iliac aneurysm. Patients with and without iliac aneurysms were compared for early failure (ie, immediate conversion or perioperative death) or late failure (ie, increase in aneurysm diameter, persisting graft-associated endoleak, late AAA rupture, or conversion).

Results.—Of 59 patients (18%) with iliac aneurysms, 19 were bilateral (total of 78 aneurysmal iliac arteries). The median diameter of the iliac aneurysms was 23 mm (range, 20-50 mm). A distal seal was attained by landing in 33 external iliac arteries, 20 ectatic CIAs, and 25 normal CIAs. Surgical times varied significantly between patients with and without CIA aneurysms (153 min vs 123 min; $P = .0001$), but no significant differences were observed among patients who had early or late failures (2% vs 3%; $P = .50$ and 14% vs 8%, $P = .11$, respectively). No incidence of buttock or colon necrosis occurred, but 7 patients had buttock claudications develop. At a median follow-up of 14 months (range, 0-46 months), the common iliac diameter diminished by 2 mm or more in 49 cases, remained stable in 25, and increased by 2 mm or more in 3 cases.

Conclusion.—The presence of an iliac aneurysm does not influence the outcome of endoluminal AAA repair but does require adjunctive procedures.

▶ These authors demonstrate that iliac artery enlargement in patients who undergo endoluminal AAA repair increases the surgical time, blood loss, and fluoroscopy time. However, the overall short-term and mid-term results appear to be similar compared with patients with nonaneurysmal iliac arteries. There are some worrisome findings within this article. One group of patients had a late 5% rate of proximal type I endoleak, something I would consider as failure of therapy. When extending to the external iliac, most surgeons/radiologists embolize the hypogastric artery to prevent a type II endoleak. Interestingly, these authors performed hypogastric embolization in only 8 of 33 cases, yet there was no difference in the incidence of type II endoleaks. Despite this finding, if I had to extend to the external iliac artery (something I try to avoid), I still would favor placing coils in the proximal hypogastric. The other treatment options used by these authors include landing in an ectatic iliac artery with a flared stent graft, or landing in a normal common iliac just distal to an ectatic/aneurysmal iliac. Of course, the other option is open aneurysm repair.

T. K. Liem, MD

Broadening the Applicability of Endovascular Aneurysm Repair: The Use of Iliac Conduits

Abu-Ghaida AM, Clair DG, Greenberg RK, et al (Cleveland Clinic Found, Ohio)
J Vasc Surg 36:111-117, 2002   2–5

Background.—Suboptimal iliac anatomy can preclude the use of endovascular techniques for the repair of abdominal aortic aneurysm (AAA). Outcomes with the use of a limited retroperitoneal approach and iliac conduit were reported for a series of patients with AAA and unsuitable iliac anatomy at high risk for standard open repair.

Methods.—A total of 312 patients underwent endovascular (AAA) repair at 1 clinic between June 1999 and November 2000. A review of charts and imaging studies identified a subgroup of 22 patients with complex iliac anatomy in whom an iliac conduit was placed. Of these procedures, 17 were planned and 5 were unplanned with the iliac conduit placed after an iliac artery injury. A group of 17 patients who underwent a standard endovascular repair without conduits was selected and matched to the 17 patients in the planned conduit group by baseline co-morbidities. The conduits used in these patients were 8 mm or 10 mm polyester grafts sewn proximally to the common iliac artery (Fig 4). After the endograft was inserted through the conduit, the distal end of the conduit was anastomosed to the external iliac or common femoral vessels.

Results.—Operative time was longer and estimated blood loss greater in the patients in whom conduits were placed, particularly when the placement was performed as an unplanned procedure. Operative time and stays in the hospital and in the ICU were longer for the patients with iliac conduits, but

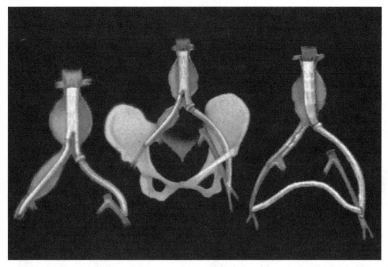

FIGURE 4.—Potential alternatives for revascularization with use of iliac conduit. (Reprinted from Abu-Ghaida AM, Clair DG, Greenberg RK, et al: Broadening the applicability of endovascular aneurysm repair: The use of iliac conduits. *J Vasc Surg* 36:111-117, 2002. Copyright 2002 by Elsevier.)

the cardiac pulmonary and renal complication rates were similar for the conduit group and the standard endovascular repair group.

Conclusion.—The applicability of endovascular repair of AAAs is increased by the use of a limited retroperitoneal approach and iliac conduit for patients with difficult iliac anatomy. This technique should be considered when an open surgical approach is contraindicated.

▶ If you want to push the indications for surgery, it is always possible to do so. The use of iliac conduits increases the number of patients who can be treated with endovascular aneurysm repair. I personally would not recommend this technique in individuals who are suitable candidates for open repair.

G. L. Moneta, MD

A Prospective Evaluation of Hypogastric Artery Embolization in Endovascular Aortoiliac Aneurysm Repair
Lin PH, Bush RL, Chaikof EL, et al (Baylor College of Medicine, Houston; Emory Univ, Atlanta, Ga)
J Vasc Surg 36:500-506, 2002   2–6

Background.—Hypogastric artery embolization (HAE) is often performed in endovascular aortoiliac aneurysm repair to prevent potential endoleaks. However, HAE can be associated with pelvic ischemic sequelae. The clinical outcome of HAE was prospectively evaluated in patients who underwent endovascular aortoiliac aneurysm repair.

Methods.—A group of 12 patients who underwent either a unilateral or bilateral HAE for endovascular aortoiliac aneurysm repair over 15 months were prospectively evaluated. All patients underwent preoperative or postoperative penile pressure measurement and pulse-volume recording evaluation. Angiographic features relating to pelvic collaterals and clinical outcomes relating to pelvic ischemia were evaluated.

Results.—Unilateral HAE was performed in 8 patients (67%), and bilateral HAE was performed in 4 patients (33%). The mean reductions in

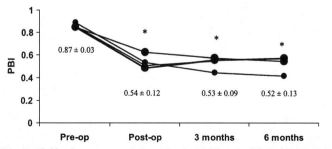

FIGURE 2.—Penile blood pressure comparison in patients undergoing bilateral HAE. *$P < .05$ when compared with preoperative PBI value. *Abbreviations: HAE*, Hypogastric artery embolization; *PBI*, penile brachial index; *Pre-op*, preoperative PBI value; *Post-op*, postoperative PBI value before discharge. (Reprinted from Lin PH, Bush RL, Chaikof EL, et al: A prospective evaluation of hypogastric artery embolization in endovascular aortoiliac aneurysm repair. *J Vasc Surg* 36:500-506, 2002. Copyright 2002 by Elsevier.)

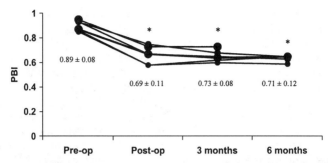

FIGURE 4.—Penile blood pressure comparison in patients in whom postoperative buttock and thigh claudication developed after either unilateral or bilateral HAE. *P < .05 when compared with preoperative PBI value. *Abbreviations: HAE*, Hypogastric artery embolization; *PBI*, penile brachial index; *Pre-op*, preoperative PBI value; *Post-op*, postoperative PBI value before discharge. (Reprinted from Lin PH, Bush RL, Chaikof EL, et al: A prospective evaluation of hypogastric artery embolization in endovascular aortoiliac aneurysm repair. *J Vasc Surg* 36:500-506, 2002. Copyright 2002 by Elsevier.)

penile brachial index (PBI) after unilateral and bilateral HAE were 13 ± 6% (not significant) and 39 ± 14%, respectively (Fig 2). Erectile dysfunction occurred in 3 patients for unilateral HAE (38%) and in 2 patients for bilateral HAE (50%), and the overall PBI reduction was 36 ± 12%. No significant change was found in the thigh brachial or ankle brachial index after HAE. Hip and buttock claudication occurred in 4 patients who underwent unilateral HAE (50%) and in 2 patients who underwent bilateral HAE (50%), and the overall PBI reduction was 18 ± 9% (Fig 4). Other associated pelvic ischemic complications after bilateral HAE included scrotal skin sloughing 3 days after aortic endografting (1 patient) and sacral decubitus that occurred 4 months after aortic endografting (1 patient). Diseased profunda femoral arteries were observed in 4 patients, all of whom had pelvic ischemic symptoms develop after HAE. However, only 4 of the remaining 8 patients with normal or mild profunda femoral artery disease had pelvic ischemic sequelae after HAE.

Conclusions.—In patients who undergo endovascular aortoiliac aneurysm repair, erectile dysfunction after HAE correlates with a significant reduction in PBI. Severe pelvic ischemic symptoms are more likely to occur after bilateral HAE. Patients with diseased profunda femoral arteries are at high risk of pelvic ischemia after HAE. Concomitant profundaplasty may have a role during aortic endografting to improve pelvic collateral flow and to reduce pelvic ischemia in this subset of patients undergoing HAE.

▶ These authors report on 12 patients who underwent either unilateral or bilateral HAE in preparation for endoluminal aortoiliac aneurysm repair. Buttock claudication occurred in 50% (consistent with several other series) and erectile dysfunction in 38% to 50%. Even Viagra was unable to overcome the coils in most of these patients. Previously, it was thought that endoluminal repair might be associated with a lower incidence of erectile dysfunction when compared with open repair. As this study suggests, we may just be replacing impotence due to splanchnic neurotrauma with vasculogenic impotence. Of note, the authors found that a diseased profunda femoris artery was associated with a higher incidence of pelvic ischemia. However, there is no evidence that routine profundoplasty will help the situation. The authors should be commended for their honest reporting of some fairly poor results.

T. K. Liem, MD

Bell-Bottom Aortoiliac Endografts: An Alternative That Preserves Pelvic Blood Flow
Kritpracha B, Pigott JP, Russell TE, et al (Jobst Vascular Ctr, Toledo, Ohio)
J Vasc Surg 35:874-881, 2002   2–7

Background.—Dilated common iliac arteries that complicate endovascular stent grafting (ESG) usually are managed with extension of the endograft across the iliac artery bifurcation combined with internal iliac artery occlusion. This study compared treatment of patients with significant common iliac artery dilation by 2 methods: endograft extension across the iliac bifurcation or a new approach using a flared cuff within the common iliac artery that preserves the internal iliac artery.

Methods.—The study group comprised 25 patients with at least 1 dilated common iliac artery. Group 1 consisted of 10 patients who underwent ESG with a standard approach using a straight extension across the iliac bifurcation and internal iliac artery coil embolization before the procedure or simultaneously with ESG. Group 2 consisted of 15 patients who underwent ESG with a flared distal cuff contained within the common iliac artery, or the "bell-bottom" procedure, which preserved the internal iliac artery (Fig 2). The main outcome measures included iliac artery dimensions, operating room times, fluoroscopy time, and postoperative complications.

Results.—The mean preoperative diameter of the abdominal aortic aneurysm (AAA) was 56.6 mm, and the mean preoperative diameter of the common iliac artery was 21.4 mm. There was no significant difference in the mean postoperative diameters of the common iliac artery for the coil embolization procedure in group 1 (mean, 19.9 mm) versus the bell-bottom procedure in group 2 (mean, 19.1 mm). However, group 2 had significantly shorter operating room time and catheter procedure time (137 minutes vs 192 minutes and 58 minutes vs 106 minutes, respectively). Neither group had any periprocedure type I endoleaks.

Nine patients in group 2 also had a second contralateral common iliac artery aneurysm, and 5 of these patients underwent treatment with extension across the iliac artery bifurcation and internal iliac artery occlusion. The use of the bell-bottom procedure on the other side allowed preservation of 1 internal iliac artery. Four patients also underwent a contralateral bell-bottom procedure. Two of these patients had complications, with severe buttock claudication in 1 and distal embolism necessitating limb salvage bypass after preoperative coil embolization of the internal iliac artery in the other.

Conclusion.—Significant ectasia or small aneurysm of the common iliac artery is often associated with AAA. In these patients, the bell-bottom procedure to preserve circulation to the internal iliac artery is a new alternative to the standard treatment of placing endograft extensions across the iliac ar-

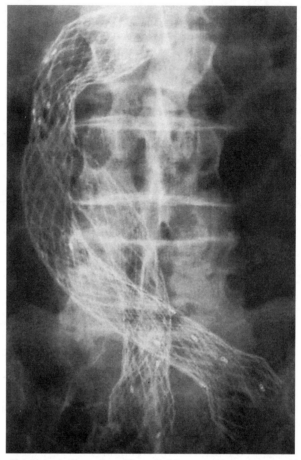

FIGURE 2.—Plain abdominal x-ray shows bilateral bell-bottom procedure. (Reprinted from Kritpracha B, Pigott JP, Russell TE, et al: Bell-bottom aortoiliac endografts: An alternative that preserves pelvic blood flow. *J Vasc Surg* 35:874-881, 2002. Copyright 2002 by Elsevier.)

tery bifurcation in patients with at least 1 common iliac artery diameter of less than 26 mm and is associated with reduced total procedure time.

▶ The authors noted a slightly decreased operating room time and catheter procedure time in the patients undergoing the bell-bottom technique. It is unclear whether this may be due to the fact that a different device was utilized for the bell-bottom procedures (AneuRx) as compared with the alternative strategy (Vanguard). With a very limited follow-up (mean, 8 months), the authors noted no differences in outcomes between the 2 groups. These results echo findings of previous authors using this technique that mild to moderately enlarged (<24 mm) iliac arteries do not mandate internal iliac artery exclusion for endovascular treatment.

D. G. Clair, MD

Identification and Implications of Transgraft Microleaks After Endovascular Repair of Aortic Aneurysms

Matsumura JS, Ryu RK, Ouriel K (Northwestern Univ, Chicago; Cleveland Clinic, Ohio)
J Vasc Surg 34:190-197, 2001   2–8

Introduction.—Endoleaks are frequent complications of endovascular repair of abdominal aortic aneurysms (AAAs), with leaks arising from patent vessels entering the aneurysm sac, from proximal and sital fixation sites and between components of modular grafts. This report describes another type of endoleak: the finding of microleaks, or tiny fabric defects, associated with persistent transgraft blood flow into the aneurysm sac.

Methods.—Four male patients who underwent endovascular repair of AAAs with modular nitinol/polyester endoprostheses were evaluated at 6 to 30 months and found to have transgraft microleaks.

Results.—Of the 4 AAAs, 3 continued to expand after the endograft repair. Standard CT scanning identified the presence but not the source of the endoleak (Fig 6). Color flow duplex US scanning was performed in 3 patients, and perigraft "jets," small areas of color flow adjacent to the endograft, were detected in each case. A microleak was observed in 1 additional patient who underwent digital subtraction arteriography with directed efforts to completely opacify the prosthesis lumen with multiple oblique projections (Fig 7). Contrast angiography with balloon occlusion of the distal endograft clearly identified midgraft microleaks that might otherwise be mistaken for graft porosity or cuff junction endoleaks. No microleaks were diagnosed with angiography when these directed efforts were not

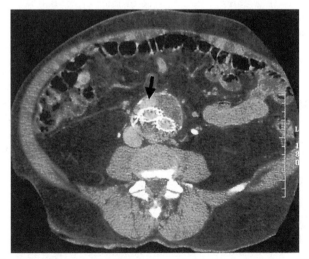

FIGURE 6.—CT scan showing endoleak (*black arrow*) intimately associated with middle segment of right iliac limb. (Reprinted from Matsumura JS, Ryu RK, Ouriel K: Identification and implications of transgraft microleaks after endovascular repair of aortic aneurysms. *J Vasc Surg* 34:190-197, 2001. Copyright 2001 by Elsevier.)

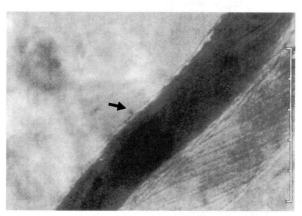

FIGURE 7.—Oblique magnified digital subtraction angiogram demonstrating microleak (*black arrow*) from midgraft. (Reprinted from Matsumura JS, Ryu RK, Ouriel K: Identification and implications of transgraft microleaks after endovascular repair of aortic aneurysms. *J Vasc Surg* 34:190-197, 2001. Copyright 2001 by Elsevier.)

undertaken. Aneurysm exploration before aortic clamping allowed conclusive determination of the presence of blood flow through the wall of the endoprostheses in 2 patients.

Conclusion.—Microleaks can occur up to 2.5 years after endovascular repair of AAAs. CT can detect the presence of an endoleak in these patients yet is not capable of identifying the exact site of origin. Doppler US scanning and directed arteriography seem to be of greater benefit in identifying the presence and location of a microleak. Balloon occlusion arteriography and aneurysm exploration without arterial clamping contribute definitive evidence of microleaks. The clinical significance of microleaks is unclear, but long-term monitoring of patients is crucial for diagnosing and treating these and other modes of endograft failure before they progress to aneurysm rupture.

▶ The "microleaks" described in this report appear to represent defects in the wall of the prosthesis. These defects arose from suture holes after breaking of the sutures used to secure the graft to the stent. Clearly, while there is a great deal of technology involved in the manufacture of aortic stent grafts, they are in many ways still "Mickey Mouse" devices that are capable of failing in more ways than we initially imagined.

G. L. Moneta, MD

Endograft Migration One to Four Years After Endovascular Abdominal Aortic Aneurysm Repair With the AneuRx Device: A Cautionary Note

Conners MS III, Sternbergh WC III, Carter G, et al (Ochsner Clinic Found, New Orleans, La)
J Vasc Surg 36:476-484, 2002   2–9

Background.—The long-term durability after endovascular aneurysm repair (EAR) is dependent on positional stability of the endograft. However, there have been few reports in the literature concerning the cumulative risk of delayed endograft migration. The incidence and risk factors for a specific failure mode—proximal endograft migration—were examined.

Methods.—Ninety-one patients underwent EAR with the AneuRx endograft. Data from a prospective database were assessed for proximal endograft migration, which was defined as a change of 5 mm or more from the initial position of the endograft. Several other anatomical characteristics were also evaluated. Of the original 91 patients, 69 were alive and had complete follow-up data at 1 year; the mean time from implantation was 33.2 ± 1.1 months.

Results.—Endograft migration developed in 15 patients, which yielded a cumulative event rate of 7.2% at 1 year, 20.4% at 2 years, 42.1% at 3 years, and 66.7% at 4 years after EAR (Fig 1). The initial aortic neck diameter did not differ between the groups; however, significant late aortic neck enlargement was observed in patients with migration but not in patients in whom no

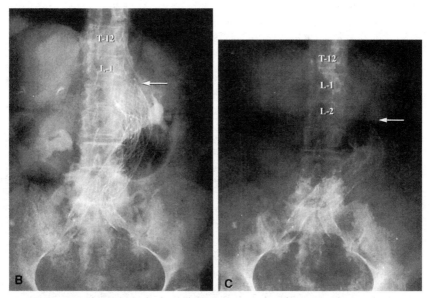

FIGURE 1.—**B,** Plain abdominal radiograph demonstrating endograft position at the L1-L2 level (*arrow*) 1-year post implantation. **C,** Plain abdominal radiograph demonstrating endograft position at the L2-L3 level (*arrow*) 2 years after implantation. (Reprinted from Conners MS III, Sternbergh WC III, Carter G, et al: Endograft migration one to four years after endovascular abdominal aortic aneurysm repair with the AneuRx device: A cautionary note. *J Vasc Surg* 36:476-484, 2002. Copyright 2002 by Elsevier.)

migration occurred. The overall risks of migration were 29.2% in patients with endografts oversized more than 20% and 18.6% in patients with endografts oversized 20% or less. Of the other anatomical characteristics assessed, aortic neck angulation, aortic neck length, initial endograft–aortic neck overlap, and the size of the abdominal aortic aneurysm were similar among patients with and without migration. Secondary endovascular treatment with aortic cuffs was required in 5 patients with device migration.

Conclusions.—A high incidence of device migration after EAR with the AneuRx endograft was found in this study. There was an increase in the incidence of migration with increasing duration of follow-up. Late aortic neck dilation was significantly associated with migration. Oversizing of the endograft by more than 20% may have accelerated this late aortic neck dilation. However, it is likely that the cause of endograft migration in this series of patients was multifactorial because the majority of patients (8 of 15) experiencing migration had endografts oversized by less than 20%. Endovascular repair of these device migrations is possible, but the long-term durability of these secondary procedures is unknown. Follow-up after EAR must include careful surveillance for proximal endograft migration.

▶ In this study, early endograft migration (1 year) tended to be related to shorter endograft/neck overlap. Endograft migration at all time points appeared to be related to increased neck diameter. While the authors did not find graft oversizing to be significantly related to endograft migration, there was clearly a trend in this direction. With these findings, the authors recommend routine measurement and recording of distance from the lowest renal artery to the top of the graft, clear documentation of neck diameter, prophylactic treatment for migrated endografts with less than 5 to 10 mm of graft/neck overlap, and close surveillance of patients treated for migration with cuff extension because of the risk of component separation. This study well documents the necessity of evaluating patients for endograft migration, especially in the setting where radial force is the only method of proximal endograft fixation.

D. G. Clair, MD

Ingrowth of Aorta Vascular Cells Into Basic Fibroblast Growth Factor–Impregnated Vascular Prosthesis Material: A Porcine and Human In Vitro Study on Blood Vessel Prosthesis Healing
van der Bas JMA, Quax PHA, van den Berg AC, et al (Gaubius Lab TNO-PG, Leiden, The Netherlands; Leiden Univ, The Netherlands)
J Vasc Surg 36:1237-1247, 2002   2–10

Background.—Endovascular aneurysm repair (EVAR) is an alternative treatment that is less invasive and provides reduced morbidity compared with conventional surgery for abdominal aortic aneurysm (AAA). However, endoleak between the aortic neck and the fabric of the endograft is a problem in EVAR and could potentially be reduced by improved healing of the endograft with the aortic neck. The hypothesis that the induction of vascular cell ingrowth into the graft material would promote better graft healing in EVAR was investigated.

Methods.—Both pig aorta and human normal and aneurysmal aortic wall were used in this study. Various growth factors (platelet-derived growth factor, vascular endothelial growth factor, and basic fibroblast growth factor [bFGF]) were evaluated for their potential to induce intimal hyperplasia. After selection of the most potent growth factor, a vascular prosthetic material (Dacron) impregnated with collagen and heparin was incubated with this growth factor. The impregnated pieces of Dacron were fixed on top of the aortic organ cultures for the study of ingrowth of the neointima formation into the graft material.

Results.—The most potent growth factor for induction of neointima in aortic organ cultures was bFGF, and the pieces of impregnated Dacron had a release of 5 ng/24 hr of bFGF for at least 28 days. When affixed to the top of the aortic organ culture, the bFGF-impregnated Dacron was capable of inducing neointima formation and ingrowth of the neointima into the graft material after 28 days.

Conclusions.—This study found that a Dacron prosthesis impregnated with collagen, heparin, and bFGF can induce graft healing in an in vitro model comprising aortic organ cultures of pig and human aortas. The indication from these findings is that the problem of endoleakage in EVAR may be obviated with a perfect proximal healing between the aortic wall and the prosthesis.

▶ The authors postulate that healing of an endograft to the aortic neck may solve the problem of delayed type I endoleak in patients with endovascular aneurysm repair. I doubt that this will be true. It appears that late type I leaks result from both graft migration and dilatation of the neck. Whereas better healing of the neck may decrease migration, it is unlikely to effect progression of aortic dilatation.

G. L. Moneta, MD

Pathogenetic Heterogeneity of In-Stent Lesion Formation in Human Peripheral Arterial Disease

Inoue S, Koyama H, Miyata T, et al (Univ of Tokyo)
J Vasc Surg 35:672-678, 2002   2–11

Background.—Intimal hyperplasia leads to in-stent restenosis after stent implantation. The major contributing factors to the development of in-stent restenosis have not been established. The authors suggest that heterogenous mechanisms coexist in the same lesion. The validity of this hypothesis was tested using resected whole arteries with in-stent lesions.

Methods.—Five patients who had had a Palmaz-Schatz stent implanted 7 to 19 months previously were included in the study. Whole arterial specimens with in-stent lesions were surgically resected and histologically analyzed. Each cross-section was divided into 3 parts: the inner intima within

250 μm of the luminal surface (zone A), the area surrounding the strent struts within 250 μm from the strut hole (zone B), and the remainder of the intimal layer (zone C). Cell density, cell replication, and cellular composition in each zone were analyzed.

Findings.—In all samples, zone A cell density was significantly greater than zone B cell density. Proliferating cell nuclear antigen staining demonstrated that cell replication in zone A was significantly greater than in other zones. However, cell-specific immunostaining revealed a substantial accumulation of leukocytes, macrophages, and T lymphocytes in zone B. Proteoglycan stained predominantly around stent struts and in the inner intima.

Conclusions.—Two different pathogenetic processes in different zones appear to contribute to in-stent lesion formation. Cell numbers in the inner intima increase because of a prolonged increase in cell replication. In addition, matrix accumulates around stent struts, possibly linked to infiltration of inflammatory cells in the same zone.

▶ Clowes et al[1] have shown formation of intimal hyperplasia consists of 3 processes: cell replication, cell migration, and accumulation of extracellular matrix in the arterial wall. Although the number of specimens analyzed in this study numbered only 5, it offers some interesting insight into the spectrum of the processes leading to in-stent stenoses. Now the real question is: how do we prevent proliferative intimal hyperplasia from occurring?

R. M. Fujitani, MD

Reference

1. Clowes AW, Reidy MA, Clowes MM: Mechanisms of stenosis after arterial injury. *Lab Invest* 49:208-215, 1983.

Five-Year Clinical Follow-up After Intracoronary Radiation: Results of a Randomized Clinical Trial
Grise MA, Massullo V, Jani S, et al (Scripps Clinic, La Jolla, Calif; Brigham and Women's Hosp, Boston; Lenox Hill, New York)
Circulation 105:2737-2740, 2002   2–12

Background.—Restenosis is a persistent problem in catheter-based vascular procedures. Evidence indicates that intracoronary brachytherapy is effective in reducing stenosis. A previous report described 6-month and 3-year results that showed significant decreases in target lesion revascularization (TLR) and angiographic restenosis after γ radiotherapy for restenotic lesions. Documented is the clinical outcome 5 years after treatment of restenotic coronary arteries with catheter-based iridium-192 (^{192}Ir).

Methods.—This double-blind, randomized trial compared ^{192}Ir to placebo in patients with restenosis after coronary angioplasty. Over 9 months, 55 patients were randomly assigned to a ^{192}Ir group (26 patients) or a placebo group (29 patients).

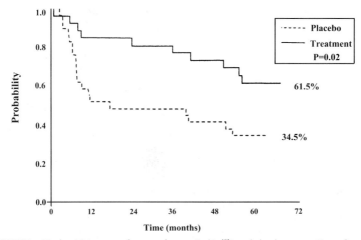

FIGURE 1.—Kaplan-Meier curves for event-free survival in ^{192}Ir and placebo groups. Event-free survival was defined as survival without myocardial infarction or repeated revascularization of target lesion. The 2 curves begin to separate at approximately 3 months, and the differences persist throughout the follow-up period. (Courtesy of Grise MA, Massullo V, Jani S, et al: Five-year clinical follow-up after intracoronary radiation: Results of a randomized clinical trial. *Circulation* 105(23):2737-2740, 2002.)

Results.—At 5 years, TLR was significantly lower in the ^{192}Ir group (23.1%) than in the placebo group (48.3%). Two cases of TLR occurred between years 3 and 5 among patients in the ^{192}Ir group compared with none in the placebo group. In addition, patients in the ^{192}Ir group had a higher 5-year event-free survival rate for freedom from death, myocardial infarction, or TLR than did patients in the placebo group (61.5% vs 34.5%) (Fig 2).

Conclusions.—These findings suggest that γ radiotherapy has durable efficacy for the treatment of restenosis after coronary angioplasty. In patients treated with ^{192}Ir, TLR was reduced by 74% at 6 months, by 68% at 3 years, and by 48% at 5 years. Thus, the early clinical benefits after intracoronary γ radiation with ^{192}Ir appear to persist at 5 years of clinical follow-up.

▶ This study highlights just how poor the results of coronary angioplasty really are. Only 34.5% of the control patients were free from death, myocardial infarction, or additional revascularization at 5 years. Improving the event-free rate to 61.5% with intracoronary radiation is therefore progress. Unfortunately, the use of drug-eluting stents may make this area of research irrelevant before it really gets started.

G. L. Moneta, MD

Gamma Radiation Induces Positive Vascular Remodeling After Balloon Angioplasty: A Prospective, Randomized Intravascular Ultrasound Scan Study

Hagenaars T, Po IFLA, van Sambeek MRHM, et al (Erasmus Med Ctr Rotterdam, The Netherlands; Leyenburg Hosp, The Hague, The Netherlands; St Franciscus Hosp, Rotterdam, The Netherlands; et al)
J Vasc Surg 36:318-324, 2002   2–13

Introduction.—Both animal and clinical trials have demonstrated that endovascular brachytherapy (EBT) prevents restenosis after percutaneous transluminal angioplasty (PTA). The effect of EBT on peripheral arteries has yet to be determined. The effect of EBT on plaque growth and vascular remodeling was evaluated at 6 months with intravascular US (IVUS) after PTA of femoropopliteal artery.

Methods.—Standard PTA was performed between September 1998 and August 2000 in 24 patients with obstructive disease of the femoropopliteal artery. The median patient age was 65 years (range, 44-85 years). Patients were randomly assigned to either additional EBT (iridium-192) or no additional therapy after PTA. IVUS was performed after PTA and at 6 months of follow-up, and patients who had or did not have EBT (8 and 16 patients, respectively) were compared for measures of change in lumen, vessel, and plaque area.

Results.—There was a significant difference in lumen area between patients without or with EBT (–9% and +23%, respectively; $P = .03$) at a 6-month follow-up. This difference resulted from a significant difference in vessel area change (+2% vs +19% in patients without vs those with EBT, respectively; $P = .05$). A similar increase in plaque area was observed in both patient groups (+12% and +16%, respectively; $P = .80$). Plaque dissections observed immediately after PTA were not present at follow-up in patients who did not undergo EBT, while 4 of 8 patients who underwent EBT had a persistent dissection.

Conclusion.—In femoropopliteal arteries, γ-radiation after PTA had a positive influence on lumen dimensions at a 6-month follow-up by inducing positive vascular remodeling (vascular dilatation). γ-Radiation did not affect plaque growth.

▶ Intravascular radiation can limit restenosis after primary angioplasty or treatment of in-stent restenosis in coronary arteries. However, in primary coronary stenting, radiation appears to prevent healing and predispose to late stent thrombosis. These mixed results, cumbersome delivery systems, and expense have limited its widespread application. This study suggests that brachytherapy will improve results of angioplasty in the femoral-popliteal segment, but small numbers (8 treated patients) and short follow-up (6 months) preclude conclusions about efficacy. However, intriguing observations were made using IVUS on structural changes within the artery wall after PTA and radiation. Consistent with the coronary literature, radiation prevented healing of dissections and caused outward remodeling of the artery wall so the lumen of treated arteries was larger. These data support my bias that lumen narrowing after PTA is due in large part to constrictive remodeling of the artery wall analogous to wound healing. Just as radiation inhibits contraction and fibrosis of cutaneous wounds, it likely limits contraction and fibrosis in the artery wall after the "wounding" from angioplasty. Curiously, and in contrast to the coronary literature, radiation did not block neointima formation in peripheral arteries. J.M.P. used to liken brachytherapy to "using a howitzer to kill a mosquito," but I believe the real challenge to its acceptance will be the drug-eluting stent.

R. L. Geary, MD

3 Vascular Laboratory

Preoperative Diagnosis of Carotid Artery Stenosis: Accuracy of Noninvasive Testing

Nederkoorn PJ, Mali WPThM, Eikelboom BC, et al (Univ Med Ctr, Utrecht, The Netherlands; Erasmus Med Ctr, Rotterdam, The Netherlands; Harvard School of Public Health, Boston)

Stroke 33:2003-2008, 2002   3–1

Background.—Digital subtraction angiography (DSA) is the reference standard for diagnosis of carotid artery stenosis. The accuracy of noninvasive testing compared with DSA was investigated.

Methods.—This prospective study included 350 consecutive symptomatic patients who underwent duplex US (DUS), MR angiography (MRA), and DSA. Stenoses were measured with the observers blinded to clinical information and other test results. Separate and combined test results of DUS and MRA were compared with the reference standard, DSA. Only the stenosis measurements of the arteries on the symptomatic side were included in the analyses.

Results.—DUS analyzed with previously defined criteria yielded a sensitivity of 87.5% and a specificity of 75.7% in identifying severe internal carotid artery stenosis. Stenosis measurements on MRA yielded a sensitivity of 92.2% and a specificity of 75.7%. Combining the MRA and DUS results yielded agreement between these 2 modalities in 84% of patients, with a sensitivity of 96.4% and a specificity of 80.2% for the identification of severe stenosis.

Conclusion.—In patients with suspected stenosis of the internal carotid artery, MRA showed a slightly better diagnostic accuracy than DUS. However, both tests should be performed to achieve the greatest diagnostic accuracy.

▶ I think this type of analysis is yesterday's news for vascular surgeons. Surgeons want to offer operations based on noninvasive testing alone. For symptomatic patients, where carotid endarterectomy has a good therapy index for lesions producing symptoms that are more than 70% diameter reducing, the goal is not to miss lesions. High negative predictive values are what are important. If the symptomatic patient actually has only a 65% stenosis, no one cares. They likely will also benefit from the procedure. With asymptomatic disease where the therapeutic index is much more narrow, you want very high positive predictive values. You do not want to offer a potentially dangerous and invasive therapy to patients with asymptomatic disease who will, as a population, derive only marginal benefit from carotid endarterectomy.

G. L. Moneta, MD

Comparison of Color-Flow Doppler Scanning, Power Doppler Scanning, and Frequency Shift for Assessment of Carotid Artery Stenosis

Müller M, Ciccotti P, Reiche W, et al (Saarland Univ, Homburg/Saar, Germany)
J Vasc Surg 34:1090-1095, 2001   3–2

Background.—Internal carotid artery stenosis is diagnosed by US on the basis of the fact Doppler shift-frequency, or blood flow velocity, increases with increasing stenosis. The application of peak shift-frequency/velocity for the diagnosis of ICA stenosis is a commonly accepted technique, but there is disagreement about the accuracy of frequency/velocity-derived data. Thus, there is a value in investigating other US techniques for diagnosis of internal carotid artery (ICA) stenosis. This study investigated the accuracy of color-flow Doppler (CD) scanning, power Doppler (PD) scanning, and peak systolic Doppler frequency shift (PSF) in the assessment of carotid artery stenosis. Angiography was used as the gold standard for comparison purposes using measurements utilized in the North American Symptomatic Carotid Surgery Trial (NASCET) and European Carotid Surgery Trial (ESCT).

Methods.—A total of 58 consecutive patients scheduled for carotid artery surgery underwent color-coded duplex sonography and angiography. The duplex examination included the assessment of PSF and videotaping of sagittal images in CD and PD mode from the proximal common carotid artery to the distal ICA. The tapes were reviewed separately by 2 experienced examiners, with kappa statistic used for interobserver agreement. For comparison with angiography (degrees of stenosis, 40%, 50%, 60%, 70%, and 80%) sensitivity, specificity, positive and negative predictive values, and overall accuracy were calculated. PSF cutoff frequencies were based on receiver operator curve analysis.

Results.—Interobserver agreement in CD and PD was good, so further analysis used the between-observer mean value for each stenosis. With the NASCET technique, the accuracy of Doppler techniques for distinguishing a 50% stenosis was 89% for PSF, 91% for CD, and 93% for PD; for a 70% stenosis, it was 86% for PSF, 84% for CD, and 81% for PDS. With the ECST measurement technique, the accuracy for distinguishing a 70% stenosis was 86% for PSF, 88% for CD, and 86% for PD, while for an 80% stenosis it was 87% for PSF, 87% for CD, and 77% for PD.

Conclusion.—CD and PD scanning measurement of carotid artery stenosis is highly reproducible In this study, accuracy was equal to that obtained with PSF.

▶ The same comments apply here as well as Abstract 3–1. Since there are no variables with PD or CD to provide positive and negative predictive values, I favor the use of velocity measurements as the primary criteria to assess the severity of carotid stenosis.

G. L. Moneta, MD

Importance of Angle Correction in the Measurement of Blood Flow Velocity With Transcranial Doppler Sonography
Krejza J, Mariak Z, Babikian VL (Bialystok Med Academy, Poland; Boston Univ)
AJNR Am J Neuroradiol 22:1743-1747, 2001   3–3

Introduction.—An important limitation in transcranial Doppler (TCD) studies is the sonographer's inability to define the angle between the long axis of the vessel and the direction of the US beam. Color flow TCD, however, permits visualization of the vessel and angle correction. The effect of angle correction on blood flow velocity was examined in patients with moderate or severe middle cerebral artery (MCA) stenosis.

Methods.—Eighteen patients with a median age of 53 years (age range, 22-72 years) who met all qualifying criteria (angiographically confirmed unilateral MCA stenosis of 50% or greater) were selected from 149 consecutive patients enrolled in a prospective investigation of color TCD sonography and cerebral digital subtraction angiography. The angle of insonation and peak systolic and mean flow velocities in both MCAs were determined from videotapes obtained at sonography.

Results.—The mean angle of insonation was 47° (range, 19°-64°) on the stenotic side and 34° on the contralateral side ($P < .05$). Angle-corrected velocities were higher, compared with uncorrected velocities. The percentage differences between angle-corrected and uncorrected peak systolic and mean flow velocities on the stenotic side were 46.6% and 45.9%, respectively, of uncorrected values. The differences between corrected and uncorrected peak systolic and mean velocities were greater on the stenotic side than on the contralateral side ($P < .05$).

Conclusion.—The angle of insonation can be significant and produce large errors when flow velocities are determined without angle correction in patients with moderate or severe MCA stenosis.

▶ This and other studies indicate that the angle of insonation of the M1 segment of the MCA can be wider in older patients with intercranial stenosis and in the setting of a mass effect. Without angle correction, MCA velocities may be falsely lower, leading to underreading of an MCA stenosis. Readers of TCD examination should be aware of this problem and whether their TCD studies are angle corrected.

G. L. Moneta, MD

Classification of Human Carotid Atherosclerotic Lesions With In Vivo Multicontrast Magnetic Resonance Imaging

Cai J-M, Hatsukami TS, Ferguson MS, et al (Univ of Washington, Seattle; PLA Gen Hosp, Beijing, China; VA Puget Sound Health Care System, Seattle; et al)
Circulation 106:1368-1373, 2002   3–4

Background.—The American Heart Association has attempted to categorize atherosclerotic lesions by creating a detailed classification scheme designed to be used as a histologic "template" for images obtained by both invasive and noninvasive techniques. Resent studies have shown that MRI can characterize the components of the carotid atherosclerotic plaque. Whether in vivo high-resolution multicontrast MRI could enable the accurate classification of human carotid atherosclerotic plaque according to the American Heart Association classification was investigated.

Methods.—Sixty consecutive patients (54 men; mean age, 70 years) who were scheduled for carotid endarterectomy were imaged with a 1.5-T scanner. A standardized protocol was used to obtain 4 different contrast-weighted images (time of flight and T1-, PD-, and T2-weighted) of the carotid arteries. The best voxel size was $0.25 \times 0.25 \times 1$ mm^3. Carotid plaques were removed intact and processed for histologic examination. Both the MR images and the histologic sections were independently reviewed, categorized, and compared.

Results.—Overall, there was good agreement between the classification obtained with the use of MRI and with the American Heart Association classification, with Cohen's κ (95% CI) of 0.74 (0.67-0.82) and weighted κ of

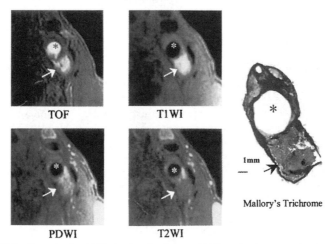

FIGURE 4.—Example of type VI lesion just distal to carotid bifurcation (acute to subacute mixed hemorrhages were detected by histology). On multicontrast-weighted MR images, acute and subacute mixed hemorrhage had high SI on both TOF and T1WI images, iso-SI to slightly high SI on PDWI and T2WI images (*arrow*). * indicates lumen. Original magnification × 10. *Abbreviations: TOF,* Time of flight; *T1WI,* T1-weighted type I; *PDWI,* PD-weighted type I; *T2WI,* T2-weighted type I; *SI,* signal intensity. (Courtesy of Cai J-M, Hatsukami TS, Ferguson MS, et al: Classification of human carotid atherosclerotic lesions with in vivo multicontrast magnetic resonance imaging. *Circulation* 106:1368-1373, 2002.)

0.79. The respective sensitivities and specificities of MR image classification were as follows: type I and II lesions, 67% and 100%; type III lesions, 81% and 98%; type IV and V lesions, 84% and 90%; type VI lesions, 82% and 91%, type VII lesions, 80% and 94%; and type VIII lesions, 56% and 100% (Fig 4).

Conclusions.—In vivo high-resolution multicontrast MRI is useful for the classification of intermediate to advanced atherosclerotic lesions in the carotid artery and can aid in distinguishing advanced lesions from early and intermediate atherosclerotic plaques.

▶ With the exception of distinguishing stenosis from occlusion, I've never been impressed that MR adds much to duplex for detection of carotid bifurcation stenosis. For characterizing plaque, however, MR may turn out to have real advantages, especially if characterizing plaque eventually turns out to predict clinical events. It will be difficult to prove whether MR evaluation of carotid plaques will be clinically useful. A very large majority of even high-grade asymptomatic plaques don't cause a problem. To prospectively determine an MR feature that correlates with adverse clinical outcomes of asymptomatic plaques is likely to require so many patients as to be an unrealistic goal.

G. L. Moneta, MD

Reproducibility of Constant-Load Treadmill Testing With Various Treadmill Protocols and Predictability of Treadmill Test Results in Patients With Intermittent Claudication

Degischer S, Labs K-H, Aschwanden M, et al (Univ of Basel, Switzerland)
J Vasc Surg 36:83-88, 2002   3–5

Background.—Both the graded-load treadmill test and the constant-load treadmill test are used internationally and have similar reliability. European investigators, however, tend to favor the constant-load protocol. However, there is no clear agreement on what treadmill settings should be used. As a result, a wide range of settings are used in clinical trials. With different settings, the claudication distances of the same patient sample will vary. It is therefore difficult to compare the results of clinical trials that use different treadmill settings. In this study, the reliability of constant-load testing with various workloads was evaluated. The various workloads were also compared with claudication distances obtained when walking at normal speed on level ground. In addition, the ability of metabolic equivalent (MET) normalization to translate the results of different treadmill tests from one to the other was also determined.

Methods.—Treadmill testing at different treadmill settings, including speeds of 2.0, 3.2, and 4.0 km/h (1.25, 2.0, and 2.5 mph) and at grades of 0% and 12%, was performed by 15 patients with claudication. Walking capacity was also tested on level ground, with the speed chosen by the individual patient. The results of virtual treadmill tests with all possible combinations of speeds and grades were predicted from real tests via MET normalization. Regression modeling was used to test the relationship between real and predicted claudication distances. Both absolute and initial claudication distances were evaluated.

Results.—Reliability coefficients (RCs) for the absolute claudication distance (ACD) were superior to RCs for the initial claudication distance. RCs for the ACD ranged from 0.61 to 0.95, and increasing values were seen with increasing workloads. The regression coefficients that best described the relationship between measured and predicted claudication distances were obtained with a model based on a power function. However, the model was only appropriate for the prediction of the group mean from clinical trials; it could not be applied to single patient data. The model was tested with 6 published studies for proof of concept. The result of the second test was predicted from the first test, and estimated and measured claudication distances were compared. The mean difference for all trials was 7.9%, and the maximum difference was 16.5%.

Conclusions.—The data indicate higher workloads should be used to achieve optimal treadmill test reliability, and the ACD should be preferred over the initial claudication distance. MET normalization allows general determination of comparability of treadmill test results obtained with different test conditions.

▶ This is an extremely important paper in that it helps provide guidelines in how treadmill tests should be performed. The use of higher workloads and ACD (the maximum distance a patient can walk) is recommended. I think if we restrict treadmill testing to patients in whom the diagnosis of claudication is open to question, or the degree of impairment is mild to moderate, the authors' suggestions will be useful.

G. L. Moneta, MD

Contrast Enhanced MR Angiography in the Assessment of Relevant Stenoses in Occlusive Disease of the Pelvic and Lower Limb Arteries: Diagnostic Value of a Two-Step Examination Protocol in Comparison to Conventional DSA

Winterer JT, Schaefer O, Uhrmeister P, et al (Univ Hosp Freiburg, Germany; Univ Hosp Bonn, Germany)
Eur J Radiol 41:153-160, 2002   3–6

Background.—The diagnostic workup for peripheral arterial occlusive disease requires exact localization and grading of stenoses. The gold standard has been catheter angiography. MR angiography (MRA), particularly contrast-enhanced MRA (ce-MRA), may be an alternative and noninvasive method. The diagnostic accuracy of ce-MRA to detect 77% stenoses was evaluated for patients with moderate and severe peripheral occlusive disease.

TABLE 2.—Assessment of Degree of Stenosis With Catheter Angiography and MR Angiography in the Iliac Arteries (n = 20)

Iliac Arteries Conventional Angiography	MR Angiography	
	Moderate Stenosis	Severe Stenosis
Moderate stenosis	7	5
Severe stenosis	2	6

Note: Grade of stenosis: moderate, ≤70%; severe, >70%.
(Courtesy of Winterer JT, Schaefer O, Uhrmeister P, et al: Contrast enhanced MR angiography in the assessment of relevant stenoses in occlusive disease of the pelvic and lower limb arteries: Diagnostic value of a two-step examination protocol in comparison to conventional DSA. *Eur J Radiol* 41:153-160, 2002. Copyright 2002 by Elsevier Science Inc.)

Methods.—The 43 patients (mean age, 67 years; range, 37-96 years) who participated had 82 stenoses that were 50% or greater and 61 stenoses that were greater than 70% as detected on catheter angiograms. All were evaluated with the use of fast gadolinium-DTPA-enhanced high resolution 3-dimensional MRA at 1.5 T; the pelvic and peripheral vascular tree was covered in 2 examination steps with the use of the body coil. Three readers judged whether stenoses were in the moderate (50%-70%) or severe (>70%) range.

Results.—On catheter angiography, moderate stenoses were found in the iliac region (12), the femoral–popliteal level (30), and the crural arteries (40). Severe stenoses were noted in these same regions: 18 were in the iliac region, 35 were at the femoral–popliteal level, and 38 were in the crural arteries. Overestimation occurred in 42% of the stenoses in the iliac level, in 27% of those in the femoral–popliteal area, and in 50% of those in the crural region; false-negative results were obtained in 25% of the iliac vessel stenoses, in 17% of those in the femoral–popliteal area, and in 11% of those in the crural arteries (Tables 2, 3, and 4). The overall sensitivity was 84%, and the specificity was 60%. The positive predictive values were a low of 44% at the crural level and a high of 78% in the femoral–popliteal area; the negative predictive values were 78% in the iliac area and 79% in the femoral–popliteal area, and the maximum was 91% in the crural vessels. Accuracy ranged from a low of 62% in the crural vessels to a high of 78% in the femoral–popliteal area.

TABLE 3.—Assessment of Degree of Stenosis With Catheter Angiography and MR Angiography in the Femoral and Popliteal Arteries (n = 65)

Femoral and Popliteal Arteries Conventional Angiography	MR Angiography	
	Moderate Stenosis	Severe Stenosis
Moderate stenosis	22	8
Severe stenosis	6	29

Note: Grade of stenosis: moderate, ≤70%; severe, >70%.
(Courtesy of Winterer JT, Schaefer O, Uhrmeister P, et al: Contrast enhanced MR angiography in the assessment of relevant stenoses in occlusive disease of the pelvic and lower limb arteries: Diagnostic value of a two-step examination protocol in comparison to conventional DSA. *Eur J Radiol* 41:153-160, 2002. Copyright 2002 by Elsevier Science Inc.)

TABLE 4.—Assessment of Degree of Stenosis With Catheter Angiography and MR Angiography in the Crural Arteries (n = 58)

Crural Arteries Conventional Angiography	MR Angiography Moderate Stenosis	Severe Stenosis
Moderate stenosis	20	20
Severe stenosis	2	16

Note: Grade of stenosis: moderate, ≤70%; severe, >70%.
(Courtesy of Winterer JT, Schaefer O, Uhrmeister P, et al: Contrast enhanced MR angiography in the assessment of relevant stenoses in occlusive disease of the pelvic and lower limb arteries: Diagnostic value of a two-step examination protocol in comparison to conventional DSA. *Eur J Radiol* 41:153-160, 2002. Copyright 2002 by Elsevier Science Inc.)

Conclusions.—The accuracy of ce-MRA in distinguishing moderate from severe stenosis was limited for these cases of peripheral occlusive disease. False grading in the crural area was significant in the direction of overestimation. The pelvic region also presented low accuracy.

▶ The authors found the MR technique employed in their study to be relatively poor in distinguishing greater than 50% to 69% stenosis from greater than 70% stenosis in peripheral arteries. While I am aware that some older studies found that 70% stenosis is required for pressure reduction, most surgeons feel that a 50% lesion in the peripheral system is hemodynamically significant. I think the authors have asked too much of the MR technique for no good clinical reason.

G. L. Moneta, MD

Comparison of Magnetic Resonance Angiography (MRA) and Duplex Ultrasound Arterial Mapping (DUAM) Prior to Infrainguinal Arterial Reconstruction

Soule B, Hingorani A, Ascher E, et al (Maimonides Med Ctr, Brooklyn, NY)
Eur J Vasc Endovasc Surg 25:139-146, 2003   3–7

Background.—Concern for complications of contrast angiography has prompted a search for less invasive imaging techniques that provide comparable accuracy and precision for vascular imaging before lower extremity arterial reconstruction. MR angiography (MRA) was compared with duplex US arterial mapping (DUAM) and intraoperative findings to determine the clinical accuracy of MRA for planning lower extremity revascularization procedures.

Methods.—MRA and DUAM evaluations were performed in 42 patients who underwent lower extremity revascularization procedures. The MRA and DUAM findings for aortoiliac, femoral-popliteal, and infrapopliteal segments were compared with intraoperative findings, and the extent of agreement was evaluated. If a disagreement between imaging modalities was discovered, it was determined whether a change in operative procedure would have resulted.

Results.—There was agreement in MRA and DUAM findings in 26 of 31 cases (83%) of aortoiliac segments, in 25 of 31 cases (81%) of femoral-popliteal segments, and in 16 of 21 cases (76%) of infrapopliteal segments. Overall, DUAM agreed with intraoperative findings in 98% of patients, whereas MRA agreed in 82% of patients. Disagreement between intraoperative findings and DUAM resulted in selection of an alternate surgical procedure in only 1 patient (2%). Disagreement with MRA resulted in a different procedure in 38% of patients ($P < .001$).

Conclusions.—MRA is not yet adequate to replace conventional angiography and is less accurate than DUAM. Further improvements in MRA are needed before it can be used as the sole modality for development of a preoperative strategy in patients with lower extremity revascularization.

▶ It is difficult to make any generalizations based on this study as 2 operator- and technology-dependent techniques are being compared. Soule et al use DUAM virtually routinely to plan vascular reconstructions. We have no idea how accurate MRA is in their institution. The most you can say from this study is that at Maimonides Medical Center, DUAM works better than MRA in planning infrainguinal arterial reconstructions. However, what really matters is what works best in your shop.

G. L. Moneta, MD

Improved Assessment of the Hemodynamic Significance of Borderline Iliac Stenoses With Use of Hyperemic Duplex Scanning
Coffi SB, Ubbink DT, Zwiers I, et al (Academic Med Ctr, Amsterdam)
J Vasc Surg 36:575-580, 2002   3–8

Introduction.—Duplex scanning is usually considered to be a reliable, noninvasive technique for evaluating arterial occlusive disease in the lower extremities. Earlier trials, however, have reported that both angiography and duplex scanning (peak systolic velocity [PSV] ratio) compared with intra-arterial pressure measurements do not identify some pressure-reducing stenoses in the aortoiliac tract. Two alternative US variables—the absolute increase in PSV across the stenosis (ΔPSV) and the end-diastolic velocity (EDV)—are both related to the flow and may be of use in improving the evaluation of the hemodynamic significance of aortoiliac stenosis by duplex scanning under conditions of increased flow. Cutoff values were defined for ΔPSV and EDV measured after physical exercise (ΔPSV$_e$ and EDV$_e$). Their capability to assess the hemodynamic significance of borderline iliac stenoses was examined.

Methods.—Borderline iliac stenoses were defined as stenoses with a PSV ratio of 1.5 to 3.5. PSV ratios lower than 1.5 were not considered hemodynamically significant. A PSV ratio above 3.5 was considered highly suggestive of a stenosis of greater than 50%. Fifty-eight legs in 53 consecutive patients with symptomatic arterial obstructive disease with borderline iliac stenosis were examined prospectively. US velocity data obtained after exercise on a bicycle ergometer at 2 W/kg for 2 minutes were judged against the assessment of the hemodynamic significance via intra-arterial pressure measurement, before and after administration of 50 mg papaverine.

Results.—Based on receiver operating characteristic curves developed from 43 iliac stenoses in 39 patients who finished the exercise, $\Delta PSV_e \geq 1.4$ m/s had an optimal sensitivity of 93% (95% CI, 0.77-0.99), specificity of 87% (95% CI, 0.06-0.98), positive predictive value of 93% (95% CI, 0.77-0.99), and negative predictive value of 87% (95% CI, 0.06-0.98) of predicting a pressure-reducing stenosis.

Conclusion.—In patients who can accomplish the workload, the assessment of the hemodynamic significance of borderline iliac artery stenosis is improved with the use of ΔPSV_e and a cutoff value of 1.4 m/s in combination with the PSV ratio.

▶ Early attempts to quantify pressure gradients in peripheral arteries by using duplex US and a modification of the Bernoulli equation were unsuccessful. This study used a different approach. It posed a binary question. Is an iliac stenosis associated with borderline resting velocity ratios between 1.5 and 3.5 hemodynamically significant or not? The authors found changes in exercise-induced peak systolic velocities across borderline iliac lesions could predict hemodynamic significance. The workload to produce the flow changes analyzed in this study is, however, probably too great for many claudicants. I doubt this technique will gain widespread acceptance outside a research setting. The authors, however, are to be congratulated for their continued attempts to advance the application of duplex techniques to the peripheral arteries.

G. L. Moneta, MD

The Additional Value of Angiography After Colour-Coded Duplex on Decision Making in Patients With Critical Limb Ischaemia: A Prospective Study

Avenarius JKA, Breek JC, Lampmann LEH, et al (St Elisabeth Hosp, Tilburg, The Netherlands; Martini Hosp, Groningen, The Netherlands)
Eur J Vasc Endovasc Surg 23:393-397, 2002   3–9

Background.—Several studies have compared color duplex imaging (CDI) and intra-arterial digital subtraction arteriography (IADSA) in the assessment of peripheral arterial status, and CDI has been found to be reliable in the detection and rating of vascular disease in the aortoiliac and femoropopliteal segments. However, controversy exists regarding the accuracy of CDI for the assessment of crural vessels. Treatment plans based on CDI were compared with those based on IADSA for the preoperative evaluation of patients with critical limb ischemia.

Methods.—A total of 98 consecutive patients with 112 legs with critical limb ischemia were investigated with both CDI and IADSA. Treatment plans based on these modalities were developed separately during a multidisciplinary meeting and retrospectively analyzed with the outcome of the operation or the endovascular procedure as a reference.

Results.—Complete analysis was possible in 88 patients (101 legs). In 91 of the legs (90%), CDI provided the same strategy as IADSA. In the remaining 10 legs, IADSA provided additional information, most of which concerned the crural vessels.

Conclusions.—CDI alone is sufficient for preoperative planning in most patients with chronic critical ischemia of the lower limb. However, additional information may be needed for treatment planning of crural revascularization. IADSA should also be performed in patients in whom severe calcification prevents adequate visualization of the crural vessels or in whom there is no patent anterior or posterior tibial artery with outflow across the ankle.

▶ The authors' conclusions are very reasonable based on their data. This study represents a middle ground between overdependence on contrast angiography and evangelic advocacy of all lower extremity reconstructions on the basis of US alone.

G. L. Moneta, MD

High-Resolution, Contrast-Enhanced Magnetic Resonance Angiography With Elliptical Centric k-Space Ordering of Supra-aortic Arteries Compared With Selective X-ray Angiography

Wutke R, Lang W, Fellner C, et al (Friedrich-Alexander Univ Erlangen-Nuremberg, Germany)
Stroke 33:1522-1529, 2002   3–10

Background.—A noninvasive method to simultaneously evaluate the entire carotid system from the aortic arch to the circle of Willis would improve the efficiency of diagnosis of carotid stenosis. The relative value of high-resolution, contrast-enhanced MR angiography (CE MRA) with elliptical centric k-space ordering was evaluated and compared with that of intra-arterial x-ray angiography for imaging the carotid arteries from the aortic arch to the circle of Willis.

Methods.—The study group comprised 30 patients with suspected stenosis of the carotid arteries. The patients were examined with CE MRA (1.5-T scanner) and x-ray angiography (ie, aortic arch survey and selective imaging of both common carotid arteries). Independent investigators assessed not only the extracranial carotid bifurcation but also all the vessel segments from the aortic arch to the circle of Willis.

Results.—A very close correlation was found between CE MRA and x-ray angiography for the internal carotid artery in the region of the extracranial carotid bifurcation: sensitivity 100% and specificity 92%. In 3 patients, the initially suspected overestimation of stenosis on CE MRA was ultimately shown to be an underestimation on x-ray angiography. CE MRA provided slightly poorer imaging of the basal vessel segments at the level of the aortic arch (because of breathing artifacts) and the intracranial vessel segments

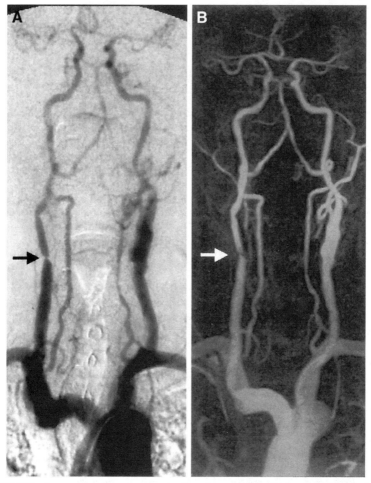

FIGURE 1.—Image of the entire vascular region from the aortic arch to the intracranial vessels. Patient had a history of endarterectomy on the left side and now exhibits high-grade stenosis of the right internal carotid artery (*arrows*). Occlusion of the external carotid artery is evident on the right side. **A**, X-ray angiography (aortic arch survey); **B**, Contrast-enhanced MR angiography. (Courtesy of Wutke R, Lange W, Fellner C, et al: High-resolution, contrast-enhanced magnetic resonance angiography with elliptical centric k-space ordering of supra-aortic arteries compared with selective x-ray angiography. *Stroke* 33:1522-1529, 2002. Reproduced with permission from *Stroke*. Copyright 2002 American Heart Association.)

(because of small vessel caliber and venous superimposition caused by delayed sequence starts, Fig 1).

Conclusions.—CE MRA provides reliable results in the diagnosis of carotid stenosis and provides an acceptable alternative to invasive conventional x-ray angiography in most patients. Improved visualization of small vessels will require additional technical developments with regard to spatial resolution.

▶ The time required for acquisition of images is one of the primary limitations of MRA. Basically, noncontrast techniques require long acquisition times while contrast-enhanced techniques need precise timing and short acquisition times to avoid superimposition of venous vessels. A minimal time of acquisition, however, is still required to achieve delineation of appropriate details of arterial anatomy. Whereas trying to time the stock market sounds great but doesn't work and never will, timing of acquisition of images with MR is required and is getting better all the time.

G. L. Moneta, MD

The Use of Color-Flow Duplex Scan for the Detection of Endoleaks
McLafferty RB, McCrary BS, Mattos MA, et al (Southern Illinois Univ, Springfield)
J Vasc Surg 36:100-104, 2002   3–11

Background.—CT is the standard for endoleak surveillance after endoluminal repair of abdominal aortic aneurysms (erAAA). Color-flow duplex scanning (CFD) may be an alternative. The accuracy of CFD scanning after erAAA was investigated.

Methods.—Seventy-nine patients underwent CFD and CT scanning during a 43-month period. Patients with CFD scans positive for endoleak had CT scanning 3 months after erAAA, and those with CFD results negative for endoleak had CT scanning 6 months after erAAA.

Findings.—Nine percent of the patients were diagnosed as having endoleak after CFD and CT scanning. All endoleaks diagnosed by CT were also detected by CFD. One patient had a CFD scan positive for endoleak at 1 month, then a CT scan negative for endoleak at 3 months. This case was considered false positive. Compared with CT, CFD had a sensitivity and specificity of 100% and 99%, respectively. The positive and negative predictive values were 88% and 100%, respectively, and the accuracy was 99%.

Conclusion.—These data show that CFD is an accurate modality for detecting endoleak after erAAA. Most endoleaks diagnosed by CFD at 1 month were again detected at 6 months. Clinicians should consider using this noninvasive test for the detection of endoleak in this patient population.

▶ The authors' conclusions should be that when an endoleak is diagnosed by CFD at 1 month, an endoleak will also be present at 6 months. Since the confirming CT studies were remote to the CFDs in this study, we really don't know if the endoleaks at 6 months are the same as those at 1 month; the authors could not identify the source of endoleak with CFD, and endoleaks do seem to come and go. In addition, we also don't know how many endoleaks were missed at the 1-month examination with CFD since CT scans were not obtained at the time.

G. L. Moneta, MD

Efficacy of Ultrasound Scan Contrast Agents in the Noninvasive Follow-up of Aortic Stent Grafts

Bendick PJ, Bove PG, Long GW, et al (William Beaumont Hosp, Royal Oak, Mich)
J Vasc Surg 37:381-385, 2003   3–12

Background.—In this study, contrast-enhanced duplex US scanning was evaluated for endoleak detection in patients after endovascular aneurysm repair.

Methods.—The study included 20 patients (mean age, 74.5 years) who had undergone endovascular repair of abdominal aortic aneurysm. After routine conventional duplex US with color Doppler imaging, the patients received 1 mL of US scan contrast agent by the antecubital vein, followed by a 5-mL flush with normal saline solution. The contrast agent was allowed to circulate, after which scanning with tissue harmonic imaging was performed. Any endoleaks were identified and classified as being graft related or arterial branch related. Within 2 weeks, all patients also underwent CT angiography.

Results.—At examination, all grafts were patent with normal aortoiliac flow hemodynamics. Eight endoleaks were detected by CT angiography: 2 graft related, 3 arterial branch related, and 3 of indeterminate origin. All 8 endoleaks were also identified by contrast-enhanced US, of which 4 were classified as graft related and 4 as arterial branch related. US with contrast also detected 2 small endoleaks at the proximal graft attachment site. These were missed with CT angiography but detected by conventional angiography at the time of endovascular revision.

Conclusions.—Duplex US scanning with intravenous contrast appears to provide a useful tool for surveillance in patients with aortic stent grafts. This US technique can sensitively detect endoleaks of various types. It may be especially valuable in patients where US is technically difficult.

▶ This study evaluating US and the follow-up of aortic stent grafts employed a more rigorous study design than that of the previous study (Abstract 3–11). Taken together, both articles suggest US will become important in the follow-up of aortic stent grafts. It may even be that with the use of US contrast agents, US will be preferred over CT scanning for follow-up of aortic stent grafts.

G. L. Moneta, MD

Duplex Scan Findings in Patients With Spontaneous Cervical Artery Dissections

Logason K, Hårdemark H-G, Bärlin T, et al (Univ Hosp, Uppsala, Sweden)
Eur J Vasc Endovasc Surg 23:295-298, 2002   3–13

Background.—Intramural hematomas associated with spontaneous dissection of the cervical internal carotid artery may lead to luminal narrowing and occlusion. Duplex scanning is frequently used as an alternative modality for diagnosis of internal carotid or vertebral artery dissection. In this experience, duplex scanning was used for the diagnosis of patients with spontaneous dissection of the internal carotid or vertebral arteries.

Methods.—This retrospective study evaluated the records of 24 patients (median age, 48 years; range, 25-68 years) who were given diagnoses of spontaneous extracranial internal carotid artery dissection (20 patients) or vertebral artery dissection (4 patients) from January 1995 to December 1999.

Results.—Four different patterns of abnormal flow were seen in patients with dissection of the internal carotid artery. An absence of flow was detected in 15% of patients, staccato flow was detected in 50% of patients, reduced flow velocity was detected in 25% of patients, and stenotic flow was detected in 10% of patients. B-mode US imaging showed a homogenous echolucent lesion in 8 patients and a double lumen in 2 patients. Staccato flow along the entire internal carotid artery was observed in only 4 patients without verified dissection. In the 4 patients with vertebral artery dissection, duplex scanning demonstrated staccato flow in 3 patients and reversed low-amplitude pulsatile flow in 1 patient.

Conclusions.—These findings indicate that duplex scanning is an important noninvasive diagnostic modality in patients with dissection of a cervical artery. Staccato flow along the extracranial internal carotid artery is a strong indicator of internal carotid artery dissection.

► It is important to recognize internal carotid artery flow patterns associated with internal carotid artery dissection. Many internal carotid artery dissections occur distal in the internal carotid artery where color-flow imaging of the narrow lumen may not be possible. Staccato flow in the proximal internal carotid artery, as defined by severely decreased systolic and absent or severely decreased diastolic velocities, appears to be a good indication of an upstream carotid dissection. This flow pattern, however, is not specific and can be associated with severe intercranial stenosis as well. In addition, the minority of dissections that do not result in severe distal luminal narrowing will not alter flow in the proximal internal carotid artery.

G. L. Moneta, MD

Hepatic Venous Pressure Gradients Measured by Duplex Ultrasound
Tasu J-P, Rocher L, Péletier G, et al (Bicêtre Hosp, Le Kremlin-Bicêtre, France)
Clin Radiol 57:746-752, 2002   3–14

Background.—Doppler US may be useful to evaluate changes in the systemic or portal circulation in patients with portal hypertension. The hepatic venous pressure gradient is an important prognostic factor in portal hypertension, but its measurement of this marker currently requires hepatic venography. In this study, the relationship between the hepatic venous pressure

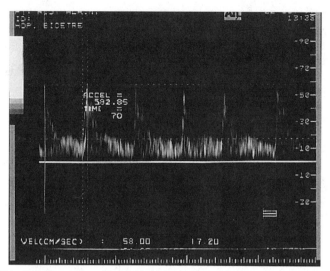

FIGURE 1.—Doppler waveforms obtained from the hepatic artery of a patient with cirrhosis. The acceleration value is 582.86 cm/s². (Courtesy of Tasu J-P, Rocher L, Péletier G, et al: Hepatic venous pressure gradients measured by duplex ultrasound. *Clin Radiol* 57:746-752, 2002.)

gradient and a number of Doppler measurements, including the arterial acceleration index, was investigated.

Methods.—The hepatic venous pressure gradient was measured in 50 fasting patients at hepatic venography. A duplex US examination of the liver was performed immediately afterward, and multiple measurements and indices of the venous and arterial hepatic vasculature were obtained.

Results.—Hepatic arterial acceleration was correlated directly with the hepatic venous pressure gradient. An acceleration index cutoff value of 1 m/s² provided a positive predictive value of 95%, a sensitivity of 65%, and a specificity of 95% for the detection of patients with severe portal hypertension (Fig 1). There was also a correlation between the hepatic venous pressure gradient and the congestion index of the portal vein velocity (portal vein cross-sectional area/0.5 [portal vein velocity])and portal vein velocity.

Conclusions.—The noninvasive evaluation of portal hypertension may be aided by duplex US measurement of the hepatic arterial acceleration index and other US-derived parameters.

▶ Very few vascular surgeons are currently involved with portal decompressive procedures. However, many do run vascular laboratories. In this study, hepatic artery acceleration index correlated with clinical and invasive determinations of portal hypertension. Before incorporating hepatic artery acceleration index into your vascular laboratory protocols, keep in mind acceleration index is a slope of a line and requires measurement of several velocities, all of which are angle dependent. Overall, the test is reasonably complex to perform and I doubt will be suitable for most vascular laboratories.

G. L. Moneta, MD

Penile Duplex Pharmaco-ultrasonography Revisited: Revalidation of the Parameters of the Cavernous Arterial Response

Speel TGW, van Langen H, Wijkstra H, et al (Univ Med Ctr, Nijmegen, The Netherlands)
J Urol 169:216-220, 2003   3–15

Background.—Duplex pharmacologic ultrasonography of the penis may be used to assess vascular functioning in men with erectile dysfunction. However, there is debate over which stimulation protocol to use and how to interpret the blood flow velocity waveforms. The cavernous arterial response, or peak systolic blood flow velocity, as a diagnostic parameter in penile duplex pharmaco-ultrasonography was re-examined.

Methods.—The study included 106 men evaluated for erectile dysfunction; their mean age was 54 years. After pharmacologic stimulation, duplex ultrasonography was performed to assess cavernous artery blood flow velocity. For comparison, common carotid artery intima media thickness was measured as part of a comprehensive clinical evaluation. Cutoff points for cavernous arterial response were set according to the clinical diagnosis.

Results.—On correlation of peak systolic velocity and acceleration time to intima media thickness, acceleration time was the strongest indicator of cavernous atherosclerotic involvement. Correlation values were $r = 0.51$ for acceleration time versus $r = -0.18$ for peak systolic velocity. As predictors of clinical diagnosis, acceleration time had an area under the curve of 0.72, compared with 0.59 for peak systolic velocity. An acceleration time of 100 msec or greater identified atherosclerotic versus nonatherosclerotic erectile dysfunction with a sensitivity of 66% and a specificity of 71%.

Conclusions.—During penile duplex pharmaco-ultrasonography for erectile dysfunction, acceleration time is a more relevant diagnostic parameter than peak systolic velocity. However, even acceleration time has relatively low diagnostic accuracy.

▶ The authors' data indicate that acceleration times are more accurate than peak systolic velocities in the evaluation of an arterial etiology of erectile dysfunction. However, the accuracy of acceleration times is still probably too low to be useful in clinical practice, and the results offer no correlation with treatment options. Furthermore, oral erectogenic drugs are now the first option for therapy of erectile dysfunction regardless of its cause. Penile duplex scanning can disappear from the clinical vascular laboratory. I doubt any vascular technologist will miss it.

G. L. Moneta, MD

Value of Dynamic Contrast-Enhanced MR Imaging in Diagnosing and Classifying Peripheral Vascular Malformations

van Rijswijk CSP, van der Linden E, van der Woude H-J, et al (Leiden Univ, The Netherlands)
AJR 178:1181-1187, 2002   3–16

Background.—Vascular malformations are presumably present at birth, increase in proportion to the growth of the child, and do not spontaneously regress. Peripheral vascular malformations may require treatment because they tend to enlarge and to cause pain, ulceration, severe deformity, and decreased function of the affected extremity. The purpose of this study was to determine whether MRI, including dynamic contrast-enhanced MR imaging, could be used to categorize peripheral vascular malformations and to identify venous malformations that do not require angiography for treatment.

Methods.—This blinded prospective study enrolled 2 observers who independently correlated MR imaging findings in 27 patients with peripheral vascular malformations with findings of diagnostic angiography and venography. The MR diagnosis of the category of vascular malformation was based on a combination of conventional MR imaging and dynamic, contrast-enhanced MR parameters and was compared with the angiographic diagnosis by means of gamma statistics. The sensitivity and specificity of conventional MR imaging and dynamic contrast-enhanced MR imaging in differentiating venous from nonvenous malformations were determined.

Results.—There was excellent agreement between the 2 observers in determining MR categories. The agreement between MR categories and angiographic categories was high for both observers (Table 5). The sensitivity of conventional MR imaging in differentiating venous and nonvenous malformations was 100%, while specificity was 24% to 33%. Specificity was increased to 95% by the addition of dynamic, contrast-enhanced MR imaging, but sensitivity decreased to 83%.

TABLE 5.—MR Diagnosis Versus Angiographic Diagnosis of Vascular Malformations

| | Angiographic Diagnosis | | | | |
MR Diagnosis	Venous ($n = 6$)	Capillary–Venous ($n = 13$)	Arteriovenous ($n = 4$)	Arterial ($n = 4$)	γ^*
Observer 1					
Venous	5	1	0	0	
Capillary–venous	1	11	2	0	0.97
Arterial or arteriovenous	0	1	2	4	
Observer 2					
Venous	5	1	0	0	
Capillary–venous	1	9	2	0	0.92
Arterial or arteriovenous	0	3	2	4	

*Gamma statistic (γ) was used to assess statistically the concordance between MR imaging and angiographic diagnosis because both of these variables are ordinal.

(From van Rijswijk CSP, van der Linden E, van der Woude H-J, et al: Value of dynamic contrast-enhanced MR imaging in diagnosing and classifying peripheral vascular malformations. *AJR* 178:1181-1187, 2002.)

Conclusion.—Vascular malformations can be categorized by a combination of conventional and dynamic contrast-enhanced MR parameters. The use of dynamic contrast-enhanced MR imaging allows the diagnosis of venous malformations with high specificity.

▶ There is increasing interest in percutaneous therapy for vascular malformations. For vascular malformations that are high flow and predominantly arterial, transarterial embolization is utilized, while for low-flow, predominantly venous malformations percutaneous US-guided induction of sclerosing agents is the preferred method of treatment when active treatment of the malformation is felt necessary. This study takes MR assessment of vascular malformations beyond just confirming the presence of the malformation and describing its anatomic extent. It appears the absence of early contrast enhancement can be used to identify pure venous malformations. They can then be treated, if necessary, without pretreatment angiography to rule out an arterial component.

G. L. Moneta, MD

4 Nonatherosclerotic Conditions

Clinical and Genetic Features of Vascular Ehlers-Danlos Syndrome
Germain DP (Hôpital Européen Georges Pompidou, Paris)
Ann Vasc Surg 16:391-397, 2001   4–1

Background.—Ehlers-Danlos syndrome (EDS) is a heterogeneous group of heritable disorders of connective tissue characterized by skin extensibility, joint hypermobility, and tissue fragility. It has an estimated prevalence ranging from 1 in 100,000 to 1 in 200,000 births, and no race is more predisposed to it than any other. EDS has been classified into 6 major types, and vascular EDS has the highest risk of arterial, intestinal, and uterine ruptures. The clinical and genetic features of vascular EDS are reported.

Overview.—EDS is an autosomal dominant inherited disorder of connective tissue that results from mutation of the *COL3A1* gene encoding type III collagen. Complications are rare during infancy but occur in up to 25% of affected individuals before age 20 years and in 80% of affected individuals before age 40 years. The median survival of patients with EDS is 48 years, and arterial ruptures account for most of the deaths. Intestinal perforations usually involve the colon and are less fatal. Pregnancy is high risk for women with EDS. The clinical diagnosis of vascular EDS is made on the basis of 4 cardinal findings, including distinctive facial features, thin translucent skin, excessive bruising/hematomas, and ruptures of vessels, viscera, or both. The diagnosis is confirmed by biochemical assays indicating qualitative or quantitative abnormalities of type III collagen secretion or by molecular biology studies that demonstrate mutation of the *COL3A1* gene. A variety of molecular mechanisms have been observed with different mutations in each family, and no correlation has been established between genotype and phenotype.

At present, no specific treatments exist for EDS; medical intervention is limited to symptomatic treatment, precautionary measures, and genetic counseling. Patients with vascular EDS should avoid strenuous physical exercise and contact sports. Arteriography, endoscopy, and the use of rectal thermometers are contraindicated in these patients, as are medications that interfere with platelet or coagulative functioning. At this time, a clinical trial is under way assessing the efficacy of beta-blockers in vascular EDS.

▶ This is a nice review of the genetic and clinical features of EDS as it pertains to vascular surgery. The article points out that spontaneous carotid dissection may be a presenting condition of EDS. This is a point not generally appreciated among vascular surgeons, at least not by me.

G. L. Moneta, MD

The Ehlers-Danlos Specter Revisited
Cikrit DF, Glover JR, Dalsing MC, et al (Indiana Univ, Indianapolis; Univ of Missouri, Columbia)
Vasc Endovasc Surg 36:213-217, 2002   4–2

Background.—Patients with Ehlers-Danlos syndrome type IV (EDS-IV) are prone to spontaneous arterial, bowel, or organ rupture. Their arteries contain decreased amounts of type III collagen. Ten members of 2 families with this inherited connective tissue disorder are described.

Methods.—The first family included 3 affected females and 2 affected males 7 to 52 years old. The proband's medical history, laboratory findings, and treatment were reviewed. The second family also had 5 involved members (3 males and 2 females) 6 to 33 years old.

Results.—The proband in the first family was a 27-year-old man who presented with spontaneous ileac artery rupture. He had also experienced spontaneous ruptures of the spleen and colon at age 20 years. Other involved family members were his father (spontaneous colon rupture at age 39 years), his sister (spontaneous spleen rupture in her 20s and subsequent spontaneous intracerebral hemorrhage), his daughter (7 years old, no hemorrhage to date), and his sister's daughter (7 years old, no hemorrhage to date). Protein gel electrophoresis of the proband's cultured skin fibroblasts revealed his type III procollagen secretion to be only about 10% that of type I secretion. Culturing confirmed that type III collagen content was low. The 3 affected females also had extremely low collagen type III levels; however, the collagen level in his father was not sufficiently low to support a diagnosis of EDS-IV. During revascularization surgery, the iliac artery had essentially no consistency for holding sutures, and many pledgetted sutures on the common iliac artery nearly at the aorta were required to control bleeding. A severe dissection of the external iliac artery was oversewn with pledgets, and femoral–femoral bypass grafting was performed. The proband is doing well at 3 years after surgery.

Three of the 5 affected members in the second family are still alive. The mother and a son died at 24 and 33 years of age of spontaneous rupture of the iliac artery. Another son had spontaneous intra-abdominal hemorrhaging. Among the 3 survivors, type III procollagen levels in the skin were only 5% to 30% of type I procollagen levels.

Conclusion.—EDS-IV should be strongly suspected in patients with spontaneous arterial or intestinal perforation, particularly in those with a family history of these events. Collagen production assays can assist in the diagnosis. Noninvasive imaging should be used to evaluate the extent of the injury. The marked friability of their vessels makes arterial repair extremely difficult.

▶ There are at least 10 varieties of EDS. Type IV is of the most concern to vascular surgeons. It is useful to be reminded of the principles of management of these patients, including use of noninvasive techniques of evaluation, and ligation, rather than arterial reconstruction, for arterial rupture.

G. L. Moneta, MD

Transesophageal Echocardiography in Patients With Recent Stroke and Normal Carotid Arteries
Mattioli AV, for the Investigators (Univ of Modena, Italy; et al)
Am J Cardiol 88:820-823, 2001   4–3

Background.—Cardiac emboli are the second most frequent cause of stroke. Transesophageal echocardiography (TEE) has been increasingly used to diagnose intracardiac thrombus as well as several other cardiac abnormalities. The evaluation of a suspected cardiac source of embolism is currently the most common indication for TEE in many centers. The clinical significance of transesophageal echocardiographic findings were evaluated in patients with normal carotid arteries who suffered cerebral ischemia.

Methods.—The study group comprised 245 patients at 3 institutions. The patients ranged in age from 36 to 86 years, with a mean of 65.7 ± 21 years. All of the patients were enrolled in the study on the basis of recent unexplained cerebral ischemia and the presence of normal carotid arteries. These patients were compared with 245 age- and sex-matched patients who underwent TEE for indications other than cerebral ischemia (the control group). All patients underwent complete transthoracic and transesophageal echocardiographic studies. The examinations were performed 1 to 7 days after the cerebral ischemic event.

Results.—The prevalence of left atrial thrombus in the study group was 10% compared with 2.8% in the control group. The prevalence of atrial septal aneurysm in the study group was 28% compared with 9.7% in the control group. The prevalence of patent foramen ovale was 22.8% in patients with stroke compared with 9.7% in the control group. Patent foramen ovale was found in 72 patients (69.2%) with atrial septal aneurysm.

Mitral valve prolapse was seen in 45 patients in the study group (18.3%) and in 43 patients in the control group (17.5%). Mitral valve prolapse was found in association with atrial septal aneurysm in 30 patients (33%) in the study group. Calcifications of the mitral annulus were found in 24 patients (9.7%) in the study group and in 5 patients in the control group (2%). Aortic atherosclerosis increased with age and was more prevalent in the descending aorta.

Conclusions.—This study identified cardiac sources in 88% of patients evaluated shortly after an embolic stroke. The presence of thrombus in the left atrium and auricola was the most significant predictor of cardiac emboli. Atrial abnormalities are common findings in patients with recent stroke and normal carotid arteries.

▶ TEE is a common diagnostic test often used in patients with nonhemorrhagic cerebral ischemia and no detectable significant carotid artery disease. In this study, a remarkable 88% of patients with cerebral ischemia and no carotid disease had a cardiac abnormality—usually an atrial abnormality such as an atrial thrombus, an atrial septal aneurysm, or a patent foramen ovale. Clearly, TEE is strongly indicated in patients with minimal carotid disease and symptoms of cerebral ischemia.

G. L. Moneta, MD

Long-term Outcome of Infrainguinal Bypass Grafting in Patients With Serologically Proven Hypercoagulability

Curi MA, Skelly CL, Baldwin ZK, et al (Univ of Chicago)
J Vasc Surg 37:301-306, 2003   4–4

Background.—Hypercoagulability is commonly found among patients with arterial insufficiency, especially those with early failure of surgical revascularization. However, there are few data on how hypercoagulability affects the long-term outcomes of infrainguinal bypass grafting. Long-term patency rates of infrainguinal bypass grafting were compared for patients with and without hypercoagulability.

Methods.—The retrospective study included 456 patients undergoing placement of 582 infrainguinal bypass grafts. Eighty-four percent were operated on because of life-threatening ischemia; the bypass operation included placement of a prosthetic conduit in 38% of the cases. Fifty-seven patients had serologically confirmed hypercoagulability of various congenital or acquired causes. Long-term patency of their 74 grafts was compared with that of the remaining grafts in patients without hypercoagulability.

Results.—The median follow-up was 19 months. Five-year primary patency rate was 28% for patients with hypercoagulability versus 35% in the comparison groups. Primary assisted patency rate was 37% for patients with and those without hypercoagulability (Fig 1); secondary patency rate was 41% versus 53%, respectively. Patients with hypercoagulability had a limb salvage rate of 55%, compared with 67% for those without hypercoagulability. Survival rate was also reduced for patients with hypercoagulability, 61% versus 74%.

Conclusions.—Patency rates and other long-term outcomes of infrainguinal bypass surgery are significantly less favorable in patients with hypercoagulability. This experience shows a 13% rate of various causes of hyperco-

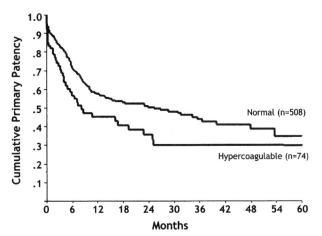

FIGURE 1.—Cumulative primary assisted patency rate in 456 patients undergoing infrainguinal bypass grafting with serologically proven hypercoagulability (hypercoagulable, n = 74 grafts) and without (normal, n = 508 grafts). Difference in patency rate was statistically significant with log-rank test ($P < .05$). All standard errors, less than 10%. (Reprinted by permission of the publisher from Curi MA, Skelly CL, Baldwin ZK, et al: Long-term outcome of infrainguinal bypass grafting in patients with serologically proven hypercoagulability. *J Vasc Surg* 37:301-306, 2003. Copyright 2003 by Elsevier.)

agulability in a referral series of patients undergoing this operation. Screening for a hypercoagulable state may be indicated, especially for patients with previous adverse events.

▶ In the authors' hands, patients with infrainguinal bypass grafts and hypercoagulable states clearly do poorly, with primary assisted graft patencies of 45% ± 6% at 5 years. The authors' use of 39% prosthetic grafts for infrainguinal bypass and their overall results are not what one would hope for from a major academic center. It is suggested that a serious effort be made to identify ways to improve performance. I have to believe that with some effort, their use of prosthetic grafts for infrainguinal bypass could be greatly reduced.

G. L. Moneta, MD

Ankle to Brachial Pressure Index in Normal Subjects and Trained Cyclists With Exercise-Induced Leg Pain
Taylor AJ, George KP (Nottingham Nuffield Hosp, England)
Med Sci Sports Exerc 33:1862-1867, 2001   4–5

Introduction.—External iliac artery endofibrosis has recently been detected in young runners, weight lifters, and competitive cyclists and can result in arterial insufficiency. Few trials have examined ankle to brachial pressure index (ABPI) responses to maximum exercise in trained athletes with exercise-induced leg pain (EILP). The ABPIs before and after maximal exercise were examined in 3 groups of research subjects to provide data regarding the normal ABPI response to maximal exercise testing in trained and untrained individuals and to establish the nature of the association between the ABPI response and EILP.

Methods.—ABPI measurements were obtained before and after cycle ergometer exercise to volitional exhaustion or reproduction of symptoms in 3 groups: (1) 10 untrained individuals (3 women, 7 men; mean age, 35 years), (2) 10 trained cyclists (3 women, 7 men; mean age, 30 years), and (3) 12 symptomatic trained cyclists with EILP (2 women, 10 men; mean age, 35 years).

Results.—No significant between-group differences were found in resting blood pressure indices. The ABPIs were diminished ($P < .05$) in all groups after exercise. No differences between right and left legs were observed in the elite and untrained groups. A significant difference ($P < .05$) was found between the nonsymptomatic and symptomatic legs (mean, 0.79 and 0.61, respectively) in participants with EILP. Only 3 participants in the symptomatic group met published criteria (index of < 0.5) for endofibrosis of the external iliac artery. All positive ABPI tests were subsequently verified by arteriograms.

Conclusion.—Maximal exercise testing combined with an ABPI measurement is a simple noninvasive method that may be beneficial in the evaluation of EILP. In patients with unilateral symptoms, a between-leg ABPI difference of 0.18 (at the first minute of recovery) may be useful as an additional diagnostic criterion.

▶ Elite athletes with EILP frequently have normal vascular laboratory findings at rest and with mild exercise. Investigation of the athlete with EILP is frustrating in that noninvasive parameters to establish arterial abnormalities are lacking in such patients. The authors have shown that with exercise of sufficient magnitude to produce symptoms, a difference in ABPIs between legs of as little as 0.18 indicates the presence of an arterial lesion in the symptomatic leg. This information should be of use to all of us who are occasionally asked to evaluate patients with claudication induced only by extreme exercise.

G. L. Moneta, MD

Popliteal Entrapment Syndrome
Turnipseed WD (Univ of Wisconsin, Madison)
J Vasc Surg 35:910-915, 2002   4–6

Background.—Popliteal entrapment syndrome is characterized by a unique set of symptoms in the lower extremity resulting from pathologic impingement behind the knee. Initially, the concept of popliteal entrapment was based on the finding of an abnormal anatomical positioning of the popliteal artery, which deviated medially around the medial head of the gastrocnemius muscle. However, it may be that popliteal impingement may also be functional with no evidence of an anatomical abnormality. Impingement then may occur as a normal physiologic variant that becomes symptomatic only with repetitive overuse or injury. Clinical similarities and differences between anatomical and functional forms of popliteal entrapment were evaluated.

Methods.—Two hundred forty patients undergoing evaluation for symptoms of atypical lower extremity claudication between 1987 and 2000 were included in the review. Most had had symptoms for more than 24 months, manifesting as paresthesias or as the swelling and cramping of isolated muscle groups.

Findings.—Only 7 of the patients (2.9%) had physical findings or noninvasive test results suggesting intrinsic vascular occlusive disease. This group included 5 men and 2 women, aged 17 to 69 years. These patients were compared with 30 patients with apparent functional popliteal entrapment. This group included 22 female and 8 male patients, aged 15 to 47 years. In the functional group, all had claudication, 43% had paresthesia, and 7% had calf swelling. None had digital swelling. In the anatomical group, 43% had claudication, 14% had paresthesia, 14% had calf swelling, and 43% had digital swelling. All patients in both groups had a positive stress test. On further assessment with digital subtraction arteriography, MRI, or MR angiography with stress testing, all patients in both groups had stress arterial displacement. However, in the anatomical popliteal entrapment group, 86% also had vascular stenosis or occlusion, 43% had static arterial displacement, and 14% had aneurysmal stenosis or occlusion.

Conclusions.—Patients with anatomical entrapment are more often male, older, and more sedentary than those with functional entrapment. Patients in the former group also have more restrictive claudication symptoms and more often have physical and noninvasive test findings suggesting peripheral occlusive disease. When anatomical entrapment is detected, surgery is indicated. In patients with functional entrapment, surgery is only indicated when symptoms develop.

▶ Dr Turnipseed places a great deal of emphasis on decreasing ankle brachial indices and flattening of plethysmographic waveforms, with planter or dorsal flexion of the foot, as a means of assisting in the diagnosis of a "functional" form of popliteal entrapment. I tell my residents that plantar and dorsal flexion is worthless in young people as many asymptomatic individuals will have a positive test. The whole thing bears a disturbing similarity to using positional arm movements to confirm a diagnosis of neurogenic thoracic outlet syndrome—a worthless test, as decreases in brachial pressure with exaggerated arm movements can be demonstrated in many asymptomatic patients.

G. L. Moneta, MD

The Utility of Color Duplex Ultrasonography in the Diagnosis of Temporal Arteritis

LeSar CJ, Meier GH, DeMasi RJ, et al (Eastern Virginia Med School, Norfolk)
J Vasc Surg 36:1154-1160, 2002   4–7

Introduction.—The diagnosis of temporal arteritis (TA) is often made from nonspecific clinical features, followed by a temporal artery biopsy to verify the presence of vasculitis. Many screening surgical biopsy specimens are negative. The potential of color duplex US scanning (CDU) as the initial screening test before surgical biopsy of the temporal artery was examined in the diagnosis of giant cell arteritis.

Methods.—Thirty-two patients with suspected TA based on clinical criteria underwent CDU before temporal artery biopsy. The presence of a hypoechoic "halo" indicating edema of the inflamed vessel and inflammatory stenoses were documented. Histologic examinations of standard temporal artery biopsy specimens were conducted. Biopsy and CDU findings were compared. A meta-analysis was also performed to identify articles concerning the use of US scanning for detection of TA.

Results.—Bilateral CDU examinations of the temporal arteries were performed in all patients. In 75% of the patients biopsied, no evidence of vasculitis was seen on histologic examination. When CDU examined for halo alone as the determinant of the presence of disease, the sensitivity, specificity, positive predictive value, and negative predictive value, versus histologic verification of TA, were 85.7%, 92.0%, 75.0%, and 95.8%, respectively. Using criteria for finding a halo sign present, an inflammatory stenosis present, or both present on CDU, sensitivity, specificity, positive predictive value, and negative predictive values were 100%, 80.0%, 58.3%, and 100%, respectively.

Conclusion.—CDU is an accurate and noninvasive technique for ascertaining the presence of vasculitis, compared with routine surgical biopsy. It can effectively predict which patients need surgical biopsy. Its high sensitivity detects patients with TA, and the high negative predictive value eliminates patients who would not benefit from biopsy.

▶ A test with 100% sensitivity and 100% negative predictive value is about as good as it gets to reduce use of a low-yield operative procedure where missing the diagnosis may be catastrophic. With more experience, this examination should probably be used more often to screen for TA. It must be kept in mind, however, that this examination is not all that easy to perform or interpret. It is suggested that each laboratory perform correlative studies before using duplex to substitute for histologic diagnosis of TA.

G. L. Moneta, MD

Evaluation of Treatment Efficacy of Raynaud Phenomenon by Digital Blood Pressure Response to Cooling

Maricq HR, for the Raynaud's Treatment Study Investigators (Med Univ of South Carolina, Charleston; et al)

Vasc Med 5:135-140, 2000   4–8

Background.—The primary measure of treatment effect in studies of patients with Raynaud phenomenon (RP) has been the change in frequency of RP attacks. The use of physiologic methods to evaluate treatment effects has produced inconsistent results. However, some studies suggest that the digital blood pressure response to cooling is closely associated with the frequency of RP attacks reported by patients. This study was conducted as part of the Raynaud's Treatment Study (RTS), a multicenter, randomized clinical trial comparing the effectiveness of sustained-release nifedipine and temperature biofeedback in the treatment of patients with primary RP.

Methods.—Data from 158 participants in the RTS trial were reviewed. All the participants had RP diagnosed by means of a standardized RP diagnostic test that included a structured interview and the use of color charts. Patients were randomly assigned to sustained-release nifedipine (42 patients), temperature biofeedback (37 patients), electromyography (38 patients), and placebo (41 patients). Digital blood pressure was determined at baseline and at 2 months and 1 year after the initiation of treatment. The response to local finger cooling was measured at 30°C, 20°C, 15°C, and 10°C. The results after 2 months of treatment were selected for use in evaluation of treatment effect. Patients recorded their RP attacks on "attack recording cards" after comparing their finger color with an "RP attack verification card."

Results.—At 15°C and 10°C local cooling temperatures, patients in the nifedipine group had a higher mean digital systolic blood pressure, a higher relative digital systolic blood pressure (RDSP), a smaller proportion of patients with an RDSP of less than 70%, and a smaller proportion of patients with a zero reopening pressure compared with patients in the 3 other treatment groups. These results were statistically significant at 10°C, with the nifedipine group being significantly different from the other 3 groups. There were no significant differences in treatment effect between the other 3 treatment groups.

Conclusions.—Nifedipine has a protective effect against finger cooling in patients with primary RP. The digital blood pressure response to cooling provides an objective measurement of the efficacy of RP treatment under standardized conditions.

▶ With the use of objective measurements of digital blood pressure response to cooling, it appears that nifedipine but not biofeedback has the potential to improve symptoms of digital ischemia in patients with Raynaud syndrome. Perhaps biofeedback provides some patients with improved tolerance of their Raynaud symptoms, but if you want improvement in digital pressures, drugs are required.

G. L. Moneta, MD

Mutations in a Novel Factor, *Glomulin*, Are Responsible for Glomuvenous Malformations ("Glomangiomas")

Brouillard P, Boon LM, Mulliken JB, et al (Université catholique de Louvain, Brussels, Belgium; Harvard Med School, Boston; Tufts Univ, Boston; et al)
Am J Hum Genet 70:866-874, 2002   4–9

Introduction.—Glomuvenous malformations (GMVs) are cutaneous venous lesions that are often present at birth and grow proportionally with the patient. Histologically, they demonstrate enlarged endothelial-lined veinlike channels with defects in the smooth muscle cell layer. Heritable GVMs link to a 4–6-cM region in chromosome 1p21-22 and have linkage disequilibrium that allows a narrowing of the VMGLOM locus to 1.48 Mb. Reported is the identification of the mutated gene, *glomulin*, localized on the basis of the YAC and PAC maps.

Findings.—Eight previously unreported families with individuals affected by GVMs and 1 patient with a sporadic case and no known family history of the disease are presented. Buccal cell samples were obtained from 2 individuals, and the remaining underwent venipuncture for blood samples. Earlier, an incomplete complementary DNA sequence for *glomulin* was designated *FAP48*, which stood for FKBP-associated protein of 48 kd. The gene is made up of 19 exons in which 14 different germline mutations were observed in patients with GVMs. In addition, a somatic "second hit" mutation was seen in affected tissue of a patient with an inherited genomic deletion.

Conclusion.—Because all except 1 of the mutations result in premature stop codons and because the localized nature of the lesions could be explained by Knudson's 2-hit model, GVMs are probably caused by complete loss of function of *glomulin*. The abnormal phenotype of vascular smooth muscle cells in GMVs indicates that *glomulin* has an important role in the differentiation of these cells and thus in vascular morphogenesis, particularly in cutaneous veins.

▶ This article details an inheritable genetic basis for one particular type of vascular malformation. By studying the genetics of vascular malformations, it is likely we will eventually have a greater understanding of the formation of normal vessels as well. It is interesting to become aware of the large number of germline mutations that can result in a phenotypically similar disease process. It appears vascular malformations will have many possible underlying defects with similar clinical presentations.

G. L. Moneta, MD

Heparin Resistance as Detected With an Antifactor Xa Assay Is Not More Common in Venous Thromboembolism Than in Other Thromboembolic Conditions

Rosborough TK, Shepherd MF (Abbott Northwestern Hosp, Minneapolis)
Pharmacotherapy 23:142-146, 2003   4–10

Background.—So-called heparin-resistant patients need extremely high doses of heparin to produce a therapeutic activated partial thromboplastin time (aPTT), and an increased frequency of heparin resistance has been noted among patients with acute venous thromboembolic disease. Whether heparin resistance is indeed more prevalent among these patients than among those with other diseases was assessed, measuring heparin activity with a chromogenic, amidolytic antifactor Xa assay.

Methods.—This cohort study involved 372 patients (182 men and 190 women) who received IV unfractionated heparin for venous thromboembolism (28% of cases) or arterial thromboembolism (72% of cases). The initial dosage was based on a protocol determined by age and estimated blood volume. The level of antifactor Xa targeted was 0.35 to 0.65 U/mL.

Results.—For the entire group, the median heparin resistance index was 0.54, with the middle 50% of individual indexes falling between 0.4 and 0.68, but the range extended from 0.22 to 2.73. Age, creatinine clearance, hemoglobin concentration, and treatment indication differed between patients with venous and arterial thromboembolism. Analysis showed that only hemoglobin concentration was linked to heparin resistance. Regardless of their indication for treatment, patients who had lower hemoglobin concentrations were more likely to exhibit heparin resistance.

Conclusions.—Venous thromboembolism was not independently associated with greater degrees of heparin resistance, but lower hemoglobin concentration was so linked.

▶ This article partially dispels the myth that increased thrombus burden leads to relative heparin resistance. It appears that decreased hemoglobin rather than increased thrombus results in the need for higher heparin doses. By careful attention to weight-based nomograms for heparin administration and increasing heparin doses in patients with decreased hemoglobin levels, heparin "resistance" in deep venous thrombosis may cease to be a problem.

G. L. Moneta, MD

Management of Cervical Ribs and Anomalous First Ribs Causing Neurogenic Thoracic Outlet Syndrome

Sanders RJ, Hammond SL (Univ of Colorado, Denver; Uniformed Services Univ of the Health Sciences, Bethesda, Md)
J Vasc Surg 36:51-56, 2002   4–11

Background.—Cervical and anomalous first ribs are rare conditions, occurring in less than 1% of the population. The management of neurogenic thoracic outlet syndrome associated with the presence of cervical and anomalous first ribs was reviewed.

Methods.—A total of 65 operations have been performed over the past 26 years for abnormal ribs producing symptoms of thoracic outlet syndrome. Of these 65 operations, 54 were for neurogenic thoracic outlet syndrome. Indications for surgery in these 54 cases were disabling pain and paresthesia and failure to respond to conservative treatment. The surgical technique for neurogenic thoracic outlet syndrome was supraclavicular cervical rib resection and scalenectomy without rib resection in 22 cases, supraclavicular cervical and first rib resection in 17 cases, supraclavicular excision of anomalous first ribs in 5 cases, and transaxillary anomalous first rib resection in 2 cases, for a total of 46 cases. The remaining 8 cases consisted of reoperations for recurrent thoracic outlet syndrome in patients who had previously undergone cervical and first rib resection.

Results.—The cause of neurogenic symptoms in 80% of patients with cervical or anomalous first ribs was neck trauma. The surgical failure rate was 28% for 46 primary operations. The etiology of symptoms was found to significantly affect the surgical outcome. The failure rate for patients in whom symptoms developed after work-related injury or repetitive stress was 42%, and the failure rate for patients in whom symptoms occurred after an auto accident or developed spontaneously were 26% and 18%, respectively.

The failure rate in each etiologic group also was affected by the type of procedure performed. Cervical rib resection without first rib resection had a failure rate of 75% in the work-related group and 38% in the non–work-related group. However, when both cervical and first ribs were resected, the failure rate dropped to 25% in the work-related group and 20% in the non–work-related group. The failure rates for the work-related and non–work-related groups were similar to the failure rates in patients without cervical ribs.

Conclusion.—The most common cause of neurogenic thoracic outlet syndrome in patients with abnormal ribs was neck trauma. Surgery for patients with neurogenic thoracic outlet syndrome should include both cervical and first rib resection. The presence of cervical or anomalous first ribs in these patients does not improve the success rate from surgery. Cervical and anomalous first ribs should be considered predisposing factors rather than the cause of neurogenic thoracic outlet syndrome.

▶ I agree that cervical ribs are of uncertain significance in patients with neurogenic thoracic outlet syndrome. However, I also believe that in the absence of electrophysiologic abnormalities, so-called neurogenic thoracic outlet syndrome probably has very little if anything to do with major nerves. A somewhat polar position would be to say that the only nervous tissue that is malfunctioning is intracranial in the surgeons who remove ribs in an attempt to treat a nonspecific disorder.

G. L. Moneta, MD

Thoracodorsal Sympathectomy for Severe Hyperhydrosis: Posterior Bilateral Versus Unilateral Staged Sympathectomy

Doblas M, Gutierrez R, Fontcuberta J, et al (Complejo Hospitalario de Toledo, Spain; Stony Brook Univ, NY)

Ann Vasc Surg 17:97-102, 2003   4–12

Background.—Hyperhidrosis can have significant psychologic and social consequences. Thoracoscopic sympathectomy is effective for patients who do not respond to medical treatment. Traditionally, the procedure is performed from an anterolateral approach with 2 separate, *unilateral* procedures. The results of a posterior *bilateral* approach to simultaneous thoracodorsal sympathectomy was evaluated.

Methods.—The investigators performed bilateral thoracodorsal sympathectomies in 101 patients with severe hyperhidrosis over a 6-year period. The patients were 79 women and 22 men, ranging in age from 19 to 65 years. Fifty-two patients were managed with staged, anterolateral sympathectomies. Unilateral procedures were performed with the patient in a supine position utilizing ipsilateral lung collapse. The other 49 patients underwent bilateral sympathectomy in a single procedure. For these procedures, the patient was placed in the prone position, without pneumothorax. Two ports were placed to give access to the thoracic cavity, allowing the surgeon to reach the sympathetic chain via the parietal pleura.

Results.—Both procedures yielded excellent immediate postoperative results. At long-term follow-up, sweating had resolved in 100% of the patients operated on by the bilateral posterior approach, compared with 92% in whom the staged anterolateral approach was used. Safety outcomes were similar between the groups; 94% of the patients were treated in the ambulatory care unit. Hospital costs were reduced by about one half in patients undergoing the bilateral procedure.

Conclusions.—For treatment of hyperhidrosis, the posterobilateral approach to thoracodorsal sympathectomy gives good results comparable with staged anterolateral procedures, with similar safety, shorter recovery time, and lower costs.

▶ Resection of the second and third thoracic ganglia provides relief from palmar and axilla hyperhidrosis, while medical therapy, except for temporary relief with botulinum toxin, has been ineffective. Patients with hyperhidrosis virtually always have bilateral symptoms, and therefore, the authors' technique of doing both sides at once with comparable complication rates to staged procedures seems a real advantage over the staged approach.

G. L. Moneta, MD

5   Perioperative Considerations

Cost Effectiveness of Aspirin, Clopidogrel, or Both for Secondary Prevention of Coronary Heart Disease

Gaspoz J-M, Coxson PG, Goldman PA, et al (Hôpitaux Universitaires, Geneva; Univ of California, San Francisco; Harvard School of Public Health, Boston; et al)

N Engl J Med 346:1800-1806, 2002   5–1

Background.—Antiplatelet therapy has been shown to reduce the rate of myocardial infarction, strokes, or death from vascular causes by about 30% in patients with prior myocardial infarction, strokes, or other high risk vascular conditions. However, the use of aspirin for these patients has lagged, despite a large volume of data and numerous recommendations for its use. Clopidogrel is a thienopyridine derivative that has been shown to reduce the relative risk of ischemic strokes, myocardial infarction, or death from vascular causes by almost 9% as compared with aspirin. The addition of clopidogrel to aspirin for patients with acute coronary syndromes reduced the risk of death from cardiovascular disease, repeated infarction, or strokes by 20% compared with aspirin alone. The cost-effectiveness of the increased use of aspirin, clopidogrel, or both for secondary prevention in patients with coronary heart disease was estimated.

Methods.—The Coronary Heart Disease Policy Model is a computer simulation of the US population. This model was used to estimate the incremental cost-effectiveness of 4 strategies in patients older than 35 years with coronary disease from 2003 to 2027. The strategies modeled were aspirin for all eligible patients, aspirin for all eligible patients plus clopidogrel for patients who were ineligible for aspirin, clopidogrel for all patients, and a combination of aspirin and clopidogrel for all patients. The cost-effectiveness was assessed in terms of dollars per quality-adjusted year of life gained.

Results.—The extension of aspirin therapy to all eligible patients for 25 years would have an estimated cost-effectiveness ratio of approximately $11,000 per quality-adjusted year of life. For the 5% of patients ineligible for aspirin, the addition of clopidogrel would cost about $31,000 per quality-adjusted year of life gained. The use of clopidogrel alone in all patients or in routine combination with aspirin would have an incremental cost of more than $130,000 per quality-adjusted year of life; this option remained financially unattractive throughout a range of assumptions. However, if the price of clopidogrel were reduced by 70% to 82%, the use of clopidogrel alone or in combination with aspirin would have a cost of less than $50,000 per quality-adjusted year of life gained.

Conclusions.—This cost-effectiveness analysis showed that the increased prescription of aspirin for the secondary prevention of coronary heart disease is an attractive course of action. Clopidogrel is more expensive than aspirin, which makes its incremental cost-effectiveness unattractive at the present time, unless its use is restricted to patients who are ineligible for aspirin because of allergies or intolerance.

▶ The authors point out in the discussion of this article that the overall cost-effectiveness of aspirin therapy was not as much as expected given the very low cost and great benefit of aspirin. The reason is that the patients live longer and therefore have other medical problems that also cost money. Eventually, costs related to coronary disease will also increase. More and more, our patients will be outliving their vascular reconstructions, and even more repeat surgery will be required unless the promised benefits of all this research on intimal hyperplasia actually make the transition from animal models to people.

G. L. Moneta, MD

Troponin T Levels in Patients With Acute Coronary Syndromes, With or Without Renal Dysfunction

Aviles RJ, Askari AT, Lindahl B, et al (Cleveland Clinic Found, Ohio; Univ of Uppsala, Sweden; Univ of North Carolina, Chapel Hill; et al)
N Engl J Med 346:2047-2052, 2002   5–2

Background.—Cardiac troponins are useful in establishing a diagnosis and prognosis in patients with suspected acute coronary syndromes. However, cardiac troponin T may be cleared by the kidney, so there is concern that renal dysfunction may compromise the diagnostic value of troponin T levels in these patients. The prognostic value of baseline cardiac troponin T levels in relation to renal functioning was investigated in patients seen with suspected acute coronary syndromes.

Methods.—Outcomes were analyzed for 7033 patients enrolled in the Global Use of Strategies to Open Occluded Coronary Arteries IV trial who had complete baseline data on troponin T levels and creatinine clearance rates. A troponin T level was considered abnormal if it was 0.1 ng/mL or higher. Creatinine clearance was assessed in quartiles. The primary end point was a composite of death or myocardial infarction within 30 days.

Results.—The primary end point of death or myocardial infarction occurred in 581 patients. An abnormally elevated troponin T level was predictive of an increased risk of myocardial infarction or death among patients with a creatinine clearance above the 25th percentile value of 58.4 mL/min. Among patients with a creatinine clearance in the lowest quartile, an elevated troponin T level was similarly predictive of increased risk (20% vs 9%). When the creatinine clearance rate was considered as a continuous variable and age, sex, ST-segment depression, heart failure, previous revascularization, diabetes mellitus, and other confounders were accounted for, an elevated troponin T level was independently predictive of risk across the entire spectrum of renal function.

Conclusions.—Cardiac troponin T levels were predictive of the short-term prognosis in patients with acute coronary syndromes, regardless of the level of creatinine clearance.

▶ In patients with acute coronary syndromes elevated troponin T levels predict short-term prognosis independent of ST-segment depression in the presence of renal failure. It would be interesting to know whether asymptomatic troponin elevations also predict short-term risk in postoperative vascular surgical patients.

G. L. Moneta, MD

Risk of Myocardial Infarction and Angina in Patients With Severe Peripheral Vascular Disease: Predictive Role of C-Reactive Protein
Rossi E, Biasucci LM, Citterio F, et al (Catholic Univ, Rome; Univ Vita-Salute, Milano, Italy)
Circulation 105:800-803, 2002   5–3

Background.—Patients with peripheral vascular disease (PVD) have an increased risk of coronary artery disease (CAD). Whether the prognostic evaluation of patients with PVD could be improved by preoperative measurements of C-reactive protein (CRP) was investigated.

Methods.—The study group included 51 patients with PVD (Fontaine Stages II to IV) without severe resting ventricular dysfunction or ischemia. The clinical and risk factor profiles, Eagle clinical scores, and preoperative CRP serum levels were assessed in these patients.

Results.—Patients were followed up for 24 months, with short-term assessment at 30 days and long-term evaluation at 24 months. Seventeen patients (34%) had fatal (11) or nonfatal (6) myocardial infarctions (MIs). On univariate logistic regression analysis, the only factors independently associated with MI were a previous history of CAD, Eagle score, and level of CRP. On multivariate analysis, only CRP levels in the upper tertile (<9 mg/L) were significantly associated with MI. CRP levels identified 65% of cases of MI.

Conclusions.—Preprocedural measurement of the serum CRP level is strongly predictive of MI for patients with PVD severe enough to require revascularization. This marker is independent of previous CAD, Eagle score index, and traditional cardiovascular risk factors. For these patients, therapy that modulates the inflammatory response may be beneficial.

▶ This is a small study with large implications. Perhaps we should be measuring CRP to decide whether our vascular surgical patients require, when possible, an extensive preoperative cardiac workup? Nothing else has proved all that useful in identifying which vascular surgical patients need extensive cardiac preoperative evaluation.

G. L. Moneta, MD

Rapid Measurement of B-Type Natriuretic Peptide in the Emergency Diagnosis of Heart Failure

Maisel AS, for the Breathing Not Properly Multinational Study Investigators (Univ of California, San Diego; et al)
N Engl J Med 347:161-167, 2002   5–4

Introduction.—B-type natriuretic peptide is a cardiac neurohormone specifically secreted from the ventricles of the heart in response to volume expansion and pressure overload. Levels have been observed to be elevated in patients with left ventricular dysfunction and correlate with New York Heart Association class and prognosis. In a prospective, 7-center, multinational trial, the use of B-type natriuretic peptide levels in the diagnosis of congestive heart failure (CHF) was validated and characterized in a broad population of patients with dyspnea.

Methods.—B-type natriuretic peptide levels were measured by means of a bedside assay in 1586 patients admitted to the emergency department with acute dyspnea. Two cardiologists reviewed all medical records and independently classified the diagnosis as dyspnea caused by CHF, acute dyspnea from noncardiac causes in a patient with a history of left ventricular dysfunction, or dyspnea not caused by CHF.

Results.—The mean age of the 883 men and 703 women was 64 years. The final diagnoses were CHF, dyspnea from noncardiac dysfunction, and no findings of CHF in 744 (47%), 72 (5%), and 770 (49%) patients, respectively. The B-type natriuretic peptide levels varied significantly between groups ($P < .001$ for each pairwise comparison). The B-type natriuretic peptide levels alone were more accurate than any historical findings or laboratory values in detecting CHF as the cause of dyspnea. The diagnostic accuracy of B-type natriuretic peptide at a cutoff of 100 pg/mL was 83.4%, and the negative predictive value at levels of less than 50 pg/mL was 96%. The levels of B-type natriuretic peptide varied significantly according to New York Heart Association functional class. Multiple logistic regression analysis revealed that measurements of B-type natriuretic peptide added significant independent predictive power to other clinical variables in models predicting which patients had CHF.

Conclusion.—The rapid determination of B-type natriuretic peptide levels is helpful in establishing or excluding the diagnosis of CHF in patients with acute dyspnea.

▶ Shortness of breath is common in vascular surgical patients and in patients with chronic obstructive pulmonary disease and possible volume overload. The test described in this article may help in clarifying the etiology of acute shortness of breath. It is important to note that the patients described in this study presented to an emergency department with shortness of breath; they were not postoperative patients. However, since B-type natriuretic peptide is released in response to increased ventricular wall tension, it theoretically could be useful in distinguishing between volume overload and other causes of shortness of breath in postoperative patients.

G. L. Moneta, MD

The Antioxidant Acetylcysteine Reduces Cardiovascular Events in Patients With End-Stage Renal Failure: A Randomized, Controlled Trial
Tepel M, van der Giet M, Statz M, et al (Freie Universität Berlin)
Circulation 107:992-995, 2003   5–5

Background.—Elevated oxidative stress is greater in hemodialysis patients with cardiovascular disease than in those patients without cardiovascular disease. There is increasing evidence that antioxidative treatment might be beneficial for these patients by reducing oxidative stress. The hypothesis that a reduction in oxidative stress might reduce cardiovascular events in hemodialysis patients was tested by investigating the effects of acetylcysteine, a thiol-containing antioxidant, on cardiovascular events in hemodialysis patients.

Methods.—A prospective, randomized, placebo-controlled study was conducted between October 1, 1999, and September 30, 2001, in 134 patients (76 men and 58 women; mean age, 62 ± 16 years) undergoing mainte-

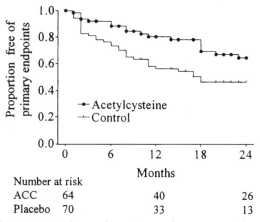

FIGURE.—Kaplan-Meier survival curves from primary end points. Hemodialysis patients were randomly assigned either to receive acetylcysteine (*ACC*, 600 mg BID) or placebo (control group). The primary end point was a composite variable consisting of cardiac events including fatal and nonfatal myocardial infarction, cardiovascular disease death, need for coronary angioplasty or coronary bypass surgery, ischemic stroke, peripheral vascular disease with amputation, or need for angioplasty. Relative risk, 0.60 (95% confidence interval, 0.38 to 0.95), P = .03. (Courtesy of Tepel M, van der Giet M, Statz M, et al: The antioxidant acetylcysteine reduces cardiovascular events in patients with end-stage renal failure: A randomized, controlled trial. *Circulation* 107:992-995, 2003.)

nance hemodialysis for a minimum of 3 months. The median follow-up was 14.5 months, with a range of 1 to 24 months. The patients were randomly assigned to receive either acetylcysteine (600 mg) twice a day or placebo. The primary end point was a composite variable consisting of nonfatal and fatal myocardial infarction, cardiovascular disease death, need for coronary angioplasty or coronary bypass surgery, ischemic stroke, peripheral vascular disease requiring amputation, or need for angioplasty. Secondary end points included each of the component outcomes, total mortality, and cardiovascular mortality.

Results.—The primary end point was obtained in 18 of 64 hemodialysis patients (28%) in the acetylcysteine group and in 33 of 70 patients (47%) in the control group (Figure). There were no significant differences between the 2 groups in secondary end points or in total mortality.

Conclusions.—Treatment with acetylcysteine (600 mg twice a day) reduced composite cardiovascular end points in patients with end-stage renal failure.

▶ No one knows why renal failure has such a dramatic effect on cardiovascular events. Oxidative stress is markedly increased in renal failure. Perhaps antioxidants will help.

G. L. Moneta, MD

Efficacy of Recombinant Human Erythropoietin in Critically Ill Patients: A Randomized Controlled Trial
Corwin HL, for the EPO Critical Care Trials Group (Dartmouth-Hitchcock Med Ctr, Lebanon, NH; et al)
JAMA 288:2827-2835, 2002   5–6

Introduction.—Anemia occurs often in critically ill patients and necessitates a large number of red blood cell (RBC) transfusions. Recent data suggest RBC transfusions may be linked with worse clinical outcome in some patients. The efficacy of a weekly dosing schedule of recombinant human erythropoietin (rHuEPO) to reduce the occurrence of RBC transfusions in critically ill patients was examined in a prospective, randomized, double-blind, placebo-controlled, multicenter trial.

Methods.—Between December 1998 and June 2001, a total of 1302 patients who had been in the ICU in 1 of 65 participating institutions for 2 days and were expected to be in the ICU for at least 2 more days were evaluated. Patients were randomly assigned to treatment with either 40,000 units of rHuEPO, or placebo, by subcutaneous injection on ICU day 3; injections were continued weekly for patients who remained in the hospital, for a total of 3 doses. Patients who remained in the ICU on study day 21 received a fourth dose. The primary outcome measure was transfusion independence, determined by comparing the percentage of patients in each treatment group who received RBC transfusions between days 1 and 28. Secondary efficacy end points were cumulative RBC units transfused per patient through day

28, cumulative mortality through day 28, change in hemoglobin level from baseline, and time to first transfusion or death.

Results.—Patients in the rHuEPO group were less likely to undergo transfusion (60.4% placebo vs 50.5% rHuEPO; $P < .001$; odds ratio [OR], 0.67; 95% confidence interval [CI], 0.54-0.83). There was a 19% decrease in the total units of RBCs transfused in the rHuEPO group (1963 units for placebo vs 1590 units for rHuEPO) and a decrease in RBC units transfused per day alive (ratio of transfusion rates, 0.81; 95% CI, 0.79-0.83; $P = .04$). The increase in hemoglobin level from baseline to completion of investigation was greater in the rHuEPO group (mean, 1.32 g/dL vs 0.94 g/dL; $P < .001$). There were no significant between-group differences in mortality (14% for rHuEPO and 15% for placebo) and adverse clinical events.

Conclusion.—The weekly administration of 40,000 units of rHuEPO decreases allogeneic RBC transfusions and increases hemoglobin levels in critically ill patients.

▶ Recent studies have indicated that overtransfusion of patients in the ICU is associated with increased mortality. This study indicates patients can be treated with erythropoietin and receive fewer transfusions and have increased hemoglobin levels compared with ICU patients not treated with erythropoietin. The problem in this study is that the comparison group may be overtransfused and therefore not really be an appropriate comparison group to the erythropoietin-treated patients. Thus, reducing blood transfusions that were not necessary in the first place is not necessarily progress.

G. L. Moneta, MD

Hemodynamic Benefits of Regional Anesthesia for Carotid Endarterectomy
Sternbach Y, Illig KA, Zhang R, et al (Strong Mem Hosp, Rochester, NY; Univ of Rochester, NY)
J Vasc Surg 35:333-339, 2002   5–7

Introduction.—The potential advantages of regional anesthesia for carotid endarterectomy (CEA) include more accurate neurologic monitoring with a reduced need for intraoperative shunting and a decrease in risk associated with general anesthesia and improved perioperative hemodynamics. Differences in perioperative hemodynamics and associated outcomes were examined in patients undergoing CEA with regional versus general anesthesia.

Methods.—The medical records of all patients who underwent nonemergent CEA using either cervical block anesthesia (CB) or general anesthetic (GA) between October 1998 and November 2000 were reviewed. Patients who were treated with combined coronary artery revascularization were excluded, as were those who needed one or the other anesthetic technique for medical reasons. Baseline intraoperative and postoperative blood pressure (BP) and heart rate were documented. Administration of vasoactive medica-

TABLE 6.—Heart Rate Variability and Systolic Blood Pressure Variability

	Cervical Block	General Anesthesia	P Value
Heart rate variability			
Preclamp	20%	34%	<.0001
Clamped	17%	19%	.02
Postclamp	14%	19%	.001
PACU	21%	24%	.02
POD 1	16%	21%	.002
Systolic blood pressure variability			
Preclamp	14%	28%	.0001
Clamped	11%	14%	.05
Postclamp	8%	15%	.0001
PACU	17%	23%	.0001
POD 1	14%	19%	.0002

Note: Heart rate variability = heart rate maximum − heart rate minimum × 100)/heart rate baseline. Systolic blood pressure variability = blood pressure maximum − blood pressure minimum × 100/blood pressure baseline.
Abbreviations: PACU, Postanesthesia unit; POD, postoperative day.
(Reprinted by permission of the publisher from Sternbach Y, Illig KA, Zhang R, et al: Hemodynamic benefits of regional anesthesia for carotid endarterectomy. *J Vasc Surg* 35:333-339, 2002. Copyright 2002 by Elsevier.)

tions was evaluated. Operative time, ICU admission, postoperative length of stay, and cardiac/neurologic morbidity were documented.

Results.—A total of 550 nonemergent CEAs were performed in 527 patients (226 had CB and 324 had GA). There were no significant between-group differences in age, presentation, or associated co-morbidities. Baseline BP and heart rate were similar in the 2 groups. Patients who underwent GA had significantly greater intraoperative and postoperative hemodynamic variability (Table 6) and received more vasoactive medications during surgery (87% vs 51%; $P < .001$) and in the recovery room (36% vs 21%; $P = .0009$).

Major postoperative BP derangements occurred more often in the GA group (18% vs 10%; $P < .05$). Patients in the GA group had more frequent ICU admissions (16% vs 7%; $P = .01$) and experienced more delays in discharge (20% vs 11%; $P = .008$, and postoperative length of stay, 2.1 vs 1.6 days; $P = .01$). There were no significant differences in neurologic morbidity rates (combined major/stroke/death rate, 1.8%). The major cardiac morbidity rate was lower in the CB group (1% vs 4%; $P = .05$). The total in-room operative time was shorter in the CB group (108 vs 122 minutes; $P < .001$).

Conclusion.—Carotid endarterectomy performed with CB is correlated with significantly less perioperative hemodynamic instability, fewer major adverse cardiac events, less use of critical care resources, and shortened length of stay, compared with GA.

▶ In the authors' hands, regional anesthesia for CEA has some measurable benefits. Like other studies on this subject and, like any other case series, we can only say that the guys at Strong Memorial Hospital should continue with regional anesthesia for CEA when possible. The rest of us have to decide whether a learning curve to institute routine regional anesthesia at our institutions is worth the effort without real evidence provided by a randomized trial.

G. L. Moneta, MD

Cost of Routine Screening for Carotid and Lower Extremity Occlusive Disease in Patients With Abdominal Aortic Aneurysms

Axelrod DA, Diwan A, Stanley JC, et al (Univ of Michigan, Ann Arbor)
J Vasc Surg 35:754-758, 2002   5–8

Introduction.—It has been reported that patients with abdominal aortic aneurysms (AAAs) may have a significant burden of atherosclerotic occlusive disease elsewhere. Diagnostic vascular laboratory and economic data were reviewed to evaluate the cost and usefulness of routine versus selective use of preoperative screening for clinically relevant nonaortic atherosclerotic occlusive disease for patients with AAAs.

Methods.—The study included 206 patients undergoing AAA repair between 1994 and 1998. All patients had routine preoperative carotid duplex scan examinations and lower-extremity Doppler scan arterial assessments, including ankle-brachial index (ABI) determinations. Medical records were reviewed to identify clinical evidence consistent with cerebrovascular or lower-extremity arterial occlusive disease. The costs of routine screening and selective screening were ascertained using Medicare reimbursement schedules.

Results.—The prevalence rate for advanced (80%-100%) carotid artery stenosis (CAS) was 3.4%; 18% had CAS between 60% and 100%. Advanced peripheral occlusive disease (PVOD [ABI, < 0.3]) was detected in 3% of patients. An ABI of less than 0.6 was determined for 12% of patients. Most patients with advanced CAS (71%) or advanced PVOD (83%) had clinical indications of disease. The absence of clinical signs of disease had a negative predictive value of 99% for both advanced CAS and PVOD. The cost of routine screening for advanced CAS of all patients was $5445 per person. The cost of routine screening for severe PVOD was $3732 per person. The costs of selective screening for advanced CAS or PVOD with appropriate history or symptoms were $1258 and $785 per patient with disease, respectively.

Conclusion.—Routine noninvasive diagnostic testing for detection of asymptomatic CAS and PVOD in patients with AAA may not be justified. Preoperative testing is indicated in patients with AAAs with clinical evidence of CAS or PVOD.

▶ Routine carotid duplex and noninvasive lower extremity arterial studies for patients with AAAs was the rule at our institution up until about 5 years ago. Based on no data, my partners and I stopped these screening studies as our impression was that the yield was too low. Now we have data.

G. L. Moneta, MD

Acute Normovolemic Hemodilution and Intraoperative Cell Salvage in Aortic Surgery

Torella F, Haynes SL, Kirwan CC, et al (Wythenshawe Hosp, Manchester, England)
J Vasc Surg 36:31-34, 2002   5–9

Background.—Autologous blood transfusion is increasingly popular. Autologous transfusion, particularly intraoperative cell salvage (ICS), has been frequently reported in aortic surgery. However, there is some controversy regarding the efficacy of ICS even with aortic surgery. Other autologous transfusion techniques, such as acute normovolemic hemodilution (ANH), are infrequently used in vascular surgery. The experience of 1 center with both ANH and ICS in infrarenal aortic surgery was reviewed. The objective of the study was to report current transfusion requirements and outcomes for patients undergoing elective aortic surgery with autologous transfusion.

Methods.—A total of 110 consecutive patients underwent infrarenal aortic surgery with a combination of ANH and INS. All patients underwent hemodilution to a target hemoglobin concentration of 11 g/dL and underwent ICS with a centrifugal device.

Results.—The median blood loss was 1140 mL in 78 aneurysm repairs and 775 mL in 32 aortobifemoral bypasses for occlusive disease. The median salvaged red cell volume was 403 mL for aneurysm repairs and 250 mL for bypass surgery. Transfusion of stored blood was required in 36 (33%) patients, for a total of 115 units. However, only 4 patients needed more than 5 units of stored blood. The mortality rate was 8% (9 of 110 patients). Multivariate analysis showed that low hemoglobin level and low platelet count were associated with transfusion of stored blood.

Conclusion.—Blood loss in surgery for occlusive disease is too small to justify the use of intraoperative cell salvage. Acute normovolemic hemodilution alone may be an acceptable strategy. With an appropriate level of experience, the combination of ANH and ICS may render cross-matching unnecessary, even in patients undergoing aortic aneurysm surgery.

▶ With attention to detail, it is possible to reduce transfusion needs in patients undergoing aortic surgery. We all need to pay more attention to details.

G. L. Moneta, MD

Transient Advanced Mental Impairment: An Underappreciated Morbidity After Aortic Surgery

Rosen SF, Clagett GP, Valentine RJ, et al (Univ of Texas, Dallas)
J Vasc Surg 35:376-381, 2002   5–10

Introduction.—Postoperative delirium may be an important complication after major surgery, especially in elderly patients. The incidence, risk factors, and associated morbidity of transient advanced mental impairment

(TAMI; defined as disorientation or confusion at 2 or more postoperative days) after aortic surgery were examined retrospectively.

Methods.—The medical records of 188 consecutive patients undergoing elective aortic reconstruction between September 1993 and July 1999 were reviewed. All patients were lucid at admission and were not intubated when assessed at least 2 days postoperatively. Preoperative, intraoperative, and postoperative clinical variables were evaluated for associations with TAMI.

Results.—Fifty-three patients (28%) had TAMI develop a mean of 3.9 days postoperatively. The following were independent predictors for TAMI: age older than 65 years (odds ratio [OR], 7.9; 95% CI, 1.3-5.9), diabetes mellitus (OR, 3.4; 95% CI, 1.2-9.8), old myocardial infarction (OR, 2.4; 95% CI, 1.2-5.3), and hypertension (OR, 2.3; 95% CI, 1.0-5.3). Alcohol consumption was not significantly correlated with TAMI. Postoperatively, patients with TAMI were significantly more likely than those without TAMI to experience hypoxia ($P = .001$), a need for reintubation ($P < .001$), pneumonia ($P < .001$), congestive heart failure ($P = .003$), and kidney failure ($P = .05$). Patients with TAMI had a longer mean duration of endotracheal intubation (3.7 vs 0.6 days; $P < .001$), stay in the ICU (8.9 vs 3.9 days; $P < .001$), and postoperative hospital stay (14.8 vs 9.2 days; $P < .001$) compared with patients who did not have TAMI. Twenty patients (38%) with TAMI were discharged to intermediate care facilities versus 11 (8%) without TAMI ($P < .001$). The largest relative risks for TAMI development postoperatively were oxygen saturation below 92% (5.4), a need for reintubation (3.3), congestive heart failure (3.3), and pneumonia (3.2). Conversely, the presence of TAMI conferred the greatest relative risks for the development of postoperative congestive heart failure (15.3), a need for reintubation (9.3), pneumonia (7.1), and a need for ICU readmission (3.8).

Conclusion.—The incidence of TAMI was 28% in patients who underwent aortic reconstruction. It is correlated with dramatically increased morbidity and postoperative hospitalization rates.

▶ Elderly postoperative patients in unfamiliar surroundings under the influence of medications and relatively sleep deprived will be frequently confused. I bet with more sophisticated psychologic testing, the incidence of transient mental impairment would be even higher than the authors have reported.

G. L. Moneta, MD

Small Bowel Motility and Transit After Aortic Surgery

Miedema BW, Schillie S, Simmons JW, et al (Univ of Missouri, Columbia; Harry S Truman VA Hosp, Columbia, Mo)
J Vasc Surg 36:19-24, 2002   5–11

Background.—Patients unable to tolerate feedings after aortic surgery have prolonged hospitalizations. The jejunal manometric and small bowel transit characteristics of ileus after transperitoneal aortic surgery were identified.

Methods.—Five men (mean age, 65 years) undergoing transperitoneal infrarenal aortobifemoral bypass were included in the study. All had a jejunal multilumen catheter placed intraoperatively. Pressure recording ports were positioned exactly at 20, 22, 24, 26, 28, and 38 cm past the ligament of Treitz. Three-hour manometric assessments were made immediately after surgery and for 3 days postoperatively.

Findings.—Between 2 and 7 days after surgery, a return of bowel sounds developed in all patients. Flatus returned at between 3 and 9 days. Jejunal motor activity was noted within 6 hours of operation. However, patients had a lower than normal motility index. Compared with control values, the patients' postoperative migrating motor complexes showed more phase I, less phase II, and more frequent phase IIIs. Phase III retrograde migration occurred commonly in the patients but not in the control subjects. All patients had a small-bowel transit time of 2 days or longer.

Conclusions.—Shortly after aortic surgery, motor activity can be observed in the jejunum. However, this activity is lower in intensity and the fasting cycles differs from control values. Phase III retrograde migration is the most common abnormality in this patient population, resulting in delayed small-bowel transit. These findings suggest a high rate of enteral feeding intolerance in the early postoperative period.

▶ The authors found that retrograde propulsions present in the duodenum suggest early feeding will be poorly tolerated in aortic surgery patients. Clinically, however, many aortic surgery patients are able to eat 3 to 5 days postoperatively and some even sooner. The discrepancy between clinical observation and the data in this study suggest the motility abnormalities do not reliably predict intolerance of oral feeding. I wish the study had addressed what appears to be a reasonably common problem of functional gastric outlet obstruction after aortic surgery. This is a condition I've attributed to a localized ileus of the duodenum, but I actually have no idea to its cause.

G. L. Moneta, MD

Intensive Diabetes Therapy and Carotid Intima–Media Thickness in Type 1 Diabetes Mellitus

Nathan DM, for the Diabetes Control and Complications Trial/Epidemiology of Diabetes Interventions and Complications Research Group (Albert Einstein College of Medicine, New York; et al)
N Engl J Med 348:2294-2303, 2003   5–12

Background.—Patients with diabetes mellitus have a significantly increased risk of cardiovascular disease. Most deaths among patients with type 2 diabetes (70%) are attributable to cardiovascular disease, and most epidemiologic and clinical trial data have been obtained from studies of type 2 diabetes. Much less is known about cardiovascular disease in patients with type 1 diabetes. Patients with type 1 disease have a lower absolute risk of cardiovascular disease than those with type 2 diabetes, but the relative risk as compared with that of nondiabetic persons of similar age may be 10-fold higher. The progression of carotid intima–media thickness, a known measure of atherosclerosis, in a group of patients with type 1 diabetes was investigated.

Methods.—This study was conducted as part of the Epidemiology of Diabetes Interventions and Complications (EDIC) study, a long-term followup of the Diabetes Control and Complications Trial (DCCT). A total of 1229 patients with type 1 diabetes underwent B-mode US of the internal and common carotid arteries in 1994 to 1996 and again in 1998 to 2000. This study assessed the intima–media thickness in 611 subjects who had been randomly assigned to undergo conventional diabetes treatment during the DCCT and in 618 subjects who were assigned to undergo intensive diabetes treatment.

Results.—At year 1 of the EDIC study, the carotid intima–media thickness was similar to that in an age- and sex-matched nondiabetic population. After 6 years, the intima–media thickness was significantly greater in the diabetic patients than in the control subjects. The mean progression of the intima–media thickness was significantly less in patients who received intensive therapy during the DCCT than in patients who received conventional therapy. The progression of carotid intima–media thickness was associated with age, and the EDIC baseline systolic blood pressure, smoking, the ratio of low-density lipoprotein to high-density lipoprotein cholesterol, and urinary albumin excretion rate as well as the mean glycosylated hemoglobin value during the mean duration of the DCCT (6.5 years).

Conclusions.—Intensive diabetes treatment during the DCCT resulted in a slowing of the progression of carotid intima–media thickness 6 years after the end of that trial.

▶ Glycemic control is crucial to decreasing manifestations of early atherosclerosis in patients with type 1 diabetes. Let's hope that this will translate into fewer clinical cardiovascular events later in life.

G. L. Moneta, MD

Wound Infections Involving Infrainguinal Autogenous Vein Grafts: A Current Evaluation of Factors Determining Successful Graft Preservation
Treiman GS, Copland S, Yellin AE, et al (Univ of Utah, Salt Lake City; Univ of California, Irvine; Univ of Southern California, Los Angeles)
J Vasc Surg 33:948-954, 2001   5–13

Background.—The treatment of infrainguinal autogenous graft infection (IAGI) has improved in recent years as a result of improvements in antibiotics and wound care and more liberal use of local or distant free tissue transfer. In addition, a better understanding of the factors that predispose to successful graft preservation has prompted some authors to recommend attempted graft preservation rather than the traditional treatment of graft ligation and excision. The purposes of this study were to review the natural history and clinical outcomes of patients with IAGI, evaluate the effectiveness of attempted graft preservation, identify variables associated with graft salvage, and better determine optimal treatment.

Methods.—A retrospective review was conducted of patients undergoing infrageniculate vein grafts at 3 hospitals from 1994 to 2000. Clinical and bacteriologic variables were analyzed and correlated with graft salvage, limb salvage, and clinical outcome.

Results.—A total of 487 patients underwent an infrageniculate vein graft; 68 (13%) had clinical evidence of IAGI. Wound cultures were positive for bacteria in 52 of 68 patients, and most of these infections resulted from *Staphylococcus aureus* (18 patients) and *Staphylococcus epidermidis* (12 patients). *Pseudomonas* was cultured from 7 infections. Twelve patients had polymicrobial infections. The time from operation to infection ranged from 7 to 180 days. All of the patients were treated with oral antibiotics, and 48 patients initially received IV antibiotics.

Operative debridement was performed in 45 patients, including 18 patients who had muscle flap coverage. Of 4 patients first seen with hemorrhage, immediate graft ligation was performed in 3 and graft excision in 1. The follow-up period ranged from 5 to 68 months, with a mean of 24.3 months, and 61 patients were alive at the publication of this report. Overall, 61 wounds healed (91%), 4 patients required below-knee amputations, and 3 wounds did not heal. Fifty-eight grafts remained patent, 6 thrombosed, and 4 required ligation to control hemorrhage. Healing time for the 61 wounds that healed ranged from 7 to 63 days.

There were no deaths from hemorrhage and no cases of delayed hemorrhage. All 18 patients treated with a muscle flap healed. The only statistically significant variables in predicting graft failure or limb loss were bleeding, elevated white blood cell count, fever, and renal insufficiency. On life-table analysis, graft patency was 94%, 72%, and 72% and limb salvage was 97%, 92%, and 92% at 1, 3, and 5 years, respectively.

Conclusion.—Most patients with an IAGI can be successfully treated with graft and limb preservation. This study found that an exposed anastomosis, interval to infection, and *Pseudomonas* infection are not associated with graft failure, a finding that contrasts with that of earlier studies. Graft salvage is less likely in the presence of fever, leukocytosis, and renal insufficiency; however, attempted graft preservation is recommended for these patients because most grafts remain patent. Graft ligation or excision should only be used in patients seen with bleeding or sepsis.

▶ Dr Linda Reilly's comments accompanying this paper are somewhat acerbic but basically correct. This really is more a series of acute wound problems accompanying autogenous grafts than a series of autogenous graft infections.

Muscle flap coverage of the grafts was uniformly associated with a good outcome.

G. L. Moneta, MD

Chlorhexidine Compared With Povidone-Iodine Solution for Vascular Catheter–Site Care: A Meta-analysis
Chaiyakunapruk N, Veenstra DL, Lipsky BA, et al (Naresuan Univ, Pitsanuloak, Thailand; Univ of Washington, Seattle; Univ of Michigan, Ann Arbor)
Ann Intern Med 136:792-801, 2002   5–14

Background.—Central venous catheter-related bloodstream infections are associated with increased morbidity, mortality, length of hospitalization, and medical costs. Several recent studies have compared the efficacy of povidone-iodine with that of chlorhexidine gluconate solutions as skin preparations for reducing catheter-related infections. However, few clinical events have been observed in these studies, so it is unclear which solution is most effective in reducing the risk of catheter-related bloodstream infections. A meta-analysis was performed to evaluate the efficacy of these 2 solutions for skin disinfection in preventing bloodstream infections associated with central venous catheters.

Methods.—A search was conducted of multiple computerized databases for the years 1966 to 2001. Data were also obtained from reference lists of identified articles and queries of principal investigators and antiseptic manufacturers. The studies included in this analysis were randomized controlled trials comparing chlorhexidine gluconate with povidone-iodine solution for central venous catheter site disinfection. Outcome measures included the study design, patient population, intervention, and incidence of catheter-related bloodstream infections.

Results.—Eight studies were identified for inclusion in this analysis. All these studies were set in a hospital, and a variety of catheter types were used. The summary risk ratio for catheter-related infections of the bloodstream was 0.49 in patients whose catheter sites were disinfected with chlorhexidine gluconate rather than povidone-iodine. In patients with central vascular catheters, the use of chlorhexidine gluconate reduced the risk of catheter-related bloodstream infections by 49%.

Conclusions.—These findings suggest that the use of chlorhexidine gluconate rather than povidone-iodine for insertion-site skin disinfection is a simple and effective method that can significantly reduce the incidence of bloodstream infections in patients with central vascular lines.

▶ We probably should change to chlorhexidine for skin prep before placement of central venous catheters.

G. L. Moneta, MD

A Single Infusion of Intravenous Ketamine Improves Pain Relief in Patients With Critical Limb Ischaemia: Results of a Double Blind Randomised Controlled Trial

Mitchell AC, Fallon MT (Western Infirmary, Glasgow, Scotland; Western Gen Hosp, Edinburgh, Scotland)
Pain 97:275-281, 2002   5–15

Background.—This study determined whether a combination of regular opioid analgesia and a single IV ketamine infusion could improve ischemia rest pain in patients with allodynia, hyperalgesia, and hyperpathia caused by critical limb ischemia.

Methods.—Thirty-five patients completed the double-blind randomized study. Seventeen patients received regular opioids plus placebo, and 18 received regular opioids plus an infusion of 0.6 mg/kg IV ketamine. The Brief Pain Inventory was used to assess levels of pain.

Findings.—The proportion of pain relief attributed to medication in the opioids plus ketamine group improved significantly from 50% immediately before infusion to 65% 24 hours after infusion and 69% 5 days after infusion. During the same period, pain relief in the placebo group increased from 58% preinfusion to 56% at 24 hours after infusion, then declined to 50% 5 days later. Between-group differences were statistically significant. The group receiving ketamine infusion also had a significant improvement 24 hours after infusion in the effect of pain on general activity and enjoyment of life.

Conclusion.—The addition of a single infusion of low-dose ketamine to regular opioid analgesia can significantly improve pain relief in patients with allodynia, hyperalgesia, and hyperpathia caused by critical limb ischemia. Such treatment should improve patients' quality of life.

▶ We all know ischemic pain is very resistant to treatment. Most of the patients in this study could be revascularized, and obviously revascularization is the treatment of choice for most patients with ischemic pain. Patients with finger ulcers and those with atheroembolism may have severe, presumably ischemic pain and yet are not candidates for revascularization. Given time, many will, however, avoid amputation. Control of ischemic pain in these patients in this interim time is something that requires improvement. It would be interesting to try the approach detailed in this paper in these types of patients.

G. L. Moneta, MD

Hyperhomocysteinaemia, Folate and Vitamin B12 in Unsupplemented Haemodialysis Patients: Effect of Oral Therapy With Folic Acid and Vitamin B12

Billion S, Tribout B, Cadet E, et al (Boulogne sur Mer Gen Hosp, France; Amiens Univ Hosp, France)
Nephrol Dial Transplant 17:455-461, 2002   5–16

Introduction.—Hyperhomocysteinemia, a well-known risk factor for atherosclerosis, commonly occurs in patients receiving dialysis, particularly those homozygous for a common polymorphism in the 5,10-methylenetetrahydrofolate reductase (MTHFR) gene (C677T transition). B-complex vitamin supplements are known to lower plasma total homocysteine (tHcy) concentrations. The effectiveness of folate and oral vitamin B12 supplementation has not, however, been demonstrated in patients receiving dialysis. The homocysteine-lowering effect of a folate supplement alone and a folate supplement with vitamin B12 was therefore examined in a cohort of patients on dialysis. Responses were stratified for the C677T genotypes of MTHFR.

Methods.—Plasma tHcy, folate, and vitamin B12 were determined in 51 patients receiving hemodialysis. All patients underwent genotyping for the C677T MTHFR mutation (homozygotes, TT; heterozygotes, CT; without mutation, CC). All patients received daily supplements of 15 mg of folic acid for 2 months; daily supplements of 1 mg of vitamin B12 were then given in addition to the folate supplements for another 2 months. Plasma tHcy, folate, and vitamin B12 were assessed after each intervention.

Results.—At baseline, folate and vitamin B12 deficiencies were identified in 10% and 6% of patients, respectively. Initial plasma tHcy concentrations were increased in all patients (mean, 38.1 µmol/L). The CC genotype subgroup tended to have a lower tHcy concentration than the pooled CT and TT groups. After 2 months of folate therapy, tHcy concentrations diminished significantly to 20.2 µmol/L ($P < .001$). There were no significant differences between the various genotype subgroups (19.4 for CC, 21.3 for CT, and 18.5 for TT).

A significant positive association was observed between the decrease in tHcy and its initial value ($P = .615; P < .0001$). The effect of the addition of vitamin B12 was negligible in all subgroups.

Conclusion.—Deficiencies in folate and vitamin B12 were observed in 10% and 6%, respectively, of unsupplemented patients receiving dialysis. After folate therapy, the tHcy levels were significantly decreased in all patients and were identical among the C677T MTHFR genotype subgroups. Vitamin B12 supplements did not lower tHcy plasma levels overall or for any MTHFR subgroups.

▶ The study indicates end-stage renal disease (ESRD) patients with hyperhomocysteinemia will not be adequately treated with the usual levels of folic acid present as a nutritional supplement in grain products. ESRD patients with hyperhomocysteinemia need approximately 15 mg/d of folic acid to lower homocysteine levels compared with approximately 1 mg/d for the general population with hyperhomocysteinemia. Patients with ESRD should be evaluated for homocysteine levels and treated if they are elevated. Note that supplemental B12 administration does not diminish homocysteine levels on its own but has other beneficial effects in the ESRD patient.

G. L. Moneta, MD

Smoking Cessation Counseling: A Missed Opportunity for General Surgery Trainees

Krupski WC, Nguyen HT, Jones DN, et al (Univ of Colorado, Denver)
J Vasc Surg 36:257-262, 2002   5–17

Background.—Smoking is the leading preventable cause of premature death and morbidity in the United States, accounting for an estimated 430,000 deaths annually, or 1 in 5 deaths. Preventive services guidelines are often targeted to primary care physicians, even though only half of office visits to physicians in the United States are to generalists. Visits to non–primary care clinicians represent additional opportunities for smoking cessation counseling. However, population-based surveys of smokers suggest that many are never counseled to stop smoking by their physicians. The attitudes, practices, technique utilization, and barrier perceptions of smoking cessation counseling in general surgery (GS) and primary care (PC) residents were evaluated and compared.

Methods.—A random survey was conducted among 100 house staff officers (45 GS and 55 PC residents). The residents were asked how frequently they asked their patients whether they smoked and how often they provided smoking cessation advice. Once the subject of smoking cessation was broached, they reported how often patients expressed an interest in quitting. The residents were also asked their opinions regarding their obligations and effectiveness in addressing smoking cessation, their role models in smoking cessation counseling, and their perceptions of their effectiveness in facilitating and achieving successful smoking abstinence in patients.

Results.—Fewer GS residents (64%) than PC residents (85%) thought that physicians were responsible for smoking cessation counseling, and fewer GS than PC residents (38% vs 58%) believed they were well-prepared to counsel their patients. However, about 85% of both groups reported a higher inclination to provide smoking cessation counseling to patients who expressed an interest in cessation. Fewer GS residents than PC residents asked new patients about smoking (64% vs 89%). In addition, GS residents used fewer smoking cessation counseling techniques than did PC residents and arranged for fewer follow-up visits for counseling. Residents from both groups perceived the main barriers to smoking cessation counseling to be time constraints, lack of patient desire, and poor patient compliance.

Conclusions.—Many GS residents agreed that physicians were responsible for smoking cessation counseling, but few of these residents followed through by arranging smoking cessation counseling follow-up visits compared with PC residents. Behavior does not appear to change as residents mature, despite greater exposure to smoking-related diseases. GS residents played a less assertive role than PC residents in every dimension of smoking cessation counseling studied. GS residents need to be more proactive in smoking cessation counseling because the diseases they treat are often related to cigarette smoking.

▶ People need to be trained in smoking cessation counseling. We have a lecture about every other year in our weekly vascular surgical lecture series that is devoted to this topic.

G. L. Moneta, MD

6 Thoracic Aorta

Surgical Treatment of Nonaneurysmal Aortic Arch Lesions in Patients With Systemic Embolization
Gouëffic Y, Chaillou P, Pillet JC, et al (Guillaume et René Laënnec Hosp, Nantes, France)
J Vasc Surg 36:1186-1193, 2002   6–1

Background.—Nonaneurysmal lesions of the aortic arch are an underappreciated source of stroke and peripheral embolization. Few patients with these lesions have undergone surgery, and the proper approach to management of these patients is not yet well established. A study was undertaken to investigate whether surgery can be proposed for treatment of nonaneurysmal atherosclerotic lesions of the aortic arch.

Methods.—A total of 38 patients (19 men and 19 women) underwent surgical treatment of nonaneurysmal aortic arch lesions from 1976 to 1996 in 17 cardiovascular surgical centers in France. The patients had an average age of 49 ±12 years at the time of surgery (range, 31-82 years). The lesions were detected with transesophageal echocardiography (19 patients), angiography of the aortic arch (16 patients), CT (9 patients), and MRI (10 patients). Surgical procedures included thrombectomy and endarterectomy (22 patients), aortic resection and graft replacement (10 patients), and patch aortoplasty (5 patients). In 1 patient the thrombus disappeared spontaneously before surgery was performed.

Results.—The average duration of the postoperative period was 30 months, with a range of 3 to 82 months. Four patients were lost to follow-up after 12 months. Examination of pathologic specimens obtained at surgery showed an atherosclerotic plaque in 73% of the patients. The aorta appeared normal in 15% of the patients, and 4 other types of lesion were identified, including 1 angiosarcoma. A thrombus was identified in 26 patients and was attached to the arterial wall in 18 patients. When mobile lesions were identified by transesophageal echocardiography (22 patients), histopathologic examination of specimens facilitated detection of a thrombus in 18 patients and an atherosclerotic plaque with a mobile projection in 4 patients. The postoperative mortality rate was 2.6%, and the morbidity rate was 28.9%. Morbidity was related to neurologic complications in 6 patients, vascular complications in 4 patients, and infection in 1 patient. Four patients (12%) underwent reoperation.

Conclusions.—In patients with nonaneurysmal aortic arch lesions, surgery can be recommended for those who are good candidates for surgery and who have experienced recurrent critical events despite medical management and who have high embolic potential.

▶ In looking for a source of artery-to-artery embolization, it is important to regard the aortic arch as a potential site, even if it is not aneurysmal. Since the lesions may be subtle, a combination of transesophageal echo and angiography should be required to exclude an aortic arch lesion in a patient with arterial embolization of unknown origin.

G. L. Moneta, MD

Effect of Treatment on the Incidence of Stroke and Other Emboli in 519 Patients With Severe Thoracic Aortic Plaque

Tunick PA, for the NYU Atheroma Group (New York Univ)
Am J Cardiol 90:1320-1325, 2002   6–2

Background.—Case-control and prospective studies since 1990 have documented the association of severe atherosclerotic thoracic aortic plaques with stroke and peripheral emboli. Thrombi have been reported in 20% to 33% of patients with severe thoracic aortic plaque. Plaque size is the most important factor in this association, with a high odds ratio for stroke when the plaque thickness is 4 mm or greater. The proper therapy for patients with severe thoracic aortic plaque in association with stroke is unknown. This observational study reports on the effect of treatment with statins, warfarin, or

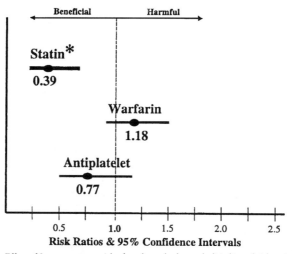

FIGURE 3.—Effect of 3 treatments on risk of stroke and other emboli (adjusted risk ratios and 95% confidence intervals). *Asterisk*, $P = .0001$. (Courtesy of Tunick PA, for the NYU Atheroma Group: Effect of treatment on the incidence of stroke and other emboli in 519 patients with severe thoracic aortic plaque. *Am J Cardiol* 90:1320-1325, 2002. Copyright 2002 by Excerpta Medica, Inc. Reprinted by permission.)

antiplatelet medications in a series of patients with severe thoracic aortic plaque evaluated with transesophageal echocardiography during a 12-year period.

Methods.—Data were obtained retrospectively for the occurrence of embolic events in 519 patients with severe thoracic aortic plaque seen on transesophageal echocardiography from 1988 to 2000. Treatment with statins, warfarin, or antiplatelet medications was noted. Treatment was not randomized. Each patient receiving each type of therapy was matched for age, gender, previous embolic event, hypertension, diabetes, congestive heart failure, and atrial fibrillation with a patient not taking that medication. Findings were subjected to multivariate analysis.

Results.—A total of 111 patients (21%) had an embolic event. Multivariate analysis indicated that the use of statins was independently protective against recurrent events (Fig 3). Matched analysis also showed a protective effect of statins. However, no protective effect was found for warfarin or antiplatelet drugs.

Conclusions.—There is a significant protective effect of statin therapy and no significant beneficial effects of warfarin or antiplatelet drugs on the incidence of stroke and other embolic events in patients with severe thoracic aortic plaque detected with transesophageal echocardiography.

▶ While this is not a randomized study, I think the suggestion that statins protect against embolization from thoracic aortic plaques is interesting. Of note is that the usual drugs used for this disease, aspirin or warfarin, had apparently no significant benefit.

G. L. Moneta, MD

Midterm Follow-up of Penetrating Ulcer and Intramural Hematoma of the Aorta
Tittle SL, Lynch RJ, Cole PE, et al (Yale Univ, New Haven, Conn; Ohio State Univ, Columbus)
J Thorac Cardiovasc Surg 123:1051-1059, 2002   6–3

Background.—Intramural hematoma and penetrating ulcer of the aorta predominantly affect women and are associated with advanced age. Most of the information currently available in the literature regarding penetrating ulcer and intramural hematoma of the aorta is limited to the initial presenting episode, with scant data on the natural history of the disease beyond the initial presentation. This study provides midterm follow-up of penetrating ulcer and intramural hematoma in an investigation to ascertain whether the aorta demonstrates radiographic healing, progressively dilates, or tends to rupture during late follow-up.

Methods.—Forty-five patients with penetrating ulcers (26 patients) or intramural hematomas (19 patients) were treated at a single institution. The 26 patients with penetrating ulcers included 10 men and 16 women ranging in age from 54 to 87 years (mean age, 72 years). The 19 patients with intra-

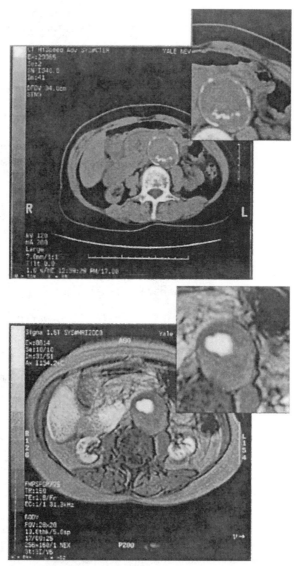

FIGURE 4.—Radiographic evidence of worsening of intramural hematoma. **Top,** Initial CT scan shows calcium in aortic wall. **Bottom,** MRI after elapsed time of 19 weeks shows marked increase in hematoma size outside aortic lumen. (Courtesy of Tittle SL, Lynch RJ, Cole PE, et al: Midterm follow-up of penetrating ulcer and intramural hematoma of the aorta. *J Thoracic Cardiovasc Surg* 123:1051-1059, 2002.)

mural hematomas included 8 men and 11 women ranging in age from 54 to 88 years (mean age, 74 years). All of the patients had symptoms of aortic disease. Patients with incidental imaging findings were not included in the analysis.

Results.—In the patients with penetrating ulcers, rupture occurred during the initial admission in 10 patients (38%). Seventeen patients (65%) underwent surgery and 22 patients (85%) survived to hospital discharge. Among the patients with intramural hematomas, rupture occurred during the initial admission in 5 patients (26%). Seven patients (37%) underwent surgery and 16 patients (84%) survived to hospital discharge. Follow-up ranged from 1 month to 12.5 years (mean, 3.4 years). There were no ischemic vascular complications. Imaging follow-up was available for 26 nonoperated patients. In these patients, 19% of lesions resolved, 23% worsened, 39% progressed to typical dissection, and 19% were unchanged (Fig 4).

There were 6 late deaths known to be caused by rupture. Among the patients with penetrating ulcers, aortic diameter increased from 4.8 to 5.1 cm over 14 months. Among patients with intramural hematomas, aortic diameter increased from 5.3 to 5.9 cm over 21 months. Overall survival was 80% at 1 year, 73% at 3 years, and 66% at 5 years.

Conclusion.—Penetrating ulcer and intramural hematoma rupture both early and late in their natural course. Radiographically documented worsening, improvement, or frank dissection may occur over time, and aortic growth does occur. However, vascular ischemic complications do not occur. In light of these findings, surgical replacement of the aorta is recommended for these virulent vascular lesions as long as co-morbidities do not preclude surgical intervention.

▶ The authors have found that even if operation can be avoided initially for penetrating ulcer and intramural hematoma, the incidence of subsequent local problems with the thoracic aorta is sufficiently high that, when possible, treatment is recommended at the time of presentation. It seems these types of lesions would be ideal to treat with an intraluminal graft.

G. L. Moneta, MD

Late Aortic and Graft-Related Events After Thoracoabdominal Aneurysm Repair

Clouse WD, Marone LK, Davison JK, et al (Harvard Med School, Boston)
J Vasc Surg 37:254-261, 2003   6–4

Background.—Thoracoabdominal aneurysm (TAA) repair is done less commonly than open abdominal aortic aneurysm (AAA) repair, and its late graft-related complications have not been as thoroughly studied. The experience of one institution with TAA repair over a period of 15 years was reviewed to define late aortic and graft-related events and pinpoint factors that may be linked to their occurrence.

Methods.—A total of 333 patients had TAA repair over the period of evaluation, with 27% having type I, 18% type II, 35% type III, and 20% type IV. Late aortic events evaluated included post-discharge aortic disease causing death or requiring further intervention, and complications related to the graft, including infection, pseudoaneurysm, and branch occlusion. Follow-up extended for 2.7 to 38.4 months (mean 26 months). Factors involved in the outcomes were analyzed statistically.

Results.—Overall survival rate at 5 years was 67.2%, with 28 patients dying in the hospital. Of the 305 patients remaining, spinal cord ischemia was found in 11.4% of patients (with complete paraplegia in 6.6%) and renal insufficiency developed in 13.5% (4.8% required hemodialysis). Pulmonary problems were noted in 44% of patients. Thirty-three patients had late aortic and graft-related events a mean of 30 months after surgery. Most were aortic disease–related events, with only 10 graft-related complications. Nine of the 33 patients died, seven as a direct result of these complications. Freedom from late aortic or graft-related event was 96% at 1 year and 71% at 5 years; freedom from aortic disease–related events was 98% at 1 year and 76% at 5 years. Survival free from graft-related complications was 95% at 2 years. The factors found to be independently predictive of the occurrence of a late event were female gender, partial resection of aortic aneurysmal disease, expansion of the remaining native aorta, and initial aneurysm rupture.

Conclusions.—Approximately 10% of patients who undergo TAA repair experience either a late aortic event or a graft-related complication. Up to a third of these occur within 5 years of their initial surgery. Progressive disease of the remaining native aorta is a primary cause for these events. Late graft-related complications are rare, occurring in only 3% of the patients evaluated. Patients who have remaining disease after surgery are at significantly higher risk for developing late aortic and graft-related events.

▶ Successful TAA grafts hold up well over time. However, we are not just talking about a piece of Dacron surrounded by a patient, but rather a patient with a piece of Dacron. Both the Dacron and the patient must do well. It looks like it is easier to get the Dacron to do well than to get the patient to do well. (See Abstract 6–5).

G. L. Moneta, MD

Functional Outcome After Thoracoabdominal Aortic Aneurysm Repair
Rectenwald JE, Huber TS, Martin TD, et al (Univ of Florida, Gainesville)
J Vasc Surg 35:640-647, 2002   6–5

Background.—The determination of patient functional outcomes, the identification of predictors of survival, and the functional recovery after thoracoabdominal aortic aneurysm (TAAA) were analyzed in a retrospective study.

Methods.—Data from the medical records of 101 consecutive patients undergoing TAAA repair between November 1993 and October 1999 were analyzed retrospectively. Fifty-eight procedures were elective, and 43 were urgent or emergent. Patient outcomes were classified as good if patients survived and were discharged home or to a rehabilitation center and were ambulatory. Poor patient outcomes included death, discharge to a long-term care facility, and being nonambulatory.

Findings.—The postoperative mortality rate was 17.8% overall—10% with elective procedures and 28% with urgent procedures. Significant postoperative complications, occurring in 77% of patients, included pulmonary complications in 41%, renal complications in 28%, and spinal cord injury in 12%. The mean length of hospital stay was 22.8 days. Eighty percent of the patients were discharged home or to rehabilitation, and 20% to long-term care facilities. By the 1-year follow-up, another 15 patients had died. Only 2 patients discharged to long-term care facilities returned home, and both were not ambulatory. Thus, at 1 year, survival rate was 67%, and only 52.4% of patients had good outcomes. Factors that independently predicted postoperative death and bad outcomes were age older than 75 years, preoperative heart disease, duration of visceral ischemia, use of left atrial femoral bypass graft, postoperative renal dysfunction, and the number of organs failing after surgery.

Conclusions.—Survival rates and functional outcomes after TAAA repair are significantly less favorable than expected. Intraoperative factors and postoperative complications are the main determinants of survival and good functional outcomes. Better outcomes may be achieved by improving operative techniques and limiting visceral ischemia reperfusion injury.

▶ Overall, in this study, only about half the patients were at home and ambulatory 1 year after TAAA repair. If the operation was elective, the patients fared a little better, but 1 in 3 still had a poor outcome at 1 year. Admittedly, the patients in this study had mostly "full-blown" TAAAs with only about 25% being type IV. Nevertheless, these sobering results should be kept in mind next time you talk to someone's grandparent about the repair of a TAAA. As always, technical success and survival are not exactly the same as a good outcome.

G. L. Moneta, MD

Type III and IV Thoracoabdominal Aortic Aneurysm Repair: Results of a Trifurcated/Two-Graft Technique
Ballard JL, Abou-Zamzam AM Jr, Teruya TH (Loma Linda Univ, Calif)
J Vasc Surg 36:211-216, 2002   6–6

Background.—A novel 2-graft technique for repair of thoracoabdominal aortic aneurysms (TAAs) was previously reported and consisted of a trifurcated graft for sequential visceral revascularization followed by a second graft for in-line aneurysm reconstruction. The intent is to minimize end-organ ischemia. In an update on the experience, the results of repair of type III and type IV TAAs are presented.

Methods.—Thirty-two patients (mean age, 70 years) underwent nonemergent repair of type III (12 patients) and type IV (20 patients) TAAs between March 1996 and October 2001. Repair was accomplished by means of a trifurcated graft for uninvolved descending thoracic aorta-to-celiac/superior mesenteric/renal artery bypass with an additional tube or bifurcated graft for in-line aneurysm reconstruction (Fig 2). The last 6 patients in

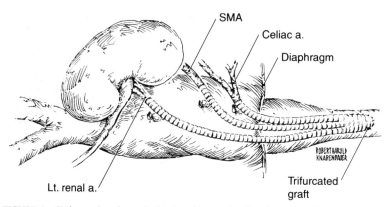

FIGURE 2.—Trifurcated graft attached end-to-side to uninvolved descending thoracic aorta with sequential end-to-end visceral and renal bypasses. (Reprinted by permission of the publisher from Ballard JL, Abou-Zamzam AM Jr, Teruya TH: Type III and IV thoracoabdominal aortic aneurysm repair: Results of a trifurcated/two-graft technique. *J Vasc Surg* 36:211-216, 2002. Copyright 2002 by Elsevier.)

this series also underwent adjunctive CSF drainage. Six patients had a solitary kidney, and 6 patients had previous infrarenal abdominal aortic aneurysm repair.

Results.—The mean visceral ischemia times were 12 minutes for the celiac artery as well as for the superior mesenteric artery, 10 minutes for the left renal artery, and 33 minutes for the right renal artery. The creatinine level at discharge was not significantly different from the preoperative level. The permanent renal failure rate was 0, but 2 patients (6.3%) had transient renal failure. None of the patients with a solitary kidney had renal dysfunction. Two patients (6.3%) had paraplegia, 1 of whom had prior abdominal aortic aneurysm repair. Neither of these patients had CSF drainage. Six patients (19%) required prolonged ventilatory support. The perioperative mortality rate was 6.5%. The mean follow-up was 22 months, and the life-table survival rate was 76% at 36 months. Preoperative functional status was maintained in 92% of long-term survivors.

Conclusions.—These results demonstrate the effectiveness of type III and IV TAA repair with a trifurcated graft for sequential visceral revascularization followed by a second graft for in-line aneurysm reconstruction. This procedure results in short visceral, renal, and spinal cord ischemia times and provides low rates of end-organ ischemic damage and paraplegia. Preoperative functional status is maintained in most survivors.

▶ The authors place a 3-limbed graft on the thoracic aorta above the aneurysm and then anastomose each limb end to end to the celiac, superior mesenteric artery, and left renal artery, respectively. The initial anastomosis is done end to side, and the aneurysm is not replaced until the viscera have been revascularized. The technique basically turns type III and type IV TAA operations into a series of small steps. I think it is a bit cumbersome for most type IV TAAs, where the viscera can, in many cases, be included in a beveled proximal anastomosis. For type III TAAs, the technique described should be given consideration.

G. L. Moneta, MD

Chronic Aortic Dissection Not a Risk Factor for Neurologic Deficit in Thoracoabdominal Aortic Aneurysm Repair
Safi HJ, Miller CC III, Estrera AL, et al (Univ of Texas, Houston)
Eur J Vasc Endovasc Surg 23:244-250, 2002   6–7

Introduction.—Chronic aortic dissection is considered a risk factor for spinal cord ischemia after thoracoabdominal aortic aneurysm (TAA) surgery. Univariate and multivariate analyses were performed of all elective cases during a 10-year period to ascertain whether chronic dissection is truly a risk factor for spinal cord ischemia after TAA and descending thoracic AAA (DTAA) repair.

Methods.—Between February 1991 and March 2001, 800 aneurysms of the descending thoracic or TAA were repaired. Of these, 33 (4.15%) were performed emergently, and 38 (4.8%) were acute dissections. Of 729 elective cases, 196 (26.9%) were for chronic dissection. Of the elective procedures, 182 (25.0%) were TAA type II. Of these, 61 (33.5%) involved chronic dissection. A detailed multivariate analyses was used to isolate the impact of chronic aortic dissection on neurologic morbidity rates, with other important risk factors considered.

Results.—Overall, 32 (4.4%) of 729 patients experienced neurologic deficit upon awakening, as did 7 (3.6%) of 196 patients in the chronic dissection group and 25 of 533 (4.7%) in the non-dissections group. Spinal cord drainage decreased the neurologic deficit in TAA extent II from 27.8% to 6.9% ($P = .001$). In univariate and multivariate analysis, chronic dissection did not increase the risk of neurologic deficit.

Conclusion.—Chronic aortic dissection was not found to be a risk factor for spinal cord ischemia after TAA repair.

▶ The authors' analysis suggests that a type II pattern of thoracoabdominal dissection, and failure to use spinal cord drainage, distal aortic perfusion, and intraoperative visceral perfusion are the real causes of spinal cord ischemia associated with chronic aortic dissections. The authors also routinely reattach intercostal arteries from T8 to T12. There appears to be no single factor that can prevent spinal cord ischemia in patients with TAAs. This problem will be minimized by attention to all the details noted above.

G. L. Moneta, MD

Cerebrospinal Fluid Drainage Reduces Paraplegia After Thoracoabdominal Aortic Aneurysm Repair: Results of a Randomized Clinical Trial

Coselli JS, LeMaire SA, Köksoy C, et al (Baylor College of Medicine, Houston)
J Vasc Surg 35:631-639, 2002   6–8

Background.—Various strategies are used to prevent spinal cord ischemia in patients undergoing thoracoabdominal aortic aneurysm (TAAA) repair, with CSF drainage (CSFD) as the most commonly used adjunct to protect the spinal cord. However, its benefits have not been established definitively. The effects of CSFD on the incidence of spinal cord injury after extensive TAAA repair were investigated in a randomized study.

Methods.—One hundred forty-five patients undergoing type I or II TAAA repair with moderate heparinization, mild hypothermia, left heart bypass, and reattachment of patent critical intercostal arteries were assigned to CSFD or no CSFD. Treatment with CSFD was begun intraoperatively and continued for 48 hours postoperatively, with a target CSF pressure of 10 mm Hg or less.

Findings.—The 2 groups were comparable in paraplegia risk factors, aortic clamp time, left heart bypass time, and number of reattached intercostal arteries. At 30 days, the mortality rate was 5.3% in the CSFD group and 2.9% in the non-CSFD group. Thirteen percent of the patients not receiving CSFD had paraplegia or paraparesis, compared with only 2.6% of the patients who had CSFD (Fig 2). None of those undergoing CSFD had immediate paraplegia. Overall, CSFD reduced the relative risk of postoperative deficits by 80%.

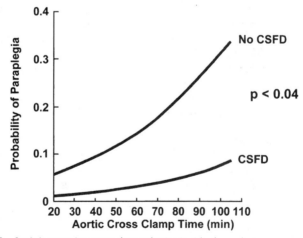

FIGURE 2.—Logistic regression curves show reduction in risk of paraplegia or paraparesis associated with CSF drainage (*CSFD*). (Reprinted by permission of the publisher from Coselli JS, leMaire SA, Köksoy C, et al: Cerebrospinal fluid drainage reduces paraplegia after thoracoabdominal aortic aneurysm repair: Results of a randomized clinical trial. *J Vasc Surg* 35:631-639, 2002. Copyright 2002 by Elsevier.)

Conclusion.—In patients undergoing type I or II TAAA repair, perioperative CSFD decreases the paraplegia rate. Further research is needed to determine whether CSFD also reduces early mortality.

▶ CSF drainage should now basically be required for open repair of extensive TAAAs. Get the CSF pressure to less than 10 mm Hg with gravity drainage, and keep it there for at least 2 days postoperatively.

G. L. Moneta, MD

Renal Perfusion During Thoracoabdominal Aortic Operations: Cold Crystalloid Is Superior to Normothermic Blood
Köksoy C, LeMaire SA, Curling PE, et al (Baylor College of Medicine, Houston; Methodist Hosp, Houston)
Ann Thorac Surg 73:730-738, 2002   6–9

Background.—Renal dysfunction continues to be a common and significant complication of thoracoabdominal aortic aneurysm (TAAA) repair. Varying studies have identified an incidence of acute renal failure ranging from 7% to 40% in patients who undergo TAAA repair, depending on how renal dysfunction is defined. Several techniques and intraoperative strategies have been developed to prevent renal dysfunction during TAAA. Two of these methods—cold crystalloid perfusion and normothermic blood perfusion—were compared to determine which technique provides the best kidney protection during thoracoabdominal aortic aneurysm repair.

Methods.—A total of 30 randomly assigned patients undergoing Crawford type II TAAA repair with left heart bypass had renal artery perfusion

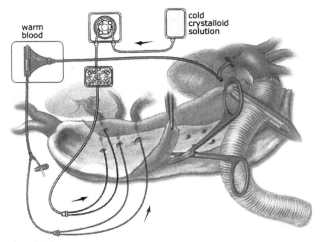

FIGURE 4.—Circuit used for left heart bypass with normothermic blood visceral perfusion and cold crystalloid renal perfusion. (Reprinted with permission from the Society of Thoracic Surgeons courtesy of Köksoy C, LeMaire SA, Curling PE, et al: Renal perfusion during thoracoabdominal aortic operations: Cold crystalloid is superior to normothermic blood. *Ann Thorac Surg* 73:730-738, 2002.)

with either 4°C Ringer's lactate solution (14 patients) or normothermic blood from the bypass circuit (16 patients) (Fig 4). Acute renal dysfunction was defined as an elevation in the serum creatinine level exceeding 50% of baseline within 10 postoperative days.

Results.—There was 1 death in each group. One patient in the blood perfusion group experienced renal failure requiring hemodialysis. Acute renal dysfunction occurred in 10 patients (63%) in the blood perfusion group and 3 patients (21%) in the cold crystalloid perfusion group. Multivariate analysis confirmed that the use of cold crystalloid perfusion was independently protective against acute renal dysfunction.

Conclusion.—In patients undergoing extensive TAAA repair, the use of selective cold crystalloid perfusion is superior to conventional normothermic blood perfusion in preserving renal function.

▶ It is clear that while the technical aspects of TAAA repair are the flash and dash portions of the operation, it is attention to all the dozens of details regarding unloading the heart, visceral perfusion, and spinal cord preservation, etc, that makes or breaks these operations. To get good results with extensive TAAA repair, these details need to be second nature to the surgeon and the surgical team. (See also Abstract 6–7.)

G. L. Moneta, MD

Vocal Cord Paralysis After Surgery for Thoracic Aortic Aneurysm

Ishimoto S, Ito K, Toyama M, et al (Univ of Tokyo; Kameda Med Ctr, Kamogawa, Japan; Tokyo Teishin Hosp)
Chest 121:1911-1915, 2002   6–10

Background.—Some patients have hoarseness after thoracic aortic aneurysm (TAA) surgery, particularly when the surgery involves the aortic arch. This complication may result from laryngeal edema, arytenoid cartilage dislocations, or vocal cord paralysis. In some patients, vocal cord paralysis occurs on the left side after TAA surgery, despite the preservation of the left recurrent laryngeal nerve. In this study, the incidence, etiology, prognosis, and treatment of vocal cord paralysis after surgery for TAA was determined.

Methods.—This retrospective study was performed in an academic tertiary care medical center and enrolled 62 of 71 patients who underwent TAA dissection or interposition surgery between 1989 and 1995.

Results.—Of the 62 patients examined for voice quality, 20 patients (32%) had hoarseness as a result of vocal cord paralysis, confirmed by laryngoscopy. The left recurrent laryngeal nerve had been sacrificed in 1 patient during surgery, but it was preserved in the remaining 19 patients. Vocal cord movement did not return to normal in 16 of 19 patients (84%), who were followed up for more than 6 months. Five patients underwent successful arytenoid adduction, and 2 patients underwent successful intracordal injection to improve voice quality.

Conclusions.—TAA is associated with a relatively high incidence of vocal cord paralysis. Paralysis occurs despite preservation of the recurrent laryngeal nerve and in the majority of cases has resolved 6 months after surgery.

▶ Vocal cord paralysis occurred surprisingly often in this series of patients with TAA repair. The main message is that the nerve does not have to be cut to lead to this complication. Every effort should therefore be made to minimize traction or compression of the recurrent nerve. Recovery of cord mobility will not occur after 6 months.

G. L. Moneta, MD

Effectiveness of Combined Blood Conservation Measures in Thoracic Aortic Operations With Deep Hypothermic Circulatory Arrest
Shibata K, Takamoto S, Kotsuka Y, et al (Univ of Tokyo)
Ann Thorac Surg 73:739-744, 2002   6–11

Introduction.—The effectiveness of blood conservation measures for thoracic aortic operations with deep hypothermic circulatory arrest (DHCA) has not been determined. The effectiveness of a blood conservation program initiated in July 1997 for thoracic aortic procedures performed using DHCA was examined retrospectively.

Methods.—Between July 1997 and December 2000, 148 thoracic aortic operations were performed. Of these, the 61 patients who underwent elective procedures with DHCA were reviewed. Homologous blood transfusion (HBT) included homologous whole blood, red blood cells, fresh-frozen plasma, and platelets. Cryoprecipitates, biological glues, and albumin were not included. Patients were evaluated postoperatively for complications including stroke, prolonged intubation, infection, and renal failure.

Results.—Seventeen patients were excluded who did not meet criteria for the blood conservation program. A total of 44 patients were evaluated. Overall, 50% of patients did not need operative HBT and 43% did not need in-hospital HBT. Smaller amounts of autologous donation, greater blood loss, and a longer surgical time were independent risk factors for need of HBT. Of 16 patients who made an autologous donation of 1600 mL or greater, 75% did not need intraoperative HBT and 69% did not need in-hospital HBT. The overall perioperative mortality rate was 4.5%. Prolonged intubation and postoperative infections were significantly more common in patients who needed in-hospital HBT.

Conclusion.—The combined blood conservation measures were effective in preventing HBT during major thoracic aortic surgeries with DHCA and may have diminished the rate of postoperative complications. The amount of the autologous donation was strongly predictive for avoiding HBT.

▶ Even given the problems with blood transfusions, I find the authors' emphasis on autologous donation to be a bit silly for operations of the magnitude described. I may be wrong, but I doubt problems secondary to transfusions are all that important compared with the others that can arise in procedures requiring hypothermic circulatory arrest.

G. L. Moneta, MD

Spinal Cord Arteriography: A Safe Adjunct Before Descending Thoracic or Thoracoabdominal Aortic Aneurysmectomy
Kieffer E, Fukui S, Chiras J, et al (Pitié-Salpétrière Univ, Paris)
J Vasc Surg 35:262-268, 2002   6–12

Background.—Spinal cord arteriography (SCA) as an adjunctive procedure before descending thoracic/thoracoabdominal aortic aneurysmectomy has been considered difficult, hazardous, and often unreliable. Those assumptions were questioned and data were presented to show that SCA can be a safe and effective procedure.

Methods.—From August 1985 to June 2000, 487 SCA procedures were performed in 480 patients during preoperative examination before surgical treatment for descending thoracic or thoracoabdominal aortic aneurysm. The study group included 381 men and 99 women with a mean age of 61.1 ±13 years. The underlying cause involved degenerative disease in 288 cases (57.8%), chronic dissection in 132 cases (26.5%), and other causes in 78 cases (15.7%).

The SCA consisted of selective catheterization, usually via the femoral route, followed by manual injection of contrast material for imaging of intercostal and lumbar arteries until the arteries supplying the anterior spinal artery were identified. Only nonionic material was used, and the study was interrupted when the dose limit of 6 mL/kg was reached.

Results.—The SCA was performed without major complications in 476 patients (97.7%). Six patients (1.2%) experienced major procedure-related complications, including spinal cord complications in 2 patients, renal complications in 2 patients, and stroke in 2 patients. Three patients experienced

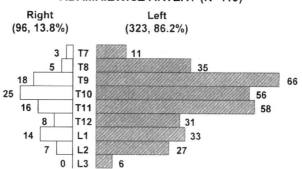

FIGURE 1.—Diagram shows origin of Adamkiewicz's artery. (Reprinted by permission of the publisher from Kieffer E, Fukui S, Chiras J, et al: Spinal cord arteriography: A safe adjunct before descending thoracic or thoracoabdominal aortic aneurysmectomy. *J Vasc Surg* 35:262-268, 2002. Copyright 2002 by Elsevier.)

complications at the puncture site. In 2 patients (0.4%), rupture of the aneurysm occurred within 3 days after SCA. Two deaths (0.4%) were directly attributable to SCA. The Adamkiewicz's artery was successfully located in 419 patients (86.2%) (Fig 1). On the basis of the extent of identification of spinal cord vasculature, the procedure was considered a complete success in 321 patients (65.9%), a partial success in 112 patients (23%), and a failure in 54 patients (11.1%). Failure rates were comparable, but the complete success rate was significantly higher in patients with degenerative rather than dissecting aneurysms and in patients with limited aneurysms.

Conclusion.—Spinal cord arteriography is a safe, effective adjunct that warrants more widespread use in the management of descending thoracic or thoracoabdominal aortic aneurysms.

▶ Professor Kieffer's group has long advocated SCA before thoracoabdominal aneurysm repair. In their hands, 98% of patients have no complications with SCA. However, the question remains as to whether it is necessary before thoracoabdominal aneurysm repair. I believe most would say no as long as attention is paid to other adjuncts of spinal cord perfusion during thoracoabdominal aneurysm repair. (See Abstracts 6–7 and 6–9.)

G. L. Moneta, MD

Self-Expandable Aortic Stent-Grafts for Treatment of Descending Aortic Dissections
Palma JH, Marcondes de Souza JA, Rodrigues Alves CM, et al (São Paulo Federal Univ, Brazil)
Ann Thorac Surg 73:1138-1142, 2002   6–13

Introduction.—Seventy consecutive nonselected patients with type B aortic dissection were treated with a self-expanding endovascular prosthesis. Outcomes and complications with this approach for type B dissection are reported.

Methods.—Between December 1996 and June 2001, 70 consecutive patients with type B aortic dissections were treated with a stent-graft introduced through the femoral artery under general anesthesia along with systemic heparinization and induced hypotension.

Results.—Fifty-eight patients had descending aortic dissections, and 12 had atypical dissections. The success rate was 92.9% (65 patients), as determined by exclusion of the false lumen in the thoracic aorta. Eleven patients (18.9%) had persistent blood flow in the false lumen as a result of distal reentries. Five procedures (7.1%) were converted to open surgery. Insertion of additional stent-grafts was necessary in 34 patients (48.6%). At 29 months' follow-up, 91.4% of the cohort was alive.

Conclusion.—Stent-grafts can be successfully placed for treatment of aortic dissections. Treatment of complicated and uncomplicated type B dissections of the aorta with stent-grafts offers a less invasive and perhaps lower-risk approach than conventional open surgery.

▶ In the comment accompanying this article, Dr Michael Grimm from the University of Vienna states, "I believe that in descending (thoracic) aortic aneurysms reduction of mortality and especially morbidity by intraluminal stent grafting is among the most impressive improvements in medicine during the last decade." Even though one half of the patients require additional intraluminal grafts to treat leak sites and long-term data are lacking, I think Dr Grimm is absolutely correct with regard to thoracic aneurysms. I believe, however, word is still out for good-risk infrarenal aortic aneurysm patients in whom the morbidity of open repair is considerably less than that for thoracic aneurysm repair.

G. L. Moneta, MD

Placement of Endovascular Stent-Grafts for Emergency Treatment of Acute Disease of the Descending Thoracic Aorta
Czermak BV, Waldenberger P, Perkmann R, et al (University Hosp, Innsbruck, Austria)
AJR 179:337-345, 2002   6–14

Background.—The surgical mortality rate associated with elective thoracic aortic aneurysm repair is relatively low, but operative mortality is almost 50% in patients needing emergent surgery. The feasibility, safety, and efficacy of endovascular stent-graft placement in patients undergoing emergent treatment of acute descending thoracic aortic disease were investigated.

Methods.—Eighteen patients undergoing emergent endovascular stent-graft placement for various types of acute descending thoracic aortic disease between January 1996 and November 2001 were included in the review. Indications for treatment were Stanford type B aortic dissection in 5 patients, traumatic thoracic aortic ruptures in 6, ruptured aortic aneurysms in 5, and penetrating atherosclerotic aortic ulcers in 2. Symptoms were life threatening in all patients, requiring stent-grafts from the emergency kit. Serious comorbidities placed all patients at high surgical risk.

Findings.—Primary placement of endovascular stent-grafts was technically successful in 78%. Primary perigraft leaks occurred in 4 patients. Secondary stent-graft placement was technically successful in 83%. Twenty hours after the intervention, 1 patient died of stent-graft-related causes. In another patient, follow-up showed stent-graft migration. Disease progressed in 1 patient treated for dissection and in both patients with penetrating ulcers. Another patient died of unknown causes 7 months after the intervention. The rest of the patients are still alive, at a mean follow-up of 17.4 months (Fig 1).

Conclusions.—Emergent repair of acute descending thoracic aortic disease with stent-graft placement is feasible and effective. This intervention may be a promising alternative to open-chest surgery, particularly in high-risk patients.

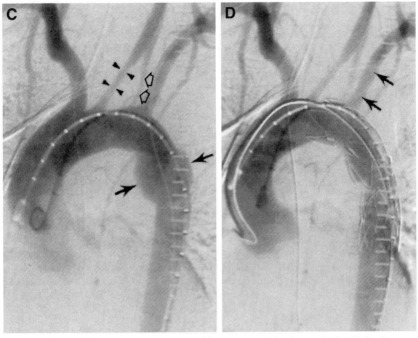

FIGURE 1.—Man, 41, with traumatic rupture of thoracic aorta. C, Angiogram obtained before intervention shows isthmic pseudoaneurysm (*solid arrows*). Mild narrowing of left lateral wall of left common carotid artery is caused by vasospasm (*arrowheads*). Left vertebral artery arises from aortic arch (*open arrows*). D, Angiogram obtained after intervention shows complete exclusion of pseudoaneurysm. Noncovered portion of stent-grafts is placed across origin of left subclavian artery. Blood flow in artery (*arrows*) remains intact. (Courtesy of Czermak BV, Waldenberger P, Perkmann R, et al: Placement of endovascular stent-grafts for emergency treatment of acute disease of the descending thoracic aorta. *AJR* 179:337-345, 2002. Reprinted with permission from the *American Journal of Roentgenology*.)

▶ I predict that in the next few years, stable patients requiring urgent or emergent descending thoracic aortic repair will preferentially be treated with endoluminal catheter–based techniques.

G. L. Moneta, MD

Endoluminal Stent Grafting of the Thoracic Aorta: Initial Experience With the Gore Excluder
Thompson CS, Gaxotte VD, Rodriguez JA, et al (Arizona Heart Inst, Phoenix)
J Vasc Surg 35:1163-1170, 2002   6–15

Background.—Presented is the experience of one group with endoluminal graft repair of a variety of pathologic processes of the thoracic aorta with the Gore Excluder thoracic stent-graft, a commercially developed device currently under investigation in a population that includes patients eligible for open surgical repair and those with prohibitive surgical risks.

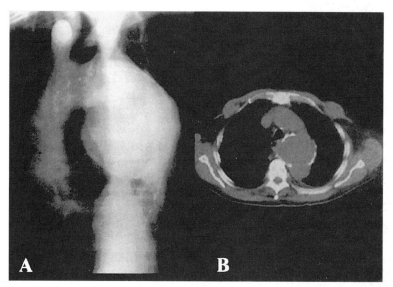

FIGURE 5.—Preoperative angiogram (A) and CT scan (B) show 7-cm aneurysm in distal aortic arch and proximal descending thoracic aorta in 72-year-old patient. (Reprinted by permission of the publisher from Thompson CS, Gaxotte VD, Rodriguez JA, et al: Endoluminal stent grafting of the thoracic aorta: Initial experience with the Gore Excluder. *J Vasc Surg* 35:1163-1170, 2002. Copyright 2002 by Elsevier.)

Methods.—From February 2000 to February 2001, endovascular stent-graft repairs of the thoracic aorta were performed in 46 patients (29 men, 17 women; mean age, 70 years) with the Gore Excluder thoracic stent-graft. Indications for endoluminal graft repair included atherosclerotic aneurysms in 23 patients (50%), dissections in 14 patients (30%), aortobronchial fistulas in 3 patients (7%), pseudoaneurysms in 3 patients (7%), traumatic ruptures in 2 patients (4%), and a ruptured aortic ulcer in 1 patient (2%). All patients were followed up with chest CT scans at 1, 3, 6, and 12 months, and follow-up ranged from 1 month to 15 months.

Results.—Technical success was attained in all procedures, and no conversions were needed. The average duration of the procedure was 120 minutes. The average length of stay in the hospital was 6 days. Sixty-four percent of the patients left the hospital within 4 days after successful endoluminal repair. The overall morbidity rate was 23%. Two patients (4%) had endoleaks that required a second procedure, and 2 patients died in the immediate postoperative period. No cases of paraplegia occurred. One patient had an endoleak that was found on the first postoperative day, and another patient had an endoleak that occurred 6 months after the procedure. Both patients were successfully treated with additional stent-grafts. No cases of migration occurred. One patient died of myocardial infarction 6 months after the graft placement. The patients treated for aneurysms had a mean aneurysm diameter of 6.8 cm (range, 5-9.5 cm) (Fig 5). The mean sac reduction at 1, 6, and 12 months was 0.59 cm, 0.77 cm, and 0.85 cm, respectively (Fig 6). The sac was unchanged in 3 patients, who had no evidence of endoleaks.

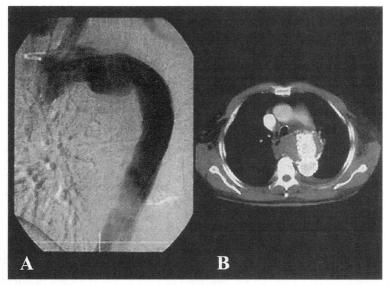

FIGURE 6.—Postoperative angiogram (**A**) and CT scan (**B**) after deployment of Gore Excluder stent-graft show adequate exclusion of aneurysm described in Figure 5. Carotid subclavian bypass procedure was performed before stent placement to allow for adequate proximal landing zone. (Reprinted by permission of the publisher from Thompson CS, Gaxotte VD, Rodriguez JA, et al: Endoluminal stent grafting of the thoracic aorta: Initial experience with the Gore Excluder. *J Vasc Surg* 35:1163-1170, 2002. Copyright 2002 by Elsevier.)

Conclusions.—This initial experience with the Gore Excluder for thoracic endoluminal grafting showed that it is a safe and feasible alternative to open graft repair. These early findings suggest that an endoluminal approach to these pathologic processes may be preferable to classic resection and graft placement.

▶ The word on the street is that, at least for stent grafting of the thoracic aorta, this device is superior to others currently in development.

G. L. Moneta, MD

7 Aortic Aneurysm

Familial Abdominal Aortic Aneurysms: Collection of 233 Multiplex Families
Kuivaniemi H, Shibamura H, Arthur C, et al (Wayne State Univ, Detroit; Dalhousie Univ, Halifax, Nova Scotia, Canada; Univ of Oulu, Finland; et al)
J Vasc Surg 37:340-345, 2003   7–1

Background.—Many reports have described abdominal aortic aneurysms (AAA) occurring in families. As a genetic disease, AAA appears to be autosomal, with either a dominant or recessive pattern of inheritance. However, it remains difficult to separate the genetic factors involved in this condition. Relations between probands with AAA and affected family members were evaluated in a large series of families with AAA.

Methods and Findings.—The analysis included 233 white families from North America and Europe with 2 or more members affected by AAA. Most families had only 2 affected members, with an average of 2.8. Brother was the most common type of relation to the proband. The pattern of inheritance appeared to be autosomal recessive in 72% of families and autosomal dominant in 25%. The remaining 8 families had evidence of autosomal dominant inheritance with incomplete penetrance.

Analysis of the 66 families with dominant inheritance identified 141 cases in which AAA was transmitted from one generation to another. Forty-six percent of these transmissions were male to male, 32% were female to male, and 11% each were male to female or female to female.

Conclusions.—This large analysis of families with AAA suggests that male first-degree relatives are at highest risk. An autosomal recessive mode of inheritance appears to predominate, but no single mode can account for AAA in all the families studied. Thus, AAA is a multifactorial disorder affected by a number of different genetic and environmental risk factors.

▶ The different modes of inheritance of AAA, along with all those patients with aneurysms and no obvious inheritance pattern, suggest the aorta, like many other organs, responds to different disease processes in the same way. It therefore seems unlikely there will be much to gain by studying the end point of the disease. Many people may assume there must be a final common factor that leads to aneurysmal degeneration in response to many different stimuli. I bet there will be many stimuli in many pathways, all of which eventually lead to the formation of an aneurysm.

G. L. Moneta, MD

The Prevalence and Natural History of Aortic Aneurysms in Heart and Abdominal Organ Transplant Patients

Englesbe MJ, Wu AH, Clowes AW, et al (Univ of Washington, Seattle)
J Vasc Surg 37:27-31, 2003   7–2

Background.—Little is known about the natural history of aortic aneurysms in heart and abdominal organ transplant recipients. The prevalence and clinical features of aortic aneurysms in heart, liver, and kidney transplant recipients were examined.

Methods.—The medical records of 1557 adult patients (82.4% men; mean age, 49.6 years) undergoing heart (n = 296), liver (n = 450), or kidney (n = 811) transplantation from 1987 through 2000 were reviewed. Imaging results and surgical reports were examined to identify aortic aneurysm (defined as an abdominal aorta >3.5 cm in diameter). The incidence of aortic aneurysms and outcomes were determined over a median follow-up of 21.6 months after transplantation.

Results.—Eighteen aortic aneurysms were identified in 13 heart recipients (4.4%), 3 liver recipients (0.7%), and 2 kidney recipients (0.2%). In 7 of these patients, the aortic aneurysm ruptured and 5 of them died. All the other 11 patients survived. At rupture, the aortic aneurysms ranged from 5.1 to 12.2 cm in diameter (mean, 6.0 cm). The rate of rupture was 22.5% per year. Eight patients underwent successful aortic aneurysm repair; all had a hospital stay of 15 days or less. The mean rate of aortic aneurysm expansion increased from 0.46 cm/y before transplantation to 1.00 cm/y after transplantation ($P = .08$). The rate of aortic aneurysm expansion was similar in heart and abdominal organ transplant patients. Early in the series (1987-1996), screening for aortic aneurysm was performed in 11% of heart recipients; 3.0% were found to have an aneurysm. In 1997, aortic aneurysm screening was performed in 87% of heart recipients, and 5.8% were found to have an aneurysm.

Conclusion.—Aortic aneurysms in heart, liver, or kidney transplant patients are aggressive: aneurysm expansion increases after transplantation, rupture rates are high, and rupture is associated with poor outcome. Elective repair of aortic aneurysms in appropriate transplant patients is generally well tolerated. Screening can detect aortic aneurysm early and thus allow repair to prevent the mortality associated with rupture. These findings support screening for aortic aneurysms in heart, liver, and kidney transplant recipients.

▶ The prevalence of aortic aneurysms in cardiac transplant patients justifies routine screening for aortic aneurysms in cardiac transplant patients. The prevalence seems too low to justify routine screening in abdominal organ transplant patients.

G. L. Moneta, MD

Long-term Outcomes of Immediate Repair Compared With Surveillance of Small Abdominal Aortic Aneurysms
Powell JT, for the United Kingdom Small Aneurysm Trial Participants (Univ Hosps of Coventry and Warwickshire, England; et al)
N Engl J Med 346:1445-1452, 2002   7–3

Introduction.—Recent trials have reported that early, prophylactic elective surgery does not improve 5-year survival rates among patients with small abdominal aortic aneurysms. This report details long-term outcomes from the United Kingdom Small Aneurysm Trial.

Methods.—A total of 1090 patients (age range, 60-76 years) with small abdominal aortic aneurysms (diameter, 4.0-5.5 cm) were randomly assigned to 1 of 2 groups. A total of 563 were assigned to undergo early elective surgery and 527 were assigned to undergo surveillance by US (Fig 2). The mean follow-up was 8 years (range, 6-10 years).

Results.—The mean survival duration was 6.5 years among patients in the surveillance group compared with 6.7 years for patients from the early-surgery group ($P = .29$). The adjusted hazard ratio for death from any cause in the early-surgery group compared with the surveillance group was 0.83 (95% CI, 0.69-1.00; $P = .05$). The 30-day surgical mortality rate was 5.5% in the early-surgery group. The survival curves crossed at 3 years; at 8 years, the mortality rate in the early-surgery group was 7.2 percentage points lower than in the surveillance group ($P = .03$) (Fig 3). There was no indication that age, sex, or the initial size of the aneurysm modified the hazard ratio or that

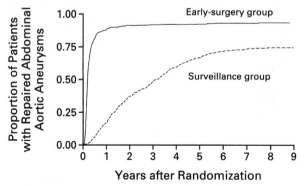

Years after Randomization

FIGURE 2.—Kaplan–Meier estimates of the cumulative proportion of patients who underwent surgery for aneurysm repair, according to treatment-group assignment. Data were not censored at the time of death. (Reprinted by permission of *The New England Journal of Medicine* from Powell JT, for the United Kingdom Small Aneurysm Trial Participants: Long-term outcomes of immediate repair compared with surveillance of small abdominal aortic aneurysms. *N Engl J Med* 346:1445-1452, 2002. Copyright 2002, Massachusetts Medical Society. All rights reserved.)

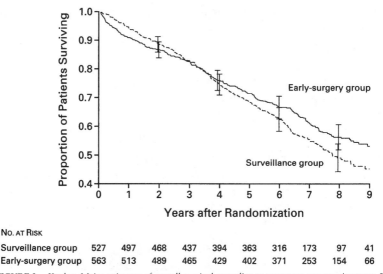

NO. AT RISK

Surveillance group	527	497	468	437	394	363	316	173	97	41
Early-surgery group	563	513	489	465	429	402	371	253	154	66

FIGURE 3.—Kaplan–Meier estimates of overall survival according to treatment group assignment. $P =$ .05 by the log-rank test. *I bars* represent the 95% CIs for the point estimates. (Reprinted by permission of *The New England Journal of Medicine* from Powell JT, for the United Kingdom Small Aneurysm Trial Participants: Long-term outcomes of immediate repair compared with surveillance of small abdominal aortic aneurysms. *N Engl J Med* 346:1445-1452, 2002. Copyright 2002, Massachusetts Medical Society. All rights reserved.)

delayed surgery in the surveillance group increased 30-day postoperative mortality. Death was caused by ruptured aneurysms in 19 of the 411 men who died (5%) and in 12 of the 85 women who died (14%) ($P = .001$). The rate of early cessation of smoking was higher in the early-surgery group compared with the surveillance cohort.

Conclusion.—No significant long-term survival differences were found between the early-surgery and the surveillance groups, although, after 8 years, total mortality was lower in the early-surgery group. This difference may partially be caused by beneficial changes in lifestyle adopted by participants in the early-surgery group. The prevalence of ruptured aneurysm may be higher in women compared with men.

▶ In this late follow-up of the United Kingdom's small abdominal aortic aneurysm trial, there is still no evidence that repair of abdominal aortic aneurysms less than 5.5 cm in diameter confer a survival advantage in men. However, 14% of all female deaths in this study were due to aneurysm rupture. The evidence is slowly accumulating that women with abdominal aortic aneurysms probably should have them repaired at slightly smaller diameters than for men.

G. L. Moneta, MD

Nonoperative Management With Selective Delayed Surgery for Large Abdominal Aortic Aneurysms in Patients at High Risk

Tanquilut EM, Veith FJ, Ohki T, et al (Albert Einstein College of Medicine, New York)
J Vasc Surg 36:41-46, 2002   7–4

Background.—Some patients with large abdominal aortic aneurysms (AAAs) have serious comorbid conditions that greatly increase operative risk. The outcomes of periods of protracted nonoperative observational management with selective delayed surgery were evaluated in patients at high risk with large infrarenal and pararenal AAAs.

Methods.—From a cohort of 226 patients with AAAs larger than 5.5 cm, 72 patients with AAAs from 5.6 to 12 cm (mean, 7 cm) were selected for periods of nonoperative management because of prohibitive surgical risk. Among the comorbid factors were a low ejection fraction of 15% to 34% in 18 patients, 1-second forced expiratory volume less than 50% in 25 patients, prior laparotomy in 10 patients, and morbid obesity in 22 patients. Follow-up examination was complete in all patients for the 6 to 76 months (mean, 23 months) of their nonoperative treatment. Surgery was subsequently performed in 53 patients because of further AAA enlargement or onset of symptoms after 6 to 72 months (mean, 19 months) of nonoperative treatment.

Results.—Of these 72 patients, 54 (75%) were living and 18 (25%) were dead at the time of this report. Seven patients who underwent only nonoperative treatment were alive at 28 to 76 months (mean, 48 months). Of the 18 deaths, AAA rupture occurred in only 3 patients (4%), who were observed for 12, 31, and 72 months, respectively, before rupture. There were 9 other deaths (13%) after 6 to 72 months from comorbidities unrelated to the AAA. Of the 53 patients who underwent delayed operation, 6 patients died within 30 days of operation, for a mortality rate of 11%. The mortality rate for the 154 good-risk patients with AAAs who underwent prompt open or endovascular repair was 2.2%.

Conclusion.—Some patients with large AAAs and serious co-morbid conditions can be satisfactorily managed for prolonged periods by nonoperative methods. Significant delays of 12 to 76 months in this series resulted in an AAA rupture rate of only 4%. These findings support the selective use of nonoperative management in some patients with large AAAs and serious comorbid conditions.

▶ The authors' results indicate that one can take his or her time with patients with large AAAs and significant comorbidities. Only a tiny minority will die from rupture while under observation. In this series, the operative mortality rate in high-risk patients exceeded death from aneurysm rupture. The discussion of the study is highly recommended. It outlines a reasonable management protocol for any patient with an AAA. It reflects the fact that the days of operating on less than 5 cm asymptomatic AAAs, at least in men, should be over. There are simply no data to support such an approach. "Ego-based" medicine needs to be flushed when evidence-based medicine is available.

G. L. Moneta, MD

The Risk of Rupture in Untreated Aneurysms: The Impact of Size, Gender, and Expansion Rate
Brown PM, Zelt DT, Sobolev B (Queen's Univ, Kingston, Ont, Canada)
J Vasc Surg 37:280-284, 2003   7–5

Background.—Several studies have shown a low risk of rupture for abdominal aortic aneurysms (AAAs) measuring less than 5.0. It is generally agreed that aneurysms measuring 6.0 cm or larger are at significant risk of rupture; yet few studies have actually examined the risk associated with aneurysms of this size. The risk of rupture for men and women with AAAs measuring 5.0 cm or larger was evaluated.

Methods.—The analysis included 476 patients with AAAs measuring 5.0 cm or larger: 377 men and 99 women with a mean age of 73 years. Because of conditions making them considered unfit for surgery, the patients were enrolled in a prospective monitoring program, including CT scans performed every 6 months. Patients were followed up until their aneurysms ruptured or until they died or were deleted from follow-up.

Results.—During a total follow-up of 982 patient-years, 50 AAA ruptures occurred. Among patients with AAAs measuring 5.0 to 5.9 cm, the average risk of rupture was 1.0% per year for men and 3.9% per year for men. For AAAs measuring 6.0 cm or larger, the risks were 14.1% per year and 22.3% per year, respectively (Table 1).

Conclusions.—For men with AAAs measuring 5.0 to 5.9 cm, the risk of aneurysm rupture is relatively low. In contrast, for women with aneurysms of similar size, the risk of rupture is 4 times higher. Thus, the threshold for surgical AAA repair may be lower for women considered fit for surgery.

TABLE 1.—Number of Patients, Ruptures, Time at Risk, Annual Rate (and Standard Error), and Relative Risk (and 95% CI) According to Gender and Aneurysm Size

Description	No. of Patients	No. of Ruptures	Time at Risk (y)	Annual Rate (Standard Error)	Relative Risk (95 CI)
Men, 5.0 to 5.9 cm	333	6	607	1.0% (0.01%)	1.0
Women, 5.0 to 5.9 cm	89	5	128	3.9% (0.15%)	4.0 (1.2,13.0)
Men, 6.0 cm or greater	186	28	198	14.1% (0.18%)	14.3 (5.9,34.5)
Women, 6.0 cm or greater	48	11	49	22.3% (0.95%)	22.6 (8.4,61.1)

▶ This is another study suggesting the risk of rupture for AAAs is higher in women than in men with similar-sized aneurysms. The weight of the evidence suggests the threshold level for consideration of repair in women should be lower than in men. Unfortunately, women may also be at higher risk with repair.

G. L. Moneta, MD

Expansion Rates and Outcomes for the 3.0-cm to the 3.9-cm Infrarenal Abdominal Aortic Aneurysm
Santilli SM, Littooy FN, Cambria RA, et al (Minneapolis VAMC; Loyola Univ, Chicago; Med College of Wisconsin, Milwaukee; et al)
J Vasc Surg 35:666-671, 2002   7–6

Background.—Disagreement continues on the best management of small abdominal aortic aneurysms (AAAs). Some of this disagreement stems from inadequate knowledge of the natural history of small AAAs. The expansion rates and patient outcomes associated with surveillance of 3- to 3.9-cm AAAs were determined.

Methods.—The study included 790 men with AAAs 3 to 3.9 cm seen at 5 Veterans Affairs Medical Centers. Eligibility requirements included at least 1 repeat US scan more than 90 days after initial screening. Patients also completed a questionnaire providing demographic and risk factor information. The mean follow-up was 3.9 years.

Findings.—The average AAA size was 3.3 cm. The median expansion was 0.11 cm/y. Expansion rates differed significantly between men with 3- to 3.4-cm AAAs and those with 3.5- to 3.9-cm AAAs. No AAA ruptures were reported during the study. However, cause of death was known in only 43% of the patients who died during observation. During the study, few AAAs 3 to 3.9 cm expanded to 5 cm or more. Patients with 3- to 3.9-cm AAAs who had operative repair were younger, had larger initial AAA diameters, and had more rapid expansion rates.

Conclusions.—AAAs of 3 to 3.9 cm expanded slowly and did not rupture. These aneurysms rarely required operative repair or expanded to 5 cm under observation for a mean of 3.9 years. Overall expansion rates and the incidence of operative repair were, however, higher in men with 3.5- to 3.9-cm AAAs than in those with 3.0- to 3.4-cm AAAs.

▶ This study annoyed me. The results section states "Table III shows that no 3.0-cm to 3.4-cm AAA expanded to 5.0 cm or more with 5 years of follow-up examination." However, Table III (see original article) seems to show 1 in 48, 1 in 90, 1 in 89, 3 in 108, and 3 in 80 3.0 cm to 3.4 cm AAAs actually reaching a 5-cm level with less than 1 year, 1 year, 2 years, 3 years, and 4 years of follow-up, respectively. Which is it?

G. L. Moneta, MD

In Vivo Analysis of Mechanical Wall Stress and Abdominal Aortic Aneurysm Rupture Risk

Fillinger MF, Raghavan ML, Marra SP, et al (Dartmouth-Hitchcock Med Ctr, Lebanon, NH)
J Vasc Surg 36:589-597, 2002   7–7

Background.—Determination of maximum abdominal aortic aneurysm (AAA) diameter helps stratify risk of rupture. However, most large aneurysms do not rupture and a few small AAAs do rupture. It is therefore important to further refine the ability to predict AAA rupture. This study calculated AAA wall stress in vivo for ruptured, symptomatic, and electively repaired AAAs with 3-dimensional computer modeling techniques, CT scan data, and blood pressure. Wall stress was then compared with clinical indices related to rupture risk.

Methods.—CT scans were analyzed for 48 patients with AAAs, subdivided as follows: 18 AAAs that ruptured (10 patients) or were urgently repaired because of symptoms (8 patients) and 30 AAAs large enough to warrant elective repair within 12 weeks of the CT scan. Three-dimensional computer models of AAAs were reconstructed from CT scan data. The stress distribution on the AAA resulting from geometry and blood pressure was computationally determined with finite element analysis with a hyperelastic nonlinear model that depicted the mechanical behavior of the AAA wall.

Results.—Peak wall stress was significantly different between groups: ruptured, 47.7 ± 6 N/cm^2; emergent symptomatic, 47.5 ± 4 N/cm^2; and elective repair, 36.9 ± 2 N/cm^2. There was no significant difference between the groups in blood pressure or AAA diameter. Because of trends toward differences in diameter, comparison was made only with diameter-matched participants. Even when the mean diameters were identical, the ruptured/symptomatic AAAs had a significantly higher peak wall stress than the electively repaired AAAs. Maximal wall stress was a better predictor of risk of rupture than the LaPlace equation or other proposed indices of rupture risk. The smallest ruptured AAA was 4.8 cm in diameter, but this aneurysm had a stress equivalent to the average electively repaired 6.3-cm AAA.

Conclusions.—Peak wall stresses in vivo for ruptured and symptomatic AAAs were significantly higher than peak stresses for electively repaired AAAs, even when matched for maximal diameters. This study suggests that calculation of wall stress with computer modeling of 3-dimensional AAA geometry can assess rupture risk more accurately than AAA diameter or other previously proposed clinical indices. Stress analysis appears to be practical and feasible and may become an important clinical tool for the evaluation of AAA rupture risk.

▶ This is one of the most interesting basic research studies in recent years. We have to assume there is a reason an AAA ruptures at a specific site. The fact that wall stress varies with the shape and topography of the aneurysm and appears to correlate with the site of rupture is fascinating. The authors' technique may allow us to stratify rupture risk based on factors other than simple diameter determinations.

G. L. Moneta, MD

Effect of Intraluminal Thrombus on Wall Stress in Patient-Specific Models of Abdominal Aortic Aneurysm
Wang DHJ, Makaroun MS, Webster MW, et al (Univ of Pittsburgh, Pa)
J Vasc Surg 36:598-604, 2002   7–8

Introduction.—The impact of intraluminal thrombus (ILT) on the rupture potential of an abdominal aortic aneurysm (AAA) is unknown. It is likely that rupture occurs when wall stress exceeds wall strength at any location along the wall. The influence of ILT on wall stress distribution and magnitude in AAA was examined with geometric models derived from 4 patients.

Methods.—The age range of 3 men and 1 woman was 73 to 86 years, and the maximal AAA diameter ranged from 6.0 cm to 6.4 cm. Patient-specific three-dimensional AAA geometric models were reconstructed with the use of CT images. Two geometric characteristics, ILT surface ratio (ie, ILT surface area divided by total AAA surface area) and ILT volume ratio (ie, ILT volume divided by the total AAA volume) were determined for each AAA. Two models were constructed for each patient: 1 with ILT and 1 without ILT. The systolic pressure determined at the time of CT imaging was applied to the internal surface of each model. Peak wall stress was compared between the 2 models for each patient.

Results.—The ILT surface ratios ranged from 0.29 to 0.72. The ILT volume ratios ranged from 0.12 to 0.66. The peak wall stress was decreased (range, 6%-38%; $P = .067$) for all models with ILT (range, 28-37 N/cm²) compared with models with no ILT (range, 30-44 N/cm²). Visual inspection also demonstrated a marked effect of ILT on the wall stress distribution.

Conclusion.—The presence of ILT alters wall stress distribution and decreases peak wall stress in AAA. ILT should be included in every patient-specific model of AAA for determination of AAA wall stress.

▶ It is impossible to make definitive conclusions from analysis of 4 patients. However, if thrombus has some elasticity, it should be able to diffuse pulsatile stress over a wider area and therefore lower stress at high stress points in the aneurysm wall. Again, mapping of stress points on the walls of the AAA is an intriguing area of research. (See also Abstract 7–7.)

G. L. Moneta, MD

Prolonged Administration of Doxycycline in Patients With Small Asymptomatic Abdominal Aortic Aneurysms: Report of a Prospective (Phase II) Multicenter Study

Baxter BT, Pearce WH, Waltke EA, et al (Univ of Nebraska, Omaha; Methodist Hosp, Chicago; Northwestern Univ, Chicago; et al)
J Vasc Surg 36:1-12, 2002   7–9

Background.—Doxycycline, proved safe in the management of certain chronic conditions, may decrease expansion of abdominal aortic aneurysm (AAA) by inhibition of matrix metalloproteinase-9 (MMP-9). Compliance, adverse effects, and the safety associated with the long-term use of doxycycline in patients with small, asymptomatic AAAs were investigated.

Methods.—Thirty-six patients with AAAs were enrolled in the 6-month, phase 2 trial. The patients were 30 men and 6 women (mean age, 69 years). Doxycycline was prescribed in an oral dose of 100 mg twice a day. The aneurysm size was measured before and after treatment. Compliance and adverse effects were also monitored, and plasma doxycycline and MMP-9 concentrations were periodically measured.

Findings.—Ninety-two percent of the patients completed the full 6 months of treatment. Five patients (13.9%) had significant treatment-related side effects, including cutaneous photosensitivity reactions in 3, tooth discoloration in 1, and a yeast infection in 1. The rate of compliance with treatment was high, despite minor but frequent adverse effects. Minor side effects were nonspecific gastrointestinal symptoms in 25%, easily managed episodes of photosensitivity in 22.2%, and reversible tooth discoloration in 5.5%. After 3 months of treatment, the mean plasma doxycycline level was 4.62 µg/mL. The median AAA diameter was not significantly changed: 42.7 mm at 6 months compared with 41 mm at baseline. The overall rate of AAA expansion was 0.63% per month. The mean plasma MMP-9 level, increased at baseline, declined to 83.8 ng/mL at 3 months and to 66.4 ng/mL at 6 months. After 6 months of treatment, 21% of the patients had an increased level of plasma MMP-9 compared with 47% at baseline.

Conclusions.—The prolonged administration of doxycycline to patients with small asymptomatic AAAs is safe and tolerable. Such treatment is associated with a gradual decline in plasma MMP-9 levels. Further research is needed to determine the long-term effects of this treatment on the rate and extent of aneurysm growth.

▶ Preventing expansion of small AAAs is one of the Holy Grails of vascular surgery. Local production of MMPs, capable of degrading collagen and elastin, are potentially associated with degeneration of the aortic wall. Tetracycline can inhibit MMPs. It therefore makes sense to investigate whether tetracycline can slow aneurysm expansion. This study is an excellent preliminary step in evaluating the effect of tetracycline on aneurysm expansion.

G. L. Moneta, MD

Response of Plasma Matrix Metalloproteinase-9 to Conventional Abdominal Aortic Aneurysm Repair or Endovascular Exclusion: Implications for Endoleak

Lorelli DR, Jean-Claude JM, Fox CJ, et al (Med College of Wisconsin, Milwaukee)

J Vasc Surg 35:916-922, 2002　　　　　　　　　　　　　　　　7–10

Background.—Matrix metalloproteinases have been implicated in the development of aneurysms. Matrix metalloproteinase-9 (MMP-9) concentrations have been found to be increased in aortic aneurysmal tissue and in patient plasma. Thus, plasma MMP-9 levels may decline significantly after conventional and endovascular infrarenal abdominal aortic aneurysm (AAA) repair. The effect of persistent endoleak on MMP-9 levels after endovascular aneurysm repair is unknown.

Methods.—Twenty-six patients with AAAs undergoing conventional repair, and 25 undergoing endovascular repair were studied. Levels of MMP-9 were determined before surgery and at 1 and 3 months after surgery with the use of a sandwich enzyme-linked immunosorbent assay. Endoleaks were identified postoperatively on CT scans in 8 patients who underwent endovascular repair.

Findings.—Preoperative plasma MMP-9 levels were not associated with age, sex, or aneurysm diameter. Patients undergoing conventional repair and those undergoing endovascular repair did not differ significantly in preop-

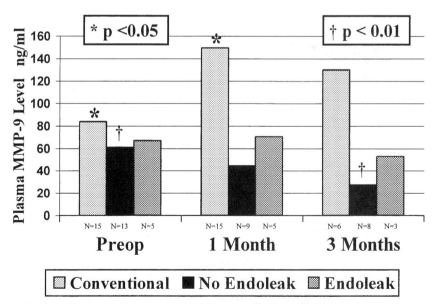

FIGURE 1.—Comparison of mean plasma matrix metalloproteinase (MMP)-9 levels (ng/mL) over time between groups. N denotes number of patients in each category. (Reprinted by permission of the publisher from Lorelli DR, Jean-Claude JM, Fox CJ, et al: Response of plasma matrix metalloproteinase-9 to conventional abdominal aortic aneurysm repair or endovascular exclusion: Implications for endoleak. *J Vasc Surg* 35:916-922, 2002. Copyright 2002 by Elsevier.)

erative plasma MMP-9 concentrations or in AAA diameter. Samples from 33 of the 51 patients were available for follow-up. The mean plasma MMP-9 concentrations were significantly increased 1 month after conventional AAA repair compared with preoperative levels: the values were 149.5 and 83.9 ng/mL, respectively. These levels remained increased, at 129.8 ng/mL, 3 months postoperatively. In patients undergoing endovascular aneurysm exclusion without endoleaks, the mean plasma MMP-9 levels were decreased significantly at 3 months compared with preoperative levels: the values were 27.4 and 60.8 ng/mL, respectively. However, patients with endoleaks did not show significant declines in plasma MMP-9 levels at 3 months (Fig 1).

Conclusions.—Plasma MMP-9 concentrations remain increased for as long as 3 months after conventional AAA repair but decrease by this time after successful endovascular exclusion of an AAA. Measuring MMP-9 levels after endovascular AAA exclusion may be a useful clinical tool for suggesting the presence of an endoleak.

▶ This study doesn't shed much light on the role of MMP-9 in aortic aneurysm disease. There is no reason MMPs should increase with conventional repair, decrease with endovascular repair without endoleak, but decrease less in endovascular repair with endoleak. I am confident postoperative MMP levels will not prove to be of any clinical value. The word is still out on the role of MMPs and AAA disease (see Abstract 7–9). Trying to make sense out of postoperative MMPs is a little like trying to reconstruct a chicken from a scrambled egg.

G. L. Moneta, MD

Ruptured Abdominal Aortic Aneurysm After Endovascular Repair
Bernhard VM, Mitchell RS, Matsumura JS, et al (Univ of Chicago; Stanford Univ, Calif; Harvard Med School, Boston; et al)
J Vasc Surg 35:1155-1162, 2002   7–11

Introduction.—Several reports have described ruptures after endograft implantation. The experience with aneurysm ruptures after deployment of Guidant/EVT endografts is described and compared with previous reported cases involving other devices.

Methods.—Medical records of all patients who received Guidant/EVT endografts from February 10, 1993, through August 31, 2000, were reviewed to identify all aneurysm ruptures that occurred after device implantation. Data regarding previously reported cases were obtained with a MEDLINE search.

Results.—Seven ruptures occurred in patients who received the Guidant/EVT devices. Five ruptures occurred among 686 patients who underwent implant insertion in US Food and Drug Administration (FDA)–approved clinical trials (group 1). These patients were followed up for a mean of 41.8 months. The ruptures occurred among 93 patients with first-generation tube endografts. The remaining 2 ruptures occurred in group 2 patients (3260 patients after market approval with limited follow-up), specifically in the sub-

TABLE 1.—Causes of Rupture*

Type and Source of Endoleaks	No. of Patients
Type I endoleak	27
Proximal attachment*	12†
Distal attachment	14
Aorta	10†
Iliac	4
Site not reported	1
Type II endoleak	2
Type III endoleak	11
Modular disconnection	5 (2‡)
Stent erosion through fabric	1
Details not reported	5
Leak present, source not reported	4

*n = 44 of 47 patients; cause not reported in 3 patients.

†Three patients met criteria for endotension (AAA enlargement in absence of detectable endoleak before AAA rupture). One had a proximal leak shown at surgery. Another was classified as having a proximal leak on the basis of known migration at the proximal neck; however, no postrupture CT scan, surgery, or autopsy was found to verify this presumption. A third had an initial increase in AAA diameter that remained stabile until rupture from distal aortic endoleak. Endoleak was recognized in retrospect.

‡Associated fabric tear in polyethylene terephthalate (Dacron) graft wall and disruption of sutures attaching it to metal frame.

Abbreviation: AAA, Abdominal aortic aneurysm.

(Reprinted by permission of the publisher from Bernhard VM, Mitchell RS, Matsumura JS, et al: Ruptured abdominal aortic aneurysm after endovascular repair. *J Vasc Surg* 35:1155-1162, 2002. Copyright 2002 by Elsevier.)

group of 166 patients who underwent treatment with second-generation tube grafts. No ruptures occurred among patients with bifurcation or unilateral iliac implants followed up for a mean of 37.5 months. All ruptures were caused by distal aortic type I endoleaks as a result of attachment system fractures (first-generation devices only), aortic neck dilatations, persistent primary endoleaks, migration, overlooked imaging abnormalities, refused reintervention, or poor patient selection. The overall mortality rate was 57% (4 of 7 patients); it was 50% for surgical repair (3 of 6 patients). The literature search identified 40 additional ruptures associated with other devices (total, 47 ruptures). All 44 ruptures with sufficient data were caused by endoleaks (26 type I, 2 type II, 11 type III, and 5 source not reported) (Table 1). Other contributing factors included graft module separation and graft wall deterioration. The overall mortality rate for the combined series was 50%; the surgical mortality rate was 41%.

Conclusion.—Ruptures after implantation of Guidant/EVT endografts have particular, unique characteristics. All occurred in patients who had tube grafts, and all were the result of a type I endoleak that developed at the distal aortic attachment site. It is recommended that tube endografts be limited to the rare patient with ideal anatomy at high risk of complications from a standard open repair.

► I remember when the initial ruptures of abdominal aortic aneurysms were first described after endovascular repair. The Portland representatives for one company's device proudly pointed out no ruptures had occurred with their device. I also remember how advocates of endovascular repair suggested ruptures with endografts were better tolerated than ruptures of unstented abdominal aortic aneurysms. With time, both of these positions proved to be wrong.

G. L. Moneta, MD

Life Expectancy After Endovascular Versus Open Abdominal Aortic Aneurysm Repair: Results of a Decision Analysis Model on the Basis of Data From EUROSTAR

Schermerhorn ML, Finlayson SRG, Fillinger MF, et al (Hitchcock Med Ctr, Lebanon, NH; Catharina Hosp, Eindhoven, The Netherlands)
J Vasc Surg 36:1112-1120, 2002   7–12

Background.—Abdominal aortic aneurysm (AAA) rupture can occur after endovascular repair in approximately 1% of cases per year, and careful long-term follow-up of all patients undergoing this method is required to detect and address complications. The risk of rupture and the need for reintervention are higher after endovascular repair than with open repair. The decision analysis method was used to examine the effect of the various risks on the quality-adjusted life expectancy (QALE) of patients having endovascular versus open repair of infrarenal AAA.

Methods.—The outcomes for hypothetic cohorts of 70-year-old men with AAA who underwent either open or endovascular repair of AAA were determined by using a Markov decision analysis model. Probabilities were gleaned from the literature, from the EUROSTAR database for endovascular repair, and from Medicare claims data for open repair. Patients moved

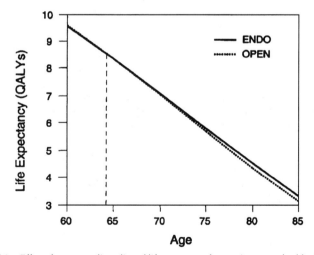

FIGURE 1.—Effect of age on quality-adjusted life expectancy for men in average health. *Abbreviation:* *QALYs*, Quality-adjusted life years. (Reprinted by permission of the publisher from Schermerhorn ML, Finlayson SRG, Fillinger MF, et al: Life expectancy after endovascular versus open abdominal aortic aneurysm repair: Results of a decision analysis model on the basis of data from EUROSTAR. *J Vasc Surg* 36:1112-1120, 2002. Copyright 2002 by Elsevier.)

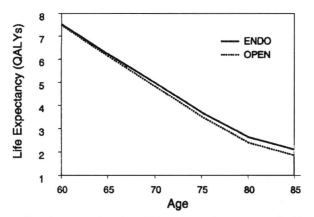

FIGURE 2.—Effect of age on quality-adjusted life expectancy for men in poor health. *Abbreviation:* *QALYs*, Quality-adjusted life years. (Reprinted by permission of the publisher from Schermerhorn ML, Finlayson SRG, Fillinger MF, et al: Life expectancy after endovascular versus open abdominal aortic aneurysm repair: Results of a decision analysis model on the basis of data from EUROSTAR. *J Vasc Surg* 36:1112-1120, 2002. Copyright 2002 by Elsevier.)

through a multistate transition model based on these data. QALE after aneurysm repair was the primary outcome measure. In addition, factors that influenced this outcome were determined by sensitivity analysis.

Results.—The QALE for 70-year-old men in average health undergoing endovascular repair averaged 7.09 years, whereas that for patients having standard repair was 7.03 years, for a difference of only 0.06 quality-adjusted life years (about 3 weeks). When the patients were in poor health, the quality-adjusted life years noted with endovascular repair was 4.98 and that for open repair was 4.82 (difference of 2 months). The effect of age was minimal (Fig 1), and operative mortality rate differed little between the 2 methods. Endovascular methods are preferred for 70-year-old men until the annual rupture rate rises above 0.7%, with a difference in QALE of less than 3 months until the annual rupture rate is greater than 1.7%. The standard technique is preferred in 60-year-old men unless the annual rupture rate is less than 0.4%. The endovascular method was preferred until the rupture rate per year exceeded 2.0% in 80-year-old men. Varying revision rates, the presence of poor health versus average health, and other parameters did not greatly influence outcome (Fig 2).

Conclusions.—Decision analysis based on the best data available did not clearly identify a superior strategy to use in the management of AAA. There was minimal difference between the endovascular and standard methods, leading to the recommendation that patient preference be considered strongly in choosing an approach. Some patients may choose the slightly higher initial operative risk of the open technique for its increased protection over the long term. Other patients may decide that the relatively long postoperative disability accompanying open repair is less desirable. The increased need for close follow-up and its attendant inconvenience may prompt some to choose open over endovascular repair. Trials comparing the 2 techniques may help to clarify the best choice for patients with AAA.

▶ This sophisticated analysis confirms what most of us think; that open repair may be best for younger, healthy patients, while endovascular repair seems more advisable for older less healthy patients with appropriate aortic anatomy. The problem is what to do with patients between the extremes. The authors suggest that a host of patient-specific factors such as employment, compliance with follow-up, and distance from appropriate centers may be important for this large middle group. Who can argue with that?

G. L. Moneta, MD

Durability of Benefits of Endovascular Versus Conventional Abdominal Aortic Aneurysm Repair

Carpenter JP, Baum RA, Barker CF, et al (Univ of Pennsylvania, Philadelphia)
J Vasc Surg 35:222-228, 2002   7–13

Background.—Previous reports have suggested that endovascular repair of an abdominal aortic aneurysm (AAA) reduces morbidity and the length of stay (LOS) compared with conventional open surgery. The durability of these benefits through midterm follow-up was assessed.

Methods.—This retrospective study included 337 patients undergoing AAA repair over a 26-month period. Of these, 174 repairs were endovascular and 163 were open; the mean follow-up was 10.6 and 12.3 months, respectively. Mortality, complications, and LOS during follow-up were compared between groups.

Findings.—The initial LOS was shorter in the endovascular group: the median was 5 days compared with 8 days in the open repair group. However,

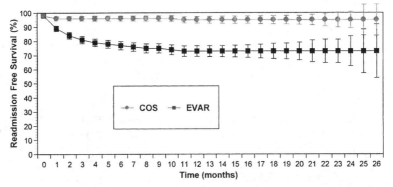

FIGURE.—Readmission-free survival rate after abdominal aortic aneurysm (AAA) repair. Readmission-free survival rate at 12 months was 95% for conventional open aneurysm surgery (COS) versus 71% for endovascular AAA repair (EVAR; *P* < .001). Patients for EVAR continued to be at risk for readmission in later follow-up period, whereas patients for COS were unlikely to be readmitted for AAA-related reasons beyond first month after AAA repair. (Reprinted by permission of the publisher from Carpenter JP, Baum RA, Barker CF, et al: Durability of benefits of endovascular versus conventional abdominal aortic aneurysm repair. *J Vasc Surg* 35:222-228, 2002. Copyright 2002 by Elsevier.)

patients undergoing endovascular AAA repair were more likely to require readmission during follow-up: the 12-month readmission-free survival rate was 71% in the endovascular group compared with 95% in the open repair group (Fig). Including readmissions, total hospital days were not significantly different between groups: 11 days for endovascular and 13.6 days for open repair. An endoleak was the most common reason for readmission in the endovascular group, followed by wound infection and graft limb thrombosis. Women undergoing open repair had a longer initial LOS than men. In the endovascular group, the readmission rate and LOS on readmission were also higher for women.

Conclusions.—In patients undergoing AAA repair, the initial LOS is shorter after endovascular repair than after conventional open repair. However, endovascular repair has a higher readmission rate, negating the advantage in terms of total hospital days. Women may have a higher rate of complications after both open and endovascular repair.

▶ Catheter-based procedures have an important role in modern vascular surgery. However, with endovascular AAA repair, it appears initial enthusiasm with this procedure as routine treatment needs to be, at least temporarily, tempered. It may be the Emperor has no clothes. The majority of papers on endovascular AAA repair now focus on the problems with the procedure. Most of the purported benefits such as decreased cost, decreased length of stay, decreased perioperative mortality rate, and increased quality of life all seem to vanish when one gets beyond the first couple of months postoperatively. Patients want the procedure because surgeons sometimes push it, the popular media pushes it, and company Web sites and advertisements also push it. However, if all the hype and advertisements went away and Web sites were replaced by abstracts, I bet patient interest would decrease substantially.

G. L. Moneta, MD

Device Migration After Endoluminal Abdominal Aortic Aneurysm Repair: Analysis of 113 Cases With a Minimum Follow-up Period of 2 Years
Cao P, Verzini F, Zannetti S, et al (Univ of Perugia, Italy)
J Vasc Surg 35:229-235, 2002   7–14

Purpose.—Device migration is a potential cause of late failure of endovascular aneurysm repair. The rate of and risk factors for device migration after endograft repair of an abdominal aortic aneurysm (AAA) were evaluated.

Methods.—One hundred forty-eight patients who underwent endoluminal AAA repair over a 2-year period were analyzed. All patients received Medtronic-AVE AneuRX modular endografts with infrarenal fixation. Patients underwent CT scanning at regular intervals. Two-year follow-up data, including a total of 418 CT scans, were available for review in 113 patients. The scans were read in a blinded fashion. Device migration was defined as a change of at least 10 mm in the distance between the lower renal artery and the first visible portion of the endograft.

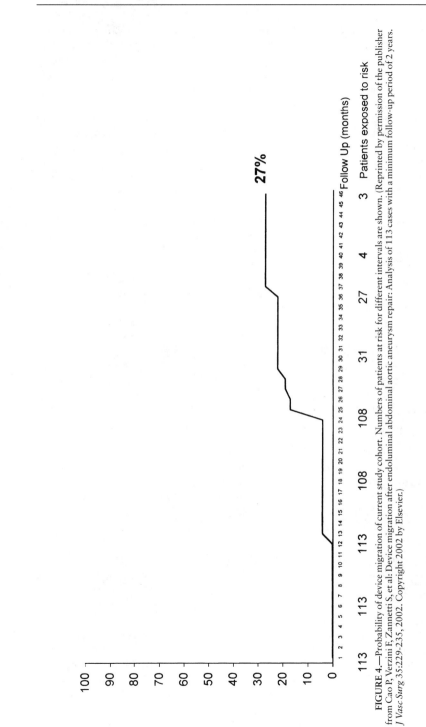

FIGURE 4.—Probability of device migration of current study cohort. Numbers of patients at risk for different intervals are shown. (Reprinted by permission of the publisher from Cao P, Verzini F, Zannetti S, et al: Device migration after endoluminal abdominal aortic aneurysm repair: Analysis of 113 cases with a minimum follow-up period of 2 years. *J Vasc Surg* 35:229-235, 2002. Copyright 2002 by Elsevier.)

Results.—One AAA ruptured. The rate of CT-detected device migration was 15%. Of these 17 patients, 8 underwent additional interventions, consisting of proximal cuff placement in 6 patients and late conversion to open repair in 2. Two independent predictors of device migration were identified: AAA neck enlargement of greater than 10% after endoluminal repair (hazard ratio, 7.3) and preoperative aneurysmal diameter of 55 mm or greater. On life-table analysis, the 36-month probability of device migration was 27% (Fig 4).

Conclusions.—Device migration is a common occurrence after endoluminal AAA repair. The risk of this complication is elevated for patients with large aneurysms or dilation of the infrarenal aortic neck.

▶ I think it is important to note 2 things from this paper. First, about one fourth of the patients treated with the AneuRx graft will have migration of the device. Second, this migration is associated with factors that are surgeon independent and disease dependent; that is, enlargement of the neck and treatment of large AAAs.

Since one might predict that device migration will lead to type I endoleak and type I endoleaks are associated with aneurysm rupture, it is clear that improved proximal fixation is urgently needed for at least the AneuRx device. That ticking sound may be getting a little louder.

G. L. Moneta, MD

Aortic Neck Angulation Predicts Adverse Outcome With Endovascular Abdominal Aortic Aneurysm Repair
Sternbergh WC III, Carter G, York JW, et al (Ochsner Clinic and Found, New Orleans, La)
J Vasc Surg 35:482-486, 2002   7–15

Introduction.—Significant aortic neck angulation may predispose patients to a suboptimal outcome after endovascular abdominal aortic aneurysm (EAAA) repair. The effect of aortic neck angulation on the incidence of early and delayed adverse events after EAAA repair was examined.

Methods.—Prospectively collected data on 148 consecutive EAAA repairs performed between December 1995 and January 2001 were supplemented with a retrospective review of medical records and radiographs. Aortic neck angulation was measured from either arteriograms or 3-dimensional CT scanning reconstructions. Twenty-four patients were excluded because their radiographs were not available for review. Because of a paucity of severe aortic neck angulation in other endograft groups, only 81 patients who were treated with a modular bifurcated device were included in the final analysis. The mean time from implantation to assessment was 26.6 months. The angle between the proximal aortic neck and the longitudinal axis of the aneurysm was used to define the aortic neck angulation (Fig 1).

Results.—The risk of a patient experiencing 1 or more adverse events was 70% for 10 patients with severe ($\geq$60°) aortic neck angulation; these rates

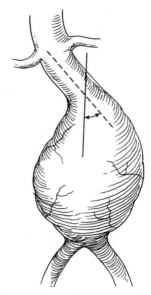

FIGURE 1.—Measurement of aortic neck angulation. (Reprinted by permission of the publisher from Sternbergh WC III, Carter G, York JW, et al: Aortic neck angulation predicts adverse outcome with endovascular abdominal aortic aneurysm repair. *J Vasc Surg* 35:482-486, 2002. Copyright 2002 by Elsevier.)

were 54.5% for 11 patients with moderate aortic neck angulation (40-59°) and 16.6% for 60 patients with mild (<40°) aortic neck angulation (*P* = .0003). The adverse events for patients with severe or moderate versus mild aortic neck angulation were death within 30 days (20% vs 0%), early conversion to open repair (20% vs 0%; *P* = .0007), aneurysm expansion (9.1%-20% vs 1.7%; *P* = .034), device migration (20%-30% vs 3.3%; *P* = .013), and a type I endoleak (23.8% vs 8.3%; *P* = .033). No significant between-group differences were found in aortic neck length and diameter, age, or medical comorbidities.

Conclusion.—Aortic neck angulation seems to be an important determinant of the outcome after EAAA repair. Patients with mild angulation had favorable outcomes in this cohort; those with moderate or severe angulation had a 54% to 70% risk of 1 or more adverse events. These outcomes occurred despite an adequate length (>2 cm) of proximal aortic neck. Great caution is needed when recommending EAAA repair in patients with an aortic neck angulation of 40° or greater.

▶ The word on the street is that the threshold for trouble with aortic neck angulation is 60%. It appears the street needs to be better informed. However, while the data here are concerning for angulation of between 40% and 59%, there are only 11 patients in this category. I don't think we can yet say neck angulations of 40% to 59% preclude EAAA repair. Neck angulation between 40% and 59%, however, clearly is a cause for concern. Neck angulation of this magnitude may tip the balance, depending on circumstances, for the thoughtful surgeon considering whether to recommend EAAA repair or open repair to an individual patient.

G. L. Moneta, MD

Conformational Changes Associated With Proximal Seal Zone Failure in Abdominal Aortic Endografts
Parra JR, Ayerdi J, McLafferty R, et al (Southern Illinois Univ, Springfield, Ill)
J Vasc Surg 37:106-111, 2003   7–16

Background.—After endovascular repair for abdominal aortic aneurysms (AAAs), the excluded aneurysm sac remains with a small risk for rupture. There are few data on conformational changes occurring in excluded AAAs. Such changes may lead to endograft failure. Patients with proximal seal zone failures occurring after endovascular repair were studied to assess the occurrence of conformational changes in the infrarenal aortas.

Methods.—The study included a series of 189 patients undergoing routine CT surveillance after aortic endograft repair of AAA. Those with type I or type III endoleaks or proximal component separation without apparent endoleak were identified. The CT scan data were used to make 3-dimensional reconstructions, and these were used to measure migration, length, volume, and angulation of the infrarenal aorta.

Findings.—Proximal seal zone failures occurred in 5 patients, for a rate of 3% (Fig 3). Aortic extender cuffs were used in 4 of these 5 patients. Measurements showed only minor alterations in AAA volume or aortic neck angle. However, mean AAA length increased by 34 mm and aortic body angulation by 17°. These changes led to proximal component separation in 4 patients, with migration in 2. Endovascular repair was performed in 2 patients and was planned in 1 other; the remaining 2 patients required removal of the endograft. One patient had recurrent proximal component separation and type III endoleak, which was managed with a custom graft.

Conclusions.—Patients with proximal seal zone failure after endovascular AAA repair show proximal angulation and lengthening of the infrarenal aorta. Most patients with this complication have aortic extender cuffs, which are a risk factor for late problems with endoleakage. The authors urge close attention to proper initial stent graft deployment to avoid the need for extender cuffs.

▶ This study emphasizes that the aorta will continue to change after endovascular AAA repair. These changes may lead to component separation. A simplistic view is that the more components used in endovascular AAA repair the more likely there will be a later problem. It all goes back to picking the patients well, not stretching the indications for endovascular AAA repair and getting it right the first time.

G. L. Moneta, MD

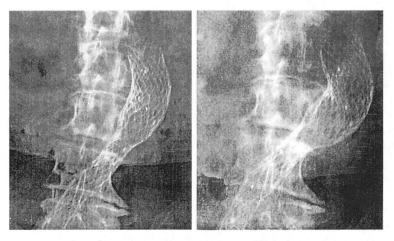

1 month   12 months

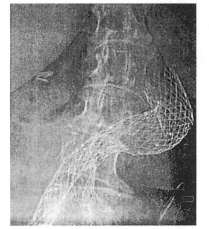

24 months

FIGURE 3.—Abdominal radiographs obtained at 1 month, 12 months, and 24 months after placement of abdominal aortic endograft. (Reprinted by permission of the publisher from Parra JR, Ayerdi J, McLafferty R, et al: Conformational changes associated with proximal seal zone failure in abdominal aortic endografts. *J Vasc Surg* 37:106-111, 2003. Copyright 2003 by Elsevier.)

Mechanical Failure of Prosthetic Human Implants: A 10-Year Experience With Aortic Stent Graft Devices

Jacobs TS, Won J, Gravereaux EC, et al (Mount Sinai School of Medicine, New York)
J Vasc Surg 37:16-26, 2003   7–17

Background.—Despite advances in endovascular stent grafting, device fatigue remains a potential complication. The incidence of device fatigue and its modes of development were examined to gain a better understanding of the clinical significance of material failure.

Methods.—The medical records of 686 patients who underwent endovascular aortic aneurysm repair during a 10-year period were examined. Follow-up radiographs and explanted stent grafts were used to determine device fatigue (ie, stent fracture, suture disruption, or graft wear). Clinical data, imaging studies, and results of scanning electron microscopy and energy dispersion spectroscopy of explanted devices were reviewed to determine the modes and consequences of graft failure.

Results.—Device fatigue was noted in 60 patients, including 49 with devices implanted in the abdominal aorta (49 of 623 devices, or 7.9%) and 11 with devices implanted in the thoracic aorta (11 of 63 devices, or 17.5%). Stent graft fatigue occurred in 7 different devices: the Vanguard, Talent, modified Parodi, EVT/Ancure, and AneuRx abdominal stents and the Gore TAG and Talent thoracic stents. In all, 43 devices had metallic stent fracture, 14 devices had suture disruption, and 3 devices had graft holes. Certain modes of failure were associated with certain stent types. For example, among the abdominal aortic devices, fatigue was detected in 16 of 22 Vanguard stents (72%), 5 of 24 modified Parodi stents (21%), 1 of 7 EVT/Ancure stents (14%), 24 of 232 Talent stents (10%), and 3 of 33 AneuRx stents (10%). Suture disruption was more frequently the cause of Vanguard stent fatigue (14 cases, or 87.5%), whereas metal fractures were responsible for fatigue in the other types of stents. Stent fatigue was recognized an average of 19 months after implantation, and patients have been followed up a mean of 8 months since stent fatigue was recognized. One patient has been lost to follow-up (2 years after device failure) and 11 patients have died 17 to 52 months after stent implantation and 2 to 26 months after stent fatigue was recognized. The remaining 48 patients are asymptomatic and continue to be monitored.

Conclusion.—Many different endovascular stents have been associated with graft fatigue after abdominal or thoracic aortic aneurysm repair. Certain modes of failure are associated with specific stent graft devices. The clinical significance of stent graft material failure is not yet clear.

▶ Given enough time, virtually every vascular intervention will fail. The questions are, how much time is acceptable and what are the consequences of the failure?

G. L. Moneta, MD

Distal Internal Iliac Artery Embolization: A Procedure to Avoid
Kritpracha B, Pigott JP, Price CI, et al (Jobst Vascular Ctr, Toledo, Ohio)
J Vasc Surg 37:943-948, 2003   7–18

Background.—As many as one third of patients with abdominal aortic aneurysm (AAA) being considered for endovascular stent grafting (ESG) have an enlarged common iliac artery. These patients often undergo stent-graft limb extension into the external iliac artery, with concurrent or prior coil embolization of the ipsilateral internal iliac artery (IIA). The reported consequences of pelvic ischemia resulting from IIA coil embolization have varied greatly in severity. Whether the placement of the coil in the IIA correlates with symptom frequency or severity was investigated.

Methods.—The subjects were 20 patients with AAA (18 men and 2 women, average age 70.5 years) who underwent ESG with unilateral coil embolization of the IIA between August 1997 and March 2002. In 8 patients the coils were placed proximal to the first branch of the IIA, while in 12 patients coils were placed distal to this point. Symptoms of pelvic ischemia and outcomes were compared between the 2 groups over a mean follow-up of 20.6 months.

Results.—Ten patients (50%) had new onset of pelvic ischemia (9 with buttock claudication, 1 with impotence) after ESG. Symptoms of ischemia were significantly more common in the patients with distal IIA embolization (9 of 12, or 75%) than in patients with proximal IIA embolization (1 of 8, or 13%). None of the patients experienced colonic ischemia. At 1-year follow-up, claudication had resolved in the 1 patient who had ischemia develop after a proximally placed coil. Of the 9 patients with ischemia after distal IIA embolization, 4 were symptom free at 12 months, but 4 had significant, persistent claudication at 1 to 2 years after embolization.

Conclusion.—In patients with AAA who require IIA coil embolization before ESG, symptoms of pelvic ischemia were significantly more common when the coil was placed distal to the first branch of the IIA than when it was placed proximally. Differences in coil placement may account for conflicting reports about the number and severity of symptoms associated with IIA coil embolization in the literature. These findings suggest that when IIA coils are necessary, they should be placed as proximally in the IIA as possible to prevent interrupting pelvic collateral circulation.

▶ If you have to embolize the internal iliac arteries before endovascular AAA repair, it appears important to keep the coils as proximal as possible. Perhaps the need to embolize the internal iliac arteries should be among the increasing number of relative contraindications to endovascular AAA repair (see also Abstract 7–19).

G. L. Moneta, MD

Internal Iliac Occlusion Without Coil Embolization During Endovascular Abdominal Aortic Aneurysm Repair

Wyers MC, Schermerhorn ML, Fillinger MF, et al (Dartmouth-Hitchcock Med Ctr, Lebanon, NH)
J Vasc Surg 36:1138-1145, 2002   7–19

Background.—From 20% to 30% of patients with abdominal aortic aneurysms (AAAs) have aneurysms involving at least one common iliac artery (CIA), making endovascular management of the internal iliac artery (IIA) an important consideration. When concomitant AAA and CIA repair is needed, endograft limb extension is often required, with the IIA often embolized to prevent endoleak (Fig 1). The authors have chosen to use coil embolization of the IIA only when there is inadequate stent graft seal in the CIA immediately proximal to the IIA origin. The outcomes of this approach were evaluated.

Methods.—Two hundred four consecutive endovascular AAA repairs performed between 1996 and 2001 were evaluated retrospectively. Most were primarily imaged by using CT angiography with 3-dimensional reconstruction. The presence before surgery of adequate graft oversizing (at least 10%-15%) in the most distal 5 mm of CIA and 15 mm of proximal external iliac artery formed the basis for choosing to cover the IIA without concomitant coil embolization. In 31 patients, 33 IIAs were occluded. For 67% of cases, the IIA was covered without coil embolization (COVER group), and for 33% of cases where the graft oversizing was inadequate in the CIA, the IIA had coil embolization (COIL group).

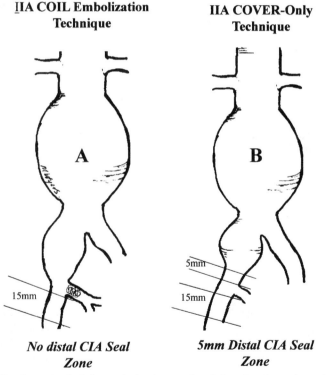

IIA COIL Embolization Technique

IIA COVER-Only Technique

No distal CIA Seal Zone

5mm Distal CIA Seal Zone

FIGURE 1.—Anatomic criteria for standard and cover only techniques in patients who need endograft extension into external iliac. **A,** Internal iliac artery (*IIA*) coil embolization is required because of absence of seal in distal common iliac artery (*CIA*). **B,** Presence of distal CIA seal zone (≥5 mm length) is needed for IIA coverage without coil embolization. (Reprinted by permission of the publisher from Wyers MC, Schermerhorn ML, Fillinger MF, et al: Internal iliac occlusion without coil embolization during endovascular abdominal aortic aneurysm repair. *J Vasc Surg* 36:1138-1145, 2002. Copyright 2002 by Elsevier.)

Results.—Technically, all the procedures in both groups were successful and showed no evidence of endoleak, stent graft migrations, or enlargements of the aneurysm on angiography. The mean follow-up was 19 months in the COVER group and 10 months in the COIL group. Four patients died of causes unrelated to endovascular repair or IIA occlusion. COIL group patients tended to have more serious postoperative lower extremity ischemic symptoms than COVER group patients. Two COIL patients had significant adverse events that most likely resulted from coil embolization.

Conclusions.—In all cases, covering the IIA without coiling excluded the CIA aneurysm effectively and carried a low rate of complications in comparison with the use of coil embolization. Coil embolization of the IIA may not be needed if detailed preoperative imaging is used and patients are carefully selected.

▶ This study serves as a nice focus of what to do with the hypogastric artery during endovascular AAA repair. A reasonable summary is as follows: (1) Save the hypogastric artery if you can. (2) If you need to take both hypogastric arteries, it appears better to stage the hypogastric occlusions. (3) If there are appropriate lengths of "normal" caliber artery proximal and distal to the origin of the hypogastric artery, then coiling of the artery may not be necessary at the time of repair. In these cases, simple coverage of the vessel by the graft seems to be sufficient.

G. L. Moneta, MD

Potential Impact of Therapeutic Warfarin Treatment on Type II Endoleaks and Sac Shrinkage Rates on Midterm Follow-up Examination
Fairman RM, Carpenter JP, Baum RA, et al (Univ of Pennsylvania, Philadelphia)
J Vasc Surg 35:679-685, 2002   7–20

Background.—Long-term postoperative anticoagulation treatment in patients with endovascular aortic aneurysm repair may delay or prevent sac thrombosis and result in endoleak fomation and altered aneurysm sac remodeling. Whether chronic warfarin treatment was associated with an increased incidence of early or delayed postoperative endoleaks or altered rates of reduction in aneurysm sac maximum diameter was investigated.

Methods.—During a 32-month period, 232 consecutive patients underwent abdominal aortic endografting. The mean follow-up was 18 months. Patients with endoleaks detected by CT angiograms 30 days after surgery subsequently had selective arteriography to characterize the source. Thirty-six patients receiving warfarin after surgery comprised the study group.

Findings.—At 30 days, 43 patients (18%) had endoleaks on CT angiograms. Thirty-nine had type II endoleaks, and 4 had type I endoleaks. None of the type I endoleaks were in warfarin recipients. All type I endoleaks were repaired with proximal or distal covered extensions. At 30 days, type II endoleaks were noted n 19.4% of the warafarin group and in 18.4% of the control group. Delayed type II endoleaks developed in 2 warfarin recipients and in 2 control group patients. Thirty-one percent of the control group had spontaneous resolution of type II endoleaks. Spontaneous endoleak thrombosis did not occur in the warfarin group. Aneurysm sac remodeling, evaluated by the mean percent reduction in maximum sac diameter at 12 months, was less in the warfarin versus control group.

Conclusions.—Warfarin treatment appears to be unrelated to increases in the incidence of early or delayed postoperative endoleaks. However, patients receiving warfarin therapy had a slower rate of reduction in maximum aneurysm sac diameter after aortic endografting at 1-year follow-up. Also, type II endoleaks appear to be less likely to thrombose spontaneously in patients taking warfarin.

▶ The authors state "aneurysm sac thrombosis with remodeling and shrinkage is the goal of endovascular aneurysm repair." I think the real goal is prevention of death from aneurysm rupture. If the aneurysms never ruptured after endovascular repair no one would care if the sac didn't shrink, thrombose, or remodel. Making up end points to get a paper on a meeting is not unique to this group. Everyone is guilty now and then. However, pointing out inconsistencies of logic is one of the duties of editing the YEAR BOOK OF VASCULAR SURGERY. By the way, it appears okay to give endovascular repair patients warfarin if they need it.

G. L. Moneta, MD

The Sac Shrinking Process After EAR Does Not Start Immediately in Most Patients

Prinssen M, Blankensteijn JD (Univ Med Ctr, Utrecht, The Netherlands)
Eur J Vasc Endovasc Surg 23:426-430, 2002   7–21

Background.—Shrinkage of the aneurysm sac an important indicator of a successful exclusion after endovascular aneurysm repair (EAR). The mechanism underlying this process is still unknown. If an aneurysm sac is not completely excluded from the arterial circulation, the pressure within the aneurysm sac may still be higher than the intra-abdominal pressure. The aneurysm may then continue to grow. However, if an aneurysm is completely excluded, it will be depressurized; in other words, the pressure in the aneurysm sac will fall to the value of the intra-abdominal pressure. The purpose of this study was to determine the pattern of shrinkage after EAR—using logarithmic, exponential, and linear models—and to calculate any lag time that may be present.

Methods.—The study group comprised 29 patients evaluated with spiral CT angiography 2 years after EAR. Six logarithmic, exponential, and linear functions, all with and without lag time, were fitted to the thrombus volume obtained by postoperative measurement and at 6, 12, and 24 months. The correlation coefficient was used to determine the association between the calculated and measured values. A correlation coefficient greater than 0.95 was considered a good fit.

Results.—The best fits were obtained with a logarithmic model. Of the 29 patients, only 2 patients could not be described by any model. The remaining 27 patients could be fitted with the use of a logarithmic function with a correlation coefficient of greater than 0.95. Of these 27 patients, 22 had a lag time ranging from 5.8 to 252.3 days (median, 63.4 days). Only 5 of the initial 44 patients (11%) showed immediate shrinkage of the aneurysm sac.

Conclusion.—Nearly all of the shrinkage processes in these EAR patients could be described by a logarithmic function. A lag time to shrinkage could be calculated in over 75% of patients. In only a small proportion of patients did the shrinking process begin immediately after EAR.

▶ The authors focus on a mathematical model to describe sac shrinkage after EAR. Sac shrinkage after EAR turns out to be like beginning a workout program after several years of inactivity. It takes a while for anything to happen. I wonder if the lag time relates to the time required for thrombus contraction to occur?

G. L. Moneta, MD

Variation in Death Rate After Abdominal Aortic Aneurysmectomy in the United States: Impact of Hospital Volume, Gender, and Age

Dimick JB, Stanley JC, Axelrod DA, et al (Univ of Michigan, Ann Arbor; Wayne State Univ, Detroit)
Ann Surg 235:579-585, 2002   7–22

Background.—Interest in regionalization of high-risk surgical procedures, such as aortic aneurysmectomy, to high-volume hospitals (HVHs) has been increasing as a method for reducing the number of perioperative deaths. A clear association has been demonstrated between hospital volume and improved outcomes for several complex vascular surgical procedures, including abdominal aortic aneurysm (AAA) repair. Several population-based studies, using state discharge data, have consistently shown lower surgical death rates at HVHs. However, the validity of these studies is questionable because in many states, there are only a few HVHs. Thus, the effect of volume on outcome may be overestimated if a single HVH has a much lower number of perioperative deaths relative to other HVHs. In contrast, the effect may be underestimated if certain low-volume hospitals (LVHs) demonstrate a much lower number of perioperative deaths compared with other LVH hospitals. To determine whether HVHs do have lower in-hospital death rates after AAA repair compared with those of LVHs, a retrospective study was conducted.

Methods.—The study included 13,887 patients undergoing repair of intact or ruptured AAAs in the Nationwide Inpatient Sample for 1996 and 1997. The Nationwide Inpatient Sample is a 20% stratified random sample representative of all US hospitals.

Results.—The overall death rate was 3.8% for intact AAA repair and 47% for ruptured AAA repair. HVHs had a lower death rate than that of

TABLE 4.—Results of the Multivariate Analysis: Independent Variables Associated With an Increased Risk of In-Hospital Death

Independent Variable	Risk of In-Hospital Death, Odds Ratio (95% CI)	P Value†
Intact Abdominal Aortic Aneurysm Repair		
Low hospital volume*	1.71 (1.37-2.14)	<.001
Emergent admission	3.48 (2.66-4.54)	<.001
Female gender	1.34 (1.04-1.73)	.02
Age >65 years	2.23 (1.94-3.34)	<.001
History of myocardial infarction	1.78 (1.11-2.85)	.02
Mild liver disease	4.86 (2.30-10.26)	<.001
Ruptured Abdominal Aortic Aneurysm Repair		
Low hospital volume*	1.43 (1.15-1.78)	.001
Urgent admission	2.06 (1.14-3.72)	.02
Emergent admission	2.39 (1.40-4.08)	.001
Female gender	1.69 (1.28-2.22)	<.001
Age >65 years	1.98 (1.41-2.76)	<.001
Nonwhite race	1.60 (1.06-2.41)	.03
History of myocardial infarction	1.64 (1.02-2.64)	.04
Mild liver disease	7.40 (1.56-35.05)	.01
Malignancy	2.76 (1.09-6.99)	.03

*Low hospital volume was considered less than 30 procedures per year.
†Statistical test for independent association of the variable to in-hospital death.
Abbreviation: CI, Confidence index.
(Courtesy of Dimick JB, Stanley JC, Axelrod DA, et al: Variation in death rate after abdominal aortic aneurysmectomy in the United States: Impact of hospital volume, gender, and age. *Ann Surg* 235:579-585, 2002.

LVHs for repair of intact AAAs. The death rate after repair of a ruptured AAA was also slightly lower at HVHs. Multivariate analysis with adjustment for case mix showed that having surgery at an LVH was associated with a 56% increased risk for in-hospital death. Other independent risk factors for in-hospital death included female sex, older than 65 years, a ruptured aneurysm, urgent or emergent admission, and the presence of co-morbid disease (Table 4).

Conclusion.—Data from a representative database reveal that HVHs have a significantly lower death rate than LVHs for repair of both intact and ruptured AAA. These findings support the regionalization of patients to HVHs for AAA repair.

▶ Administrators of small hospitals probably hate volume-related papers. I doubt they put them on their Web sites. One also is curious as to what the American Board of Surgery thinks.

G. L. Moneta, MD

Open Infrarenal Abdominal Aortic Aneurysm Repair: The Cleveland Clinic Experience From 1989 to 1998

Hertzer NR, Mascha EJ, Karafa MT, et al (Cleveland Clinic Found, Ohio)
J Vasc Surg 35:1145-1154, 2002   7–23

Background.—The safety and durability of traditional open surgical treatment for asymptomatic infrarenal abdominal aortic aneurysms (AAAs) was investigated in a large series of patients who underwent open operation before the commercial availability of stent graft devices for endovascular AAA repair.

Methods.—From 1989 to 1998, 1135 consecutive patients (985 men and 150 women) underwent elective graft replacement of infrarenal AAAs. Computerized perioperative data, hospital charts and outpatient records, and a telephone canvass were used to calculate the survival rates and the incidence rate of subsequent graft-related complications. The median follow-up for the entire series was 57 months, during which time 74 patients (6.5%) were lost to follow-up.

Results.—The 30-day mortality rate was 1.2%. The hospital course was completely uneventful for 939 patients (83%), and the median length of stay overall was 8 days. Single or multiple postoperative complications occurred in 196 patients; these complications were more likely to occur in men and in patients with a history of congestive heart failure, chronic pulmonary disease, or renal insufficiency. Kaplan-Meier survival estimates were 75% at 5 years and 49% at 10 years (Fig 1).

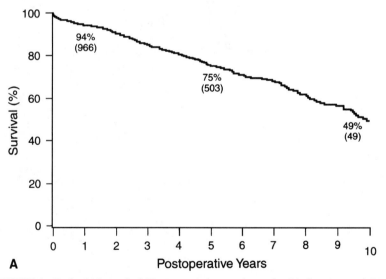

FIGURE 1.—Kaplan-Meier method 10-year survival rate estimates for (**A**) all patients and (**B**) age quartiles. (Reprinted by permission of the publisher from Hertzer NR, Mascha EJ, Karafa MT, et al: Open infrarenal abdominal aortic aneurysm repair: The Cleveland Clinic experience from 1989 to 1998. *J Vasc Surg* 35:1145-1154, 2002. Copyright 2002 by Elsevier.)

Long-term mortality rate was influenced primarily by age more than 75 years, a previous history of congestive heart failure, chronic pulmonary disease, or renal insufficiency. A total of 1047 patients survived their operation and were available for follow-up study; only 4 (0.4%) of these patients have had late complications related to their aortic replacement grafts.

Conclusion.—The success of open infrarenal AAA repair is confirmed by these findings. The use of stent grafts should be justified by the presence of serious surgical risk factors until the long-term outcome of the current generation of stent grafts is adequately documented.

▶ Open AAA repair works very well at the Cleveland Clinic. The mortality rate of 1.2% in this series will be difficult for most centers to duplicate. Note particularly that only 4 (0.4%) of 1047 patients surviving open repair had late complications related to their aortic grafts. This seems unbelievably low and certainly contrasts with recent results of endovascular aneurysm repair. If these results with open repair are correct, one wonders how all but the highest risk patients at the Cleveland Clinic can be ethically offered an endovascular aneurysm repair.

G. L. Moneta, MD

Outcome in Patients at High Risk After Open Surgical Repair of Abdominal Aortic Aneurysm
Menard MT, Chew DKW, Chan RK, et al (Brigham and Women's Hosp, Boston)
J Vasc Surg 37:285-292, 2003   7–24

Background.—Endovascular therapy has been proposed as an alternative to surgical repair of abdominal aortic aneurysm (AAA) in patients considered at high risk. However, the outcomes after surgery in high-risk AAA patients remain unclear. The short-term and long-term outcomes of open infrarenal AAA repair were compared for high- and low-risk patients.

Methods.—The study included 572 consecutive patients undergoing open surgery to repair nonruptured infrarenal AAA from 1990 to 2000. According to criteria of age 80 or older, creatinine concentration 3.0 mg/dL or higher, severe pulmonary insufficiency, severe cardiac dysfunction, or liver failure, 22% of the patients were considered to be at high risk. These patients' short-term and long-term outcomes were compared with those of the low-risk patients.

Results.—The 30-day operative mortality rate was much higher in the high-risk group: 4.7%, compared with 0 in the low-risk group. Overall morbidity was 29% for high-risk patients and 17% for low-risk patients; rates of serious morbidity were 14% versus 5%, respectively. The 5-year survival rate was 46% for high-risk patients versus 74% for the low-risk cohort. All patients with 3 high-risk factors died within 3 years after AAA repair (Fig 2).

Conclusions.—This experience shows relatively good safety and short-term results in high-risk patients undergoing open surgical AAA repair. However, fewer than half of the high-risk patients are still alive 5 years after

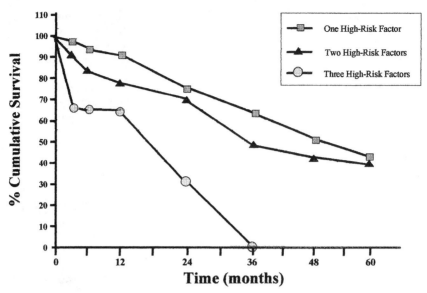

FIGURE 2.—Five-year cumulative survival rate after infrarenal AAA repair in patients with 1, 2, and 3 high-risk factors. (Reprinted by permission of the publisher from Menard MT, Chew DKW, Chan RK, et al: Outcome in patients at high risk after open surgical repair of abdominal aortic aneurysm. *J Vasc Surg* 37:285-292, 2003. Copyright 2003 by Elsevier.)

surgery. The findings have important implications for patient selection; the short-term postoperative mortality rate for high-risk patients appears at least as good as that following endovascular repair.

▶ It is difficult to know what is high risk anymore. The definitions of high risk used in this study are reasonable but, as the authors admit, there is no information about patients turned down for surgery. These types of studies are often used for comparison of outcomes with endovascular aneurysm repair patients. Such studies, however, are of no use in that regard in that issues of operative risk and outcome of different procedures are nearly impossible to address in retrospective studies. What we can conclude is that good surgeons, exercising good judgment, will get good results with open aneurysm repair across a wide spectrum of patients. We can't conclude much more.

G. L. Moneta, MD

Postoperative Regression of Retroperitoneal Fibrosis in Patients With Inflammatory Abdominal Aortic Aneurysms: Evaluation With Spiral Computed Tomography

Pistolese GR, Ippoliti A, Mauriello A, et al (Univ of Rome "Tor Vergata")
Ann Vasc Surg 16:201-209, 2002   7–25

Background.—A new series evaluating regression of aortic and retroperitoneal fibrosis after surgery for inflammatory abdominal aortic aneurysm (AAA) is presented.

Methods and Findings.—Nineteen consecutive men and 2 women (mean age, 66 years) with inflammatory AAA were operated on at one center. The patients underwent preoperative CT angiography, abdominal US, and aortoiliac angiography. No perioperative deaths occurred. The perioperative morbidity rate was 9.5%. The aortic wall was studied histologically in 95.2% of the patients, and an inflammatory index was calculated. Postoperatively, all patients were reassessed with spiral CT angiography. Patients with higher intraoperative determination of inflammatory indices in the aneurysmal wall had significantly more improvement postoperatively. The time course and progression of regression varied. Overall, improvement was more marked in the early months after surgery, with significant slowing after the second or third year.

Conclusions.—In most patients, retroperitoneal fibrosis associated with inflammatory AAAs regresses after surgery. Spiral CT angiography provides detailed information on the aneurysmal wall and adjacent structures in the monitoring of postoperative evolution of the fibrotic process.

▶ This study is included to point out it is possible to get very good results repairing inflammatory abdominal aortic aneurysms by a transperitoneal approach. The surgical approach to an inflammatory aneurysm should be individualized based on the pattern of fibrosis and surgeon familiarity with technique. In addition, whereas improvement of perianeurysmal fibrosis following repair generally occurs, complete resolution is unusual (24%), and a few patients show no improvement (10%).

G. L. Moneta, MD

Minimally Invasive Vascular Surgery for Repair of Infrarenal Abdominal Aortic Aneurysm With Iliac Involvement

Matsumoto M, Hata T, Tsushima Y, et al (Sakakibara Hosp, Okayama, Japan)
J Vasc Surg 35:654-660, 2002   7–26

Introduction.—A minimally invasive vascular surgery (MIVS) technique for repair of infrarenal abdominal aortic aneurysms (AAAs) with iliac involvement was examined and its outcome compared with conventional open repair.

Methods.—Twenty patients with AAAs with iliac involvement underwent treatment with bifurcated graft replacement and the use of the MIVS approach. The procedure was performed with the use of a mini-laparotomy. The incision length was made according to the extent of the AAA, as determined by US scanning; the small incision was confined completely within the abdominal cavity. The proximal and distal surgical field are accessed by changing the patient's position and arranging for the abdominal incision to be retracted cephalad and caudad (Fig 1). The perioperative courses in these 20 patients (the MIVS group) were examined in comparison with 14 patients who underwent conventional open repair, performed through a full midline laparotomy.

Results.—A mean incision length of 8.4 cm (range, 6.5-11.2 cm) was used for the MIVS technique for AAA repair. Patients in the MIVS group had an earlier resumption of oral intake and ambulation than did the conventional group (liquid diet: 1.1 vs 2.9 days, $P < .01$; solid diet: 2.0 vs 3.9 days, $P < .01$; ambulation: 2.1 vs 4.3 days, $P < .01$). Mortality and morbidity rates were similar for both groups. Patients in the MIVS group were discharged earlier than were patients in the conventional group (20.7 vs 33.9 days; $P < .01$), and their total hospitalization cost was significantly lower (¥2,232,791 vs ¥2,640,441; $P < .01$).

Conclusion.—The MIVS technique was associated with earlier postoperative recovery, but rates of morbidity and mortality were comparable to the conventional technique. The MIVS group had significantly shorter hospital lengths of stay and total hospital charges than did the conventional group. The MIVS technique may be considered an effective minimally invasive approach for open AAA repair.

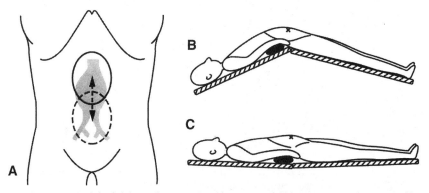

FIGURE 1.—**A,** Shift of abdominal incision. Suitable operating field for aneurysm neck is acquired by retracting abdominal incision together with retroperitoneum cephalad, with patient in arched back position. Conversely, operating field for iliac region is obtained by retracting abdominal incision together with retroperitoneum caudad with patient in reversed jackknife position. **B,** Arched back position. In supine position, patient arched both legs and upper back downwards about 10° on either side (arched back position). Placing water bag against patient's back (*black ellipse*) helped in projecting upper abdomen further, where aneurysm neck exists. **C,** Reversed jackknife position. Both upper and lower halves of patient's body were slightly elevated from horizontal level to relax abdominal skin and release muscle tension. In this position, caudal retraction was performed more effectively. (Reprinted by permission of the publisher from Matsumoto M, Hata T, Tsushima Y, et al: Minimally invasive vascular surgery for repair of infrarenal abdominal aortic aneurysm with iliac involvement. *J Vasc Surg* 35:654-660, 2002. Copyright 2002 by Elsevier.)

▶ The Japanese can also do mini-laparotomies for repair of AAAs. Dr Turnipseed should be proud. However, the amazingly long length of stays permitted by the Japanese health system are what impressed me the most. A large majority of patients stayed in the hospital for 2 weeks, with the median length of stay for patients undergoing standard open repair being more than 1 month! It seems to me the benefits of mini-laparotomy for AAA repair should be evident early in the postoperative course. Why mini-laparotomies should affect hospital stays at greater than 2 weeks when both standard and mini-laparotomy repair patients were eating and ambulating by 4 days postoperatively makes no sense. Observational bias may be the primary reason for the authors' results.

G. L. Moneta, MD

8 Aortoiliac Disease

Evidence for Heritability of Abdominal Aortic Calcific Deposits in the Framingham Heart Study
O'Donnell CJ, Chazaro I, Wilson PWF, et al (Natl Heart Lung and Blood Inst's Framingham Heart Study, Mass; Harvard Med School, Boston; Boston Univ; et al)
Circulation 106:337-341, 2002   8–1

Introduction.—Radiographic findings of abdominal aortic calcific (AAC) deposits are indicative of aortic atherosclerosis and are independently predictive of cardiovascular disease events. Data regarding the heritability of aortic calcification are sparse and were examined in the original cohort of the Framingham Heart Study.

Methods.—A total of 2151 participants from 1109 extended pedigrees underwent lateral lumbar radiographs. The presence and severity of AAC deposits at the level of the first through fourth lumbar vertebrae were graded with a previously validated rating scale. Correlation coefficients were determined in pairs of siblings, parents–offspring, and spouses.

Results.—Age-, sex-, and multivariable-adjusted correlation coefficients for AAC deposits in spouse pairs was –0.02. The estimated heritability for age-, sex-, and multivariable-adjusted AAC was 0.49 ($P < .001$). Thirty-one percent of overall variance in the AAC deposits was the result of measured covariates, and 49% was the result of heritable factors.

Conclusion.—Heritable factors had an important role in the presence and extent of AAC deposits. A marked portion of the variation in AAC deposits is caused by additive effects of genes, which have not yet been characterized. Measures of aortic atherosclerosis may provide heritable quantitative phenotypes for assessment of atherosclerosis in human populations.

▶ Measurements of aortic wall calcification on plain x-rays is an insensitive and antiquated method of detecting the presence of early atherosclerosis. The authors suggest their data provide a measure of the heritability of atherosclerosis. However, what they really have shown is only heritability of atherosclerotic plaques that produce calcium in the abdominal aorta, nothing more in my opinion.

G. L. Moneta, MD

Prospective Comparison of MRA With Catheter Angiography in the Assessment of Patients With Aortoiliac Occlusion Before Surgery or Endovascular Therapy

Torreggiani WC, Varghese J, Haslam P, et al (Beaumont Hosp, Dublin; Vancouver Gen Hosp, British Columbia, Canada)
Clin Radiol 57:625-631, 2002   8-2

Introduction.—Three-dimensional (3D) gadolinium-enhanced MR angiography (CE MRA) allows ultrafast acquisition of volumetric data during gadolinium-induced T1 shortening of blood. This results in a study with high signal-to-noise and contrast-to-noise ratios with minimal movement or flow artifacts traditionally observed with time-of-flight and phase-contrast MRA. The usefulness of CE MRA as an alternative to translumbar or brachial angiography was examined in the preoperative workup of patients with aortoiliac occlusion.

Methods.—Nineteen patients (14 men, 5 women; mean age, 62 years; range, 45-77 years) with contraindications for transfemoral angiography (18, aortoiliac occlusion; 1, infected femorofemoral graft with femoral artery pseudoaneurysm) underwent preoperative CE MRA and catheter angiography (5, translumbar; 14, brachial). For CE MRA, a 3D fast spoiled gradient-recalled pulse sequence was used during a 32-second breath-hold with IV injection of 40 mL of gadolinium diethylenetriaminepentaacetic acid. All patients underwent subsequent surgical or percutaneous transluminal treatment (13 and 6 patients, respectively). The accuracy of CE MRA was assessed by means of catheter angiography as the gold standard.

Results.—Accurate information was provided by CE MRA regarding the occlusive lesion, flow, and distal run-off in most patients. Accuracy in detecting occlusive lesions of the aorta, iliac segment, and common femoral segment was 94.7%, 98.7%, and 100%, respectively. The arterial segments distal to the common femoral artery were not totally visualized in 4 patients; however, CE MRA provided adequate information for planning either surgical or percutaneous transluminal therapy in all except 1 patient.

Conclusion.—The CE MRA approach was highly accurate in identifying the presence and extent of aortoiliac occlusions.

▶ Diagnostic contrast angiography for aortoiliac disease is rapidly heading for the crapper.

G. L. Moneta, MD

Surgical Reconstruction Without Preoperative Angiography in Patients With Aortoiliac Occlusive Disease

Ardin AB, Karacagil S, Hellberg A, et al (Univ Hosp, Uppsala, Sweden)
Ann Vasc Surg 16:273-278, 2002   8–3

Introduction.—The feasibility of performing surgical reconstructions in patients with aortoiliac disease with duplex scanning findings alone was examined retrospectively.

Methods.—Between January 1995 and December 1999, the medical records of 112 patients undergoing lower extremity arterial duplex scanning that demonstrated aortoiliac occlusive disease or inconclusive findings were reviewed. Of these patients, 44 underwent surgery with the use of findings obtained solely from preoperative duplex scanning. The median age of these 26 men and 18 women was 68 years (range, 49-88 years). The results of preoperative duplex scanning were compared with surgical findings.

Results.—In the subgroup of 44 patients who had surgery based only on duplex scanning findings, 17 underwent aortobifemoral/iliac bypass, 6 underwent iliofemoral bypass, 19 underwent femorofemoral bypass, and 2 underwent axillobifemoral bypass. In patients undergoing aortobifemoral/iliac bypass grafting, no deviations from preoperatively planned surgical reconstructions occurred. The technical details of the interventions in limbs undergoing iliofemoral and femorofemoral grafting based on duplex scanning were also in agreement with surgical findings in all but 1 patient. In the 2 patients who underwent axillobifemoral bypass grafting, the sites of distal anastomoses were correctly selected with the use of duplex scanning.

Conclusion.—Duplex scanning offers valuable information concerning therapeutic decision making in patients with aortoiliac occlusive disease. Surgical reconstructions without preoperative angiography can be safely performed with the use of duplex scanning as the sole preoperative diagnostic modality in patients with conclusive duplex findings of aortoiliac occlusive disease.

▶ All types of nails are closing the coffin of diagnostic arteriography for atherosclerotic aortoiliac disease. RIP. (See also Abstract 8–2.)

G. L. Moneta, MD

Long-term Results 10 Years After Iliac Arterial Stent Placement

Schürmann K, Mahnken A, Meyer J, et al (Univ of Technology of Aachen, Germany; Clinic of Ingolstadt, Germany)
Radiology 224:731-738, 2002   8–4

Background.—Iliac artery stent placement has been in clinical use for approximately 15 years, with no long-term results thus far reported. Long-term results may help improve treatment strategies and preinterventional patient information. A series of patients treated with stents for iliac arterial occlusive disease before 1991 was retrospectively evaluated.

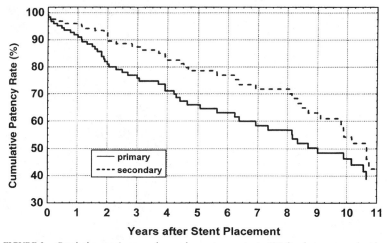

FIGURE 2.—Graph shows primary and secondary patency rates in 126 iliac lesions treated with stent placement. Data constituting the basis of this Figure are given in Table 2. (Courtesy of Schürmann K, Mahnken A, Meyer J, et al: Long-term results 10 years after iliac arterial stent placement. *Radiology* 224:731-738, 2002. Radiological Society of North America.)

Methods.—One hundred ten patients (88 men, 22 women) with occlusive disease of the iliac arteries were treated with percutaneous transluminal angioplasty and stent placement from January 1987 to December 1990. The mean age of the patients was 57 years (range, 40-73 years). Stenoses were treated after failed angioplasty in 66 patients, and occlusions in 60 patients were treated with primary stent placement. Follow-up was by angiography or color duplex US and clinical examination with ankle-brachial index measurement. Patients lost to follow-up were interviewed by means of dedicated questionnaires administered by telephone and mail. In the case of a deceased patient, the relatives and attending physicians were interviewed.

Results.—The fates of all but 1 patient were determined. There were 46 deaths overall: 39 patients died within 10 years—including 18 who died within 5 years—and 7 more patients died after 10 years. The 5-year survival rate was 83%, and the 10-year survival rate was 64%. Cardiovascular disease was the cause of death in 23 patients, and 15 patients died of malignant tumor. In 5 patients, the cause of death was unknown. Primary stent patency rates were 66% ± 4.8 (SD) after 5 years and 46% ± 5.9 after 10 years (Fig 2). Secondary patency rates were 79% ± 4.2 after 5 years and 55% ± 6.3 after 10 years. Seventeen patients (16%) underwent surgical bypass of the aortoiliac arteries that involved the segment with the stent, 14 because of stent restenosis and 3 because of stenosis in other iliac arterial segments.

Conclusion.—Long-term results after iliac arterial stent placement reveal iliac arterial stent placement has a moderate long-term patency.

▶ The authors have provided 10-year results of iliac stents placed primarily for claudication. Analysis of the data indicates extensive lesions greater than 10 cm did poorly and probably should be treated with bypass when feasible, while results with shorter lesions are okay but not great long term. There are no real surprises here, but I was impressed by the clinical results. It would have been nice to have seen a correlation between patency and relief of clinical symptoms. There are so many other things that can effect mobility in patients with claudication other than the status of the iliac artery.

G. L. Moneta, MD

Predictors for Adverse Outcome After Iliac Angioplasty and Stenting for Limb-Threatening Ischemia

Timaran CH, Stevens SL, Freeman MB, et al (Univ of Tennessee, Knoxville)
J Vasc Surg 36:507-513, 2002   8–5

Introduction.—Several observational trials have attempted to identify risk factors after placement of iliac stents in patients with limb-threatening ischemia (LTI). The influence of risk factors on the outcome of iliac artery angioplasty and stenting (IAS) placement was examined in 74 patients with LTI.

Methods.—Between 1996 and 2001, 85 IAS placement procedures (107 stents) were performed in 31 women and 43 men. Patients with claudication were excluded. Variables were defined with the use of criteria prepared by the

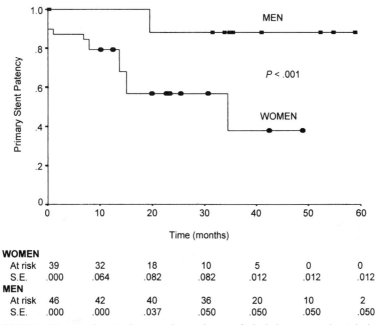

WOMEN							
At risk	39	32	18	10	5	0	0
S.E.	.000	.064	.082	.082	.012	.012	.012
MEN							
At risk	46	42	40	36	20	10	2
S.E.	.000	.000	.037	.050	.050	.050	.050

FIGURE 1.—Women undergoing iliac angioplasty and stenting for limb-threatening ischemia had significantly lower primary stent patency rates than did men (KM, log-rank test, $P < .001$). (Reprinted by permission of the publisher from Timaran CH, Stevens SL, Freeman MB, et al: Predictors for adverse outcome after iliac angioplasty and stenting for limb-threatening ischemia. *J Vasc Surg* 36:507-513, 2002. Copyright 2002 by Elsevier.)

Ad Hoc Committee on Reporting Standards (Society for Vascular Surgery/International Society for Cardiovascular Surgery). The TransAtlantic Inter-Society Consensus classification was used for classification of the type of iliac lesions. The associations among variables, cumulative patency, limb salvage, and survival were examined by both univariate (Kaplan-Meier) and multivariate (Cox proportional hazards model) analyses.

Results.—The indications for IAS included ischemic rest pain in 56% and tissue loss in 44%. Stents were placed selectively after iliac angioplasty primarily for residual stenosis or pressure gradient (43%). Thirty-six patients (42%) underwent primary stenting. The overall primary stent patency rates at 1, 2, and 3 years were 90%, 74%, and 69%, respectively. The primary stent patency rate was significantly decreased in women versus men ($P <$ .001) (Fig 1). The primary patency rates for women at 1, 3, and 5 years were 79%, 57%, and 38%, respectively. For men, the rates were 92%, 88%, and 88% at 1, 3, and 5 years, respectively. The primary stent patency rate was also significantly diminished in patients with renal insufficiency (creatinine level, >1.5 mg/dL; $P <$ .001). Female sex (relative risk [RR], 5.1; 95% CI, 1.8-7.9; $P =$ .002) and renal insufficiency (RR, 6.6; 95% CI, 1.6-14.2; $P =$ .01) were independent predictors of reduced primary stent patency. No independent predictors for limb salvage or survival were found.

Conclusion.—Women undergoing iliac angioplasty and IAS for LTI have significantly reduced primary stent patency rates after IAS, as do patients with renal insufficiency and critical ischemia. Limb salvage is not influenced by previous iliac stent failure.

▶ There continues to be controversy about the results of arterial reconstruction procedures in women. In this study, females have poorer patency of iliac stents than males when the indication for stenting was critical limb ischemia. Overall, the weight of evidence seems to suggest poor results of angioplasty in females in terms of patency but not limb salvage. Since limb salvage is the real goal, there seems to be no reason not to recommend angioplasty and stenting when technically feasible and indicated in female patients with arterial limb ischemia.

G. L. Moneta, MD

Intravascular Ultrasound Scanning Improves Long-term Patency of Iliac Lesions Treated With Balloon Angioplasty and Primary Stenting
Buckley CJ, Arko FR, Lee S, et al (Texas A & M Univ, Temple; Stanford Univ, Calif)
J Vasc Surg 35:316-323, 2002   8–6

Background.—Intravascular US (IVUS) provides an accurate measurement of the diameter of both diseased and true lumens of arteries. Whether the use of IVUS improves the anatomical and clinical results of stenting was determined.

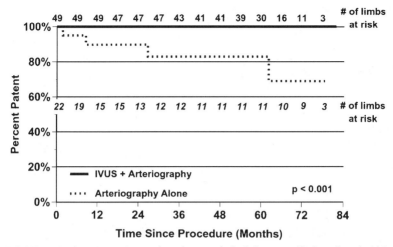

FIGURE 1.—Kaplan-Meier estimates of vessel patency for both the group of limbs evaluated with intravascular US scanning (*IVUS*) and the group of limbs not evaluated with IVUS (*P* < .001). (Reprinted by permission of the publisher from Buckley CJ, Arko FR, Lee S, et al: Intravascular ultrasound scanning improves long-term patency of iliac lesions treated with balloon angioplasty and primary stenting. *J Vasc Surg* 35:316-323, 2002. Copyright 2002 by Elsevier.)

Methods.—Fifty-two patients (71 consecutive limbs) with aortoiliac occlusive disease had balloon angioplasty and primary stenting of symptomatic iliac lesions performed at a single center multispecialty clinic. As a means of evaluating stent deployment, IVUS and arteriography were used in 49 limbs and arteriography alone in 22 limbs. All patients received at least 162 mg of aspirin preoperatively and 162 mg of aspirin and 150 mg of dipyridamole postoperatively.

Results.—In 40% (20/49) limbs, IVUS demonstrated inadequate stent development at the original procedure. In the IVUS plus arteriography group, there were no re-stenoses or occlusions, and a sustained improvement in the ankle-brachial index of all 49 limbs was reported at last follow-up (Fig 1). In the arteriography alone group, early re-stenosis or occlusion of stented lesions occurred in 18% (4 of 22) of limbs after 5.5 months follow-up, and there was a sustained mean ankle-brachial index improvement of 0.37 in 17 of 22 patients after 3 years. No secondary procedures were performed in the limbs evaluated and treated in the IVUS plus arteriography group; however, a secondary intervention rate in the arteriography alone group was 23% (5 of 22 limbs).

Conclusion.—IVUS, as used to define the appropriate arterial diameter for an angioplasty procedure and for assessing adequacy of stent deployment, should be considered for improving the long-term patency of iliac arterial occlusive lesions that are treated with balloon angioplasty and stenting.

▶ It has always been an axiom of vascular surgery that technical perfection improves results. What has become apparent is that the means of evaluating technical perfection is also important. IVUS appears to provide a better assessment of the technical adequacy of iliac stent placement than angiography alone. Assessment of the technical adequacy of angioplasty with IVUS and retreatment of residual lesions may improve the long-term clinical outcome of balloon angioplasty and primary stenting of iliac arteries. If this study can be duplicated, IVUS should become the standard of care in the peri-procedure assessment of the technical adequacy of iliac stent placement.

G. L. Moneta, MD

Early Results of External Iliac Artery Stenting Combined With Common Femoral Artery Endarterectomy

Nelson PR, Powell RJ, Schermerhorn ML, et al (Dartmouth Med School, Lebanon, NH)
J Vasc Surg 35:1107-1113, 2002   8–7

Background.—Endarterectomy for treatment of occlusive disease of the common femoral artery has been standard practice for more than 50 years. Treatment is complex in patients with a diseased segment extending proximally into the external iliac artery. A pure endovascular approach to external iliac artery disease extending into the common femoral artery has been avoided because of problems with placement of the stent across the inguinal ligament. Surgical treatment in these patients has included extensive endarterectomy or bypass procedures or a combination of both. This report describes a combined open and endovascular approach to patients with extensive external iliac and common femoral artery occlusive disease.

Methods.—A retrospective analysis was performed of all patients who underwent intraoperative external iliac artery stenting after common femoral artery endarterectomy/patch angioplasty between 1997 and 2000. Stents were positioned to end at the proximal endarterectomy end point, without crossing the inguinal ligament. The main outcome measures were technical success, hemodynamic success, and clinical success according to criteria from the Society of Vascular Surgery/International Society of Cardiovascular Surgery. Life-table analysis was performed for evaluation of patency.

Results.—A total of 34 patients (mean age, 68 years; 23 men and 11 women) underwent combined endovascular and open treatment for iliofemoral occlusive disease. The indications for treatment were claudication in 41% and critical limb ischemia in 59%. Endarterectomy with patch angioplasty was performed in all patients, and the stent deployment in the external iliac artery incorporated the stenotic iliac segment and the proximal end point of the endarterectomy in all patients. Four patients (12%) also underwent concurrent common iliac angioplasty for proximal iliac disease, and 14 patients (41%) also required distal revascularization for associated femoropopliteal or tibial disease. Technical and hemodynamic successes were attained in all patients. The overall complication rate was 15%. Over a mean follow-up period of 13 months (range, 0.5-28 months), the 1-year primary patency rate was 84% and the primary-assisted patency rate was 97% (Fig). No perioperative mortality occurred.

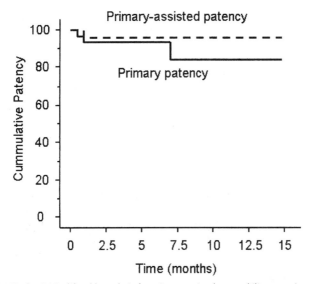

FIGURE.—Kaplan-Meier life-table analysis for primary-assisted external iliac artery/common femoral artery patency rates. Primary patency rate depicted with *solid line*, and primary-assisted patency rate depicted with *dashed line*. Standard error was less than 10% for both curves over time period shown. (Reprinted by permission of the publisher from Nelson PR, Powell RJ, Schermerhorn ML, et al: Early results of external iliac artery stenting combined with common femoral artery endarterectomy. *J Vasc Surg* 35:1107-1113, 2002. Copyright 2002 by Elsevier.)

Conclusions.—Stenting of the external iliac artery as an adjunct to endarterectomy/patch angioplasty of the common femoral artery allows more localized surgery than does a conventional bypass. This technique provides for a better interface between the stent and the endarterectomy than does staged perioperative stenting and achieves excellent technical success and early patency rates.

▶ I'm going to hold back on recommending this approach to combined common femoral and external iliac artery stenosis. There is sufficient doubt about the durability of external iliac stenting, and the follow-up in this paper is so short that a "wait and see" position is appropriate. If one chooses to do this procedure, be sure and note that the authors recommend placing the guidewire for angioplasty before performance of the common femoral endarterectomy.

G. L. Moneta, MD

Late Complication of Aortoiliac Stent Placement–Atheroembolization of the Lower Extremities

Lin PH, Bush RL, Conklin BS, et al (Emory Univ, Atlanta, Ga; Atlanta Veterans Affairs Med Ctr, Decatur, Ga; Baylor College of Medicine, Houston)

J Surg Res 103:153-159, 2002   8–8

Background.—Aortoiliac stent placement can rarely result in atheroembolization. The risk factors associated with lower-extremity atheroembolization and its management after aortoiliac stent placement for occlusive disease were retrospectively analyzed.

Methods.—Data from the hospital records of all 8 patients who experienced thromboembolic events after aortoiliac stent placement between March 1993 and February 2001 were analyzed. Data from a control group of 493 patients who underwent aortoiliac stent placement during that period with no atheroembolic complications were analyzed for comparison.

Findings.—The 8 patients underwent placement of 12 iliac artery stents and 1 aortic stent. Atheroembolization occurred 9 to 43 months after aortoiliac stent placement. On arteriography, the stented artery was identified as the source of atheroembolism in all patients. Five patients successfully underwent 5 corrective operations, including 2 aortobifemoral bypasses, 1 ileofemoral bypass, and 2 aortoiliac endarterectomies. Two concomitant femoropopliteal thrombectomies were also required. In the remaining 3 patients, thrombolysis and/or additional stents were placed, resulting in iliac occlusion or recurrent embolic symptoms. These 3 patients were treated eventually with bypass procedures. None of the patients died perioperatively. At a mean 16-month follow-up, 2 patients needed minor amputations and 1 required a major leg amputation. After surgical bypass, no further episodes of atheroembolism were noted in the involved limbs. Risk factor analysis did not identify potential correlates of atheroembolism after aortoiliac stent placement.

Conclusions.—Aggressive examination is warranted for patients with atheromatous embolization after aortoiliac stent placement. Surgical correction or bypass with exclusion of the offending embolic source is the treatment of choice. Intra-arterial stent placement in an atheroembolic stented iliac artery is possible but may produce a less durable outcome.

▶ Stenotic embolizing native iliac arteries are effectively treated with stents. This small series suggests that when the stents themselves are the source of embolization, a bypass procedure rather than restenting is more likely to produce a durable result.

G. L. Moneta, MD

Obstructive External Iliac Arteriopathy in Avid Bicyclists: New and Variable Histopathologic Features in Four Women

Kral CA, Han DC, Edwards WD, et al (Mayo Clinic, Rochester, Minn)
J Vasc Surg 36:565-570, 2002   8–9

Background.—Competitive bicyclists may experience obstruction of the external iliac arteries. The mechanism of injury is thought to be injury secondary to the shear stresses of very high blood flow coupled with the mechanical stress to the artery from the cyclist's body position. The end result of this process is referred to as endofibrosis. European studies of this injury found that endofibrosis primarily affected young men. The histopathologic features of obstructed external iliac arteries resected from competitive bicyclists were reviewed.

Methods.—Medical records and microscopic slides were reviewed from competitive bicyclists who underwent resection and graft placement for segmental external iliac artery disease.

Results.—Four patients underwent resection and graft placement and had specimens available for histopathologic review. These patients, all women, ranged in age from 31 to 40 years (mean age, 36 years). Claudication was the primary symptom. Five iliac arteries were involved in the 4 women. Preoperative arteriography demonstrated stenotic disease, ranging from subtle stenosis to occlusion (Fig 6). Gross examination of the resected arteries showed wall thickening and luminal narrowing, without aneurysm formation. A luminal thrombus was observed on microscopic examination in 2 arteries (1 old and 1 recent). Four specimens had intimal thickening. Thicken-

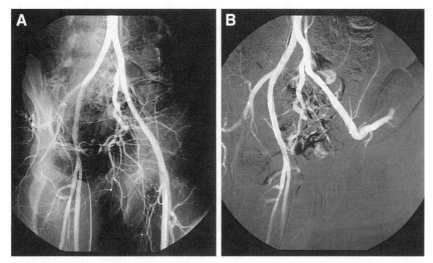

FIGURE 6.—**A**, Angiogram revealing subtle stenosis of proximal left external iliac artery with patient in supine position. **B**, Angiogram with patient in hyperflexed, "racing" position accentuating stenosis. (Reprinted by permission of the publisher from Kral CA, Han DC, Edwards WD, et al: Obstructive external iliac arteriopathy in avid bicyclists: New and variable histopathologic features in four women. *J Vasc Surg* 36:565-570, 2002. Copyright 2002 by Elsevier.)

ing was the result of smooth muscle hyperplasia, and only mild collagen or elastin deposition was present. Three specimens also showed medial hypertrophy, and 1 of these specimens also contained focal calcification. Adventitial thickening was prominent in 4 specimens and resulted from smooth muscle hyperplasia. None of the specimens showed intimal, medial, or adventitial inflammation.

Conclusions.—Iliac arteriopathy in competitive bicyclists may occur in women, and the microscopic lesions responsible for stenosis are more varied than previously reported. This study demonstrated medial and adventitial responses to repetitive trauma in addition to the intimal fibrosis and luminal thrombosis noted in previous studies. The term *external iliac arteriopathy* is proposed for this disease entity.

▶ From surgical specimens, we are learning more about the pathology of external iliac artery damage secondary to the high iliac artery flows combined with hyperflexion of the thigh in competitive cyclists. I am not in favor of placing prosthetic grafts in young patients so they can continue to cycle 400 miles per week. This seems to be a bit of misplacement of priorities.

G. L. Moneta, MD

Isolated Dissection of the Abdominal Aorta: Clinical Presentation and Therapeutic Options
Farber A, Wagner WH, Cossman DV, et al (Cedars-Sinai Med Ctr, Los Angeles; Dartmouth-Hitchcock Med Ctr, Lebanon, NH)
J Vasc Surg 36:205-210, 2002   8–10

Introduction.—Dissection of only abdominal aorta without thoracic aortic involvement is rare. Because the natural history and treatment strategies of isolated abdominal aortic dissection (IAAD) are based only on case reports and small case series. Described is the largest published case series of IAAD.

Methods.—Data from medical records, imaging studies, and telephone interviews were obtained for all patients treated for IAAD between January 1996 and July 2001. Only patients definitely shown by contrast-enhanced chest CT scans not to have a concomitant thoracic dissection were included. The degree of aortic calcification in the area of the dissection was quantified by means of the aortic calcification index.

Results.—Ten patients were treated for IAAD during the evaluation period. The mean patient age was 62 years; 60% were men. Initial symptoms were abdominal pain in 7 patients and lower extremity ischemia in 1 patient. For 2 patients, dissection was asymptomatic. Hypertension, smoking history, remote trauma, and claudication were recorded in 4, 3, 2, and 2 patients, respectively. Three, 3, and 5 patients, respectively, had abdominal tenderness, a pulsatile mass, or benign abdominal examination findings. The diagnosis of dissection was determined on abdominal CT scans in 8 patients (Fig 1), with angiography in 1 patient, and at surgery in 1 patient. The dis-

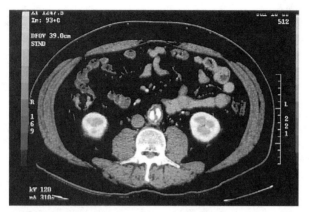

FIGURE 1.—Abdominal CT scan of patient 5 shows double-barrel appearance of dissected infrarenal aorta. (Reprinted by permission of the publisher from Farber A, Wagner WH, Cossman DV, et al: Isolated dissection of the abdominal aorta: Clinical presentation and therapeutic options. *J Vasc Surg* 36:205-210. Copyright 2002 by Elsevier.)

section flap originated below or at the renal arteries in 9 patients and at the superior mesenteric artery in 1 patient. The length of the dissection ranged between 21 and 110 mm. In 3 patients, the dissection flap extended beyond the aortic bifurcation into the common iliac arteries. In 3 patients who underwent aortograms, evidence of flow limitation was identified on the basis of the presence of aortic stenosis or occlusion. One patient was treated by aortic stent graft deployment, 3 were treated by direct aortic reconstruction, and 6 were treated by observation.

Conclusion.—In patients with IAAD, aneurysmal degeneration may occur, and close surveillance is needed if definitive treatment is not used initially. Patients with ischemic symptoms and those with intractable pain need intervention that is based on their risk profile and aortoiliac anatomy.

▶ The overall take on this paper is that the mere presence of an IAAD does not mandate intervention at the time of presentation. Patients who have abdominal aortic dissection and clinical indications for treatment such as coexisting aneurysm, ischemia, or unrelenting pain should be treated. Those without a mandate for treatment generally have resolution of pain within 1 month and little short-term change in the follow-up CT appearance of their infrainguinal aorta. However, the data beyond 1 year are virtually nonexistent for this condition. Regular CT follow-up of untreated patients seems indicated.

G. L. Moneta, MD

9 Visceral Renal Artery Disease

Long-term Outcome After Mesenteric Artery Reconstruction: A 37-Year Experience
Cho J-S, Carr JA, Jacobsen G, et al (Henry Ford Hosp, Detroit)
J Vasc Surg 35:453-460, 2002   9–1

Background.—The late results and factors determining morbidity and mortality after mesenteric artery reconstruction (MAR) for atherosclerotic mesenteric ischemia were investigated.

Methods.—A retrospective review identified 48 consecutive patients (66 arteries) who underwent MAR for acute mesenteric ischemia (AMI) of nonembolic origin (23 patients, 12 with and 11 without prior symptoms) and chronic mesenteric ischemia (CMI, 25 patients) between 1963 and 2000 in a tertiary care referral center. The 29 women (60%) and 19 men (40%) had a mean age of 64 years (range, 40 to 87 years). The operative procedures included bypass grafting in 36 arteries, local endarterectomy in 16 arteries, and transaortic endarterectomy in 14 arteries. Follow-up in the 34 survivors was complete in all but 4 patients and averaged 5.3 years (range, 30 days to 36 years). Radiographic documentation of graft patency was available in 33 of 34 survivors.

Results.—Single-vessel revascularization was performed more frequently in the AMI group than in the CMI group (91% vs 48%). The CMI group had a lower perioperative (<30 days) mortality rate (0%) than the AMI group (52%). Nine patients died of bowel infarction. Major complications occurred in 60% of cases. There were 15 late graft failures, for a cumulative patency rate of 57% at 5 years and 46% at 10 years. Transaortic endarterectomy was associated with improved patency rates as compared with local endarterectomy.

Eight patients had symptomatic recurrence develop, all involving superior mesenteric artery thrombosis. Among the survivors, the freedom-from-recurrence rates were 79% at 5 years and 59% at 10 years (Fig 6). Late survival rates were 54% at 5 years and 20% at 10 years. Excluding the perioperative deaths, the probability of long-term survival was 77% at 5 years and 29% at 10 years and did not differ between AMI and CMI.

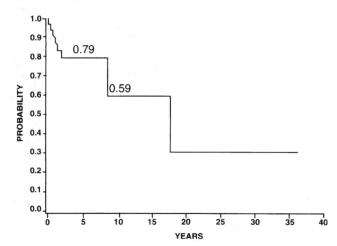

FIGURE 6.—Long-term freedom-from-recurrence rate (Kaplan-Meier method). (Reprinted by permission of the publisher from Cho J-S, Carr JA, Jacobsen G, et al: Long-term outcome after mesenteric artery reconstruction: A 37-year experience. *J Vasc Surg* 35:453-460, 2002. Copyright 2002 by Elsevier.)

Conclusion.—MAR for CMI carries a low mortality rate, but AMI continues to be a highly lethal problem. MAR for AMI provides long-term patency and symptom-free survival, with rates comparable to those obtained from MAR for CMI. The patency of the superior mesenteric artery is important in the prevention of symptomatic recurrence.

▶ The authors' results with mesenteric artery reconstruction are comparable to those published previously. They emphasize that patency of the superior mesenteric artery is the most important factor in preventing symptomatic recurrence. The authors noted that a patent celiac artery reconstruction does not reliably prevent symptomatic recurrence when the superior mesenteric artery reconstruction fails. This makes sense, as virtually all postprandial intestinal hyperemia is via the superior mesenteric artery, not the celiac artery. The bottom line is that maintaining patency of the superior mesenteric artery is most important in preventing recurrence of ischemic symptoms after visceral revascularization.

G. L. Moneta, MD

Current Results of Open Revascularization for Chronic Mesenteric Ischemia: A Standard for Comparison
Park WM, Cherry KJ Jr, Chua HK, et al (Mayo Clinic and Found, Rochester, Minn)
J Vasc Surg 35:853-859, 2002   9–2

Background.—Chronic mesenteric ischemia (CMI) is usually treated with operative revascularization of the stenotic or occluded mesenteric vessels.

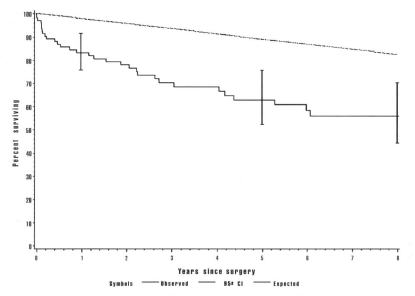

FIGURE 1.—Survival rates. (Reprinted by permission of the publisher from Park WM, Cherry KJ Jr, Chua HK, et al: Current results of open revascularization for chronic mesenteric ischemia: A standard for comparison. *J Vasc Surg* 35:853-859, 2002. Copyright 2002 by Elsevier.)

However, questions remain as to the optimal site of graft origin and the extent of revascularization necessary to achieve excellent surgical results.

Methods.—The study included 76 women and 22 men (average age, 66 years) who underwent surgery for CMI from 1989 to 1998. Abdominal pain was present in 95 patients (97%), and weight loss was present in 92 patients (94%). The superior mesenteric artery was severely diseased in 92% of patients, the celiac artery was severely diseased in 83% of patients, and both arteries were diseased in 78% of patients. Bypass grafts were performed in 91 patients; among the remaining 7 patients, 1 reimplantation, 1 patch angioplasty, and 5 endarterectomies were performed.

Results.—Five hospital deaths occurred, of which all were in patients older than 70 years. The median follow-up period was 1.9 years. The 1-year, 5-year, and 8-year survival rates were 83%, 63%, and 55%, respectively, which were worse than rates in the age- and sex-matched control subjects. Survival was unaffected by the number of vessels revascularized or by graft orientation (Fig 1).

Conclusions.—In this review of outcomes from open revascularizations for CMI, operation was successful for most patients, with low operative mortality and excellent long-term results. Mortality rates were not increased by selective concomitant aortic procedures. No differences were found in symptomatic recurrence rates for single- versus multiple-vessel reconstruction or for antegrade versus retrograde grafts. Patients older than 70 years had increased operative mortality and decreased survival rates.

▶ It is interesting and somewhat gratifying that a series of visceral revascularizations from 2 very different institutions—Henry Ford (see Abstract 9–1) and this from the Mayo Clinic—achieve similar results and conclusions regarding visceral revascularization. The issues of what vessel to revascularize, the numbers of vessels to revascularize, and what graft configuration to use (antegrade vs retrograde) don't really matter all that much. The main thing is the importance of patency of the superior mesenteric artery reconstruction in preventing recurrence.

Successful splanchnic revascularization depends on technical performance and whether the operation is done for acute or chronic symptoms. The authors argue for a potentially greater role for endovascular treatment of chronic mesenteric ischemia in higher-risk patients. I think this is already happening in many practices, including our own. A more interesting question will be whether to extend stents to better-risk patients with chronic mesenteric ischemia. Operative mortality for chronic mesenteric ischemia in good-risk patients is near 0 in many institutions with excellent durability of results. However, the allure of minimally invasive therapy will surely lead to liberalization of the use of stents in the superior mesenteric artery as it has in other vessels.

G. L. Moneta, MD

Revascularization of the Superior Mesenteric Artery After Acute Thromboembolic Occlusion
Björck M, Acosta S, Lindberg F, et al (Uppsala Univ Hosp, Sweden; Blekinge County Hosp, Karlskrona, Sweden; Skellefteå District Hosp, Sweden)
Br J Surg 89:923-927, 2002   9–3

Background.—The prognosis for patients with acute thromboembolic occlusion of the superior mesenteric artery (SMA) is dismal. The clinical course of patients undergoing revascularization for acute thromboembolic occlusion of the SMA was reviewed, and factors associated with survival in patients who undergo revascularization were identified.

Methods.—A retrospective analysis was performed with the use of data obtained from the Swedish Vascular Registry. A total of 60 patients with acute thromboembolic occlusion of the SMA underwent revascularization procedures at 21 hospitals from 1987 to 1998.

Results.—The patients had a median age of 76 years. Most of the patients (73%) had cardiac disease, and 23% had previously undergone vascular surgery. The onset of symptoms was sudden in 30% of patients, severe in 33% of patients, and insidious in 37% of patients. The diagnosis was suspected on initial examination in 32% of patients, and the median time to surgery was shorter in these patients. Exploratory laparotomy and subsequent revascularization were performed in 58 patients, and 2 of these patients were treated with thrombolysis alone. A secondary laparotomy was performed in

41 patients, and a third-look procedure was performed in 8 patients. Nineteen patients required an additional bowel resection. The overall mortality rates were 43% at 30 days, 52% at discharge, 60% at 1 year, and 67% at 5 years. None of the patients required IV nutrition after 1 year. Previous vascular surgery resulted in a higher institutional mortality rate (79%). The outcome was better for patients who had a sudden onset of symptoms (27%).

Conclusions.—This retrospective analysis of revascularization in patients with acute thromboembolic occlusion of the SMA demonstrated a frequent need for bowel resection with "second-look" laparotomy. Revascularization for patients with thromboembolic acute occlusion of the SMA followed by routine "second-look" laparotomy may improve mortality rates in these patients.

▶ This paper was selected for the YEAR BOOK not because it demonstrates a high mortality rate for acute intestinal ischemia. Even my 14-year-old daughter can deduce that. What is interesting is that it documents the yield of a second-look laparotomy. Thirty-eight percent of the time, more bowel will need to be resected. In addition, while some survivors are dependent on IV nutrition when they initially leave the hospital, by 1 year none remain dependent on IV nutrition. The bottom line is, second-look laparotomies are important, and there is hope for those initially dependent on hyperalimentation.

G. L. Moneta, MD

Superior Mesenteric Artery Pseudoaneurysm Successfully Treated With Polytetrafluoroethylene Covered Stent

Cowan S, Kahn MB, Bonn J, et al (Jefferson Med College, Philadelphia; Miami Cardiac and Vascular Inst, Fla)
J Vasc Surg 35:805-807, 2002   9–4

Introduction.—Reported is the first superior mesenteric artery (SMA) pseudoaneurysm associated with a pancreatic pseudocyst complicating aortic surgery successfully treated with a polytetrafluoroethylene (PTFE) covered stent.

> *Case Report.*—Man, 61, underwent repair of a 6.9-cm infrarenal abdominal aortic aneurysm. The repair was complicated by proximal suture line disruption, for which he underwent multiple revisions that culminated in supraceliac aortic clamping and a proximal anastomosis beveled under the SMA and celiac arteries. He had a fever and abdominal distention 10 days postoperatively. CT scanning revealed a pancreatic phlegmon. An exploratory laparotomy was performed. Intraoperative cultures of abdominal fluid and peripancreatic tissue were negative. An additional CT scan 30 days later revealed a 14- × 9- × 4.7-cm pancreatic pseudocyst, which was drained percutaneously. A catheter check 10 weeks later revealed a

communication with the SMA. Selected angiograms revealed a 1.5-cm proximal SMA pseudoaneurysm. Drain cultures grew enterococcus. IV vancomycin was started. The pseudoaneurysm was treated with the use of 2 balloon-expandable Palmaz P204 stents covered with 3-mm thin wall PTFE from which the external reinforcement had been removed. The PTFE was secured to the stent with the use of two 5-0 polypropylene sutures. Postprocedural imaging with the use of helical CT scanning verified successful treatment of the pseudoaneurysm. The drain catheter was removed 1 month later. The patient continued taking ciprofloxacin on a long-term basis and had no signs of ongoing sepsis. He did well clinically and ultimately died 5.5 years later of end-stage cardiac disease.

Conclusion.—For patients considered to be at high risk for traditional open repair, a PTFE covered stent for repair of an SMA pseudoaneurysm should be considered.

▶ Patients with visceral pseudoaneurysms associated with pancreatitis are not high on any life insurance salesman's prospective client list. This paper demonstrates a clever way out of a bad problem. Although this patient eventually recovered, I think a stent covered with an autogenous vein would make better therapeutic sense, given the risk of infection in patients with postoperative pancreatic phlegmons.

G. L. Moneta, MD

Celiac Arterial Aneurysms: A Critical Reappraisal of a Rare Entity
Stone WM, Abbas MA, Gloviczki P, et al (Mayo Clinic, Scottsdale, Ariz; Mayo Clinic, Rochester, Minn)
Arch Surg 137:670-674, 2002   9–5

Background.—Overall, celiac artery aneurysms are rare, but they are the fourth most common visceral artery aneurysm. The risk of ruptures is reported to range from 10% to 20%. The majority of historical series have described infections as the most common cause of celiac arterial aneurysms, but more recent series have indicated a declining incidence of infectious causes. It would seem that rare true aneurysms of the celiac artery are at a definite risk of rupturing, but there are no definite indications for elective repair of celiac artery aneurysms, and their management has varied. Indications, risks of surgical repair, and morbidity of rupture therefore were assessed for celiac artery aneurysms in an institutional review.

Methods.—A retrospective chart review was conducted of all patients with true celiac arterial aneurysms at 1 institution from January 1, 1980, through December 31, 1998. Study participants were followed up via medical records and/or telephone calls to the patient or a relative. Patients were excluded if they had thoracoabdominal aneurysms and pseudoaneurysms.

Results.—True celiac arterial aneurysms were seen in 18 patients. These patients comprised 5.9% of true visceral artery aneurysms diagnosed during the study period. These 12 men and 6 women had a mean age of 64.2 years. Concomitant associated aneurysms were present in 12 patients (67%) at the time of presentation. The size of the celiac aneurysms ranged from 1.5 to 4.0 cm in diameter. Only 1 patient in this series had a ruptured aneurysm (6%). Of the 17 patients with intact aneurysms, 9 underwent surgical intervention, including revascularization in 8 patients (2 saphenous vein grafts, 2 artery-to-artery anastomoses, and 4 prosthetic grafts). No operative deaths occurred. Both saphenous vein grafts occluded within 6 months. Among 9 patients treated nonoperatively, 1 late rupture resulted in death. Eight patients (44%) were alive without symptoms after a mean follow-up of 91 months.

Conclusions.—Celiac arterial aneurysms are rare. Elective repair should be considered for aneurysms larger than 2 cm but saphenous vein grafts may be inadequate. There is a frequent association with nonvisceral aneurysms.

▶ Even though, comparatively speaking, this is a very large series of celiac aneurysms, perhaps even the largest, the numbers are still too small to make definitive statements. We can, however, infer the following: most celiac aneurysms will be found incidentally, a few will be associated with infection, and about half will be calcified. Rupture is bad, and the patient is likely to die; aneurysms less than 2.5 cm in diameter can rupture; calcified celiac aneurysms may rupture less frequently; prosthetic grafts seem to work better than veins grafts, and elective repair in good-risk patients by skilled surgeons has essentially no operative mortality. So there you have it, a summary of what is known about celiac artery aneurysms in one little paragraph.

G. L. Moneta, MD

Prospective Multicentre Study of the Natural History of Atherosclerotic Renal Artery Stenosis in Patients With Peripheral Vascular Disease
Pillay WR, for the Joint Vascular Research Group, UK (St Mary's Hosp, London)
Br J Surg 89:737-740, 2002   9–6

Background.—Renal artery stenosis (RAS) is common in patients with peripheral vascular disease. Revascularization may decrease progression of ischemic nephropathy and improve renovascular mediated hypertension. However, which patients benefit most from "prophylactic" revascularization remains unclear. Thus, the course of disease, treatments, and outcomes of patients with RAS diagnosed during angiography for peripheral vascular disease were prospectively studied.

Methods.—The research subjects were 85 patients 51 to 87 years old with peripheral artery disease and significant RAS (>50% RAS). Unilateral RAS was present in 52 patients (group 1) and was managed conservatively. Of the 33 patients with bilateral disease, 21 were managed conservatively (group 2), and 12 underwent intervention to improve renal artery blood flow (group 3). Renal size, blood pressure, and serum creatinine levels were measured at baseline and every 6 months for a minimum of 2 years.

Results.—After 2 years of follow-up, mortality rates in groups 1, 2, and 3 did not differ significantly (33%, 29%, and 33%, respectively; overall mortality rate, 32%). Only 3 deaths were directly related to RAS; most deaths were caused by coronary disease. All 3 patients requiring dialysis died within 1 year. Among the 58 survivors, the median blood pressure did not change significantly during follow-up. Creatinine clearance increased significantly in groups 1 and 3 at follow-up, but the increase in group 2 was not significant. Kaplan-Meier analyses indicated that overall survival times did not differ significantly among patients with unilateral or bilateral disease or among patients with bilateral disease who were managed conservatively or who underwent intervention.

Conclusion.—Patients with peripheral vascular disease and RAS have a poor prognosis, and about one third were dead after 2 years of follow-up. Most deaths were attributable to coronary disease, not renal failure. Intervention to improve renal artery blood flow does not seem to improve survival duration or overall renal functioning (as evaluated by serum creatinine levels).

▶ RAS is a frequent "incidental" finding in patients undergoing angiography for peripheral vascular disease. In this paper, the outcomes of patients with unilateral and bilateral disease were analyzed. Basically, cardiac and not renal-related events drove mortality, and mortality was high—32% at 2 years. We can't say much about the patients with bilateral disease as 1 in 3 had a renal artery intervention. However, only 2 of 52 patients with unilateral disease progressed to dialysis, and none underwent intervention for RAS. Mortality was no different than that of those with bilateral disease. Based on these data, it simply makes no sense to treat an incidentally discovered, unilateral RAS in a patient with peripheral arterial disease.

G. L. Moneta, MD

Surgical Management of Atherosclerotic Renovascular Disease
Cherr GS, Hansen KJ, Craven TE, et al (Wake Forest Univ, Winston-Salem, NC)
J Vasc Surg 35:236-245, 2002   9–7

Background.—The indications and methods for treatment of atherosclerotic renovascular disease (ASO-RVD) have changed during the past 50 years. Little attention, however, has been paid to the management of ASO-RVD as it relates to dialysis-free survival. The data from 1 center's experience with ASO-RVD in consecutive adults with hypertension who underwent surgical intervention during a recent 12-year period were reviewed retrospectively.

Methods.—626 patients underwent operative renal artery repair at 1 center. From this group, a subgroup of 500 patients with hypertension and atherosclerotic renal artery repair were selected for detailed dialysis.

Results.—203 patients underwent unilateral renal artery procedures, 297 underwent bilateral renal artery procedures, and 205 underwent combined renal and aortic reconstruction. After surgery, 23 deaths (4.6%) were recorded in the hospital or within 30 days of surgery. Significant and independent predictors of perioperative death included advanced age and clinical congestive heart failure. Among patients who survived surgery, hypertension was considered cured in 12%, improved in 73%, and unchanged in 15%. Renal function increased significantly for the entire group after surgery. Forty-three percent had improved renal function (with a 20% or more change in estimated glomerular filtration rate [EGFR] considered significant), 47% had no change in function, and 10% had worsened function.

Preoperative renal insufficiency, diabetes mellitus, prior stroke, and severe aortic occlusive disease were significantly and independently associated with death or dialysis during follow-up. After surgery, improved blood pressure and improved renal function were shown to be significantly and independently associated with an improved dialysis-free survival rate (Figs 3 and 4). All categories of patients' functional response and time to death or dialysis showed significant interactions with perioperative EGFR

Conclusion.—Surgical correction of atherosclerotic renovascular disease improved blood pressure and renal function in selected patients with hyper-

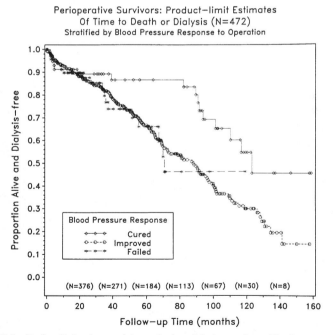

FIGURE 3.—Product-limit estimates of time to death or dialysis according to blood pressure response to operation. (Reprinted by permission of the publisher from Cherr GS, Hansen KJ, Craven TE, et al: Surgical management of atherosclerotic renovascular disease. *J Vasc Surg* 35:236-245, 2002. Copyright 2002 by Elsevier.)

FIGURE 4

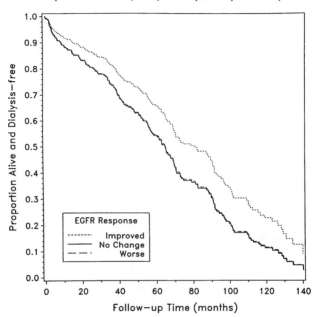

Predicted Survival Estimates of Time to Death or Dialysis
Preop EGFR = 25 ml/min/m**2 (25-th percentile)

(Continued)

tension. Patients with hypertension cured or EGFR improved after operation showed increased dialysis-free survival compared with that of other patients who underwent surgery.

▶ Since there are no randomized trials, this paper is as good as it gets to evaluate surgical therapy for ASO-RVD. A large number of patients were treated by a group of recognized experts. Unfortunately, it is not good enough to convince anyone who thinks above the level of a flatworm. Why? A 4.6%, 30-day mortality is one reason. Another is only 12% of the patients were cured of hypertension, and only these patients had improved dialysis-free survival. Also, improvement (ie, decreased number of antihypertensive medications) did not correlate with increased survival. Clearly, there is not much "bang for the buck" when operating for hypertension. Finally, only patients with low preoperative estimated glomerular filtration rates (<25%) could be predicted to have improved survival postoperatively. Some day we are all going to realize that the shotgun approach to surgical treatment of atherosclerotic renal artery stenosis is inefficient and a waste of resources. We need to move away from case series on this subject and concentrate on

FIGURE 4 (cont.)

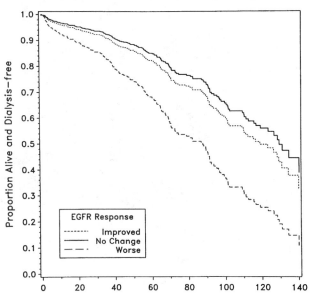

Predicted Survival Estimates of Time to Death or Dialysis
Preop EGFR = 38 ml/min/m**2 (Median)

FIGURE 4.—Predicted dialysis-free survival rate according to postoperative renal function response for patients with preoperative estimated glomerular filtration rate of 25 mL/min/m² (**A**, 25th percentile) or 39 mL/min/m² (**B**, median value). Interaction between preoperative estimated glomerular filtration rate and renal function response for dialysis-free survival rate was significant and independent. *Abbreviation: EGFR,* Estimated glomerular filtration rate. (Reprinted by permission of the publisher from Cherr GS, Hansen KJ, Craven TE, et al: Surgical management of atherosclerotic renovascular disease. *J Vasc Surg* 35:236-245, 2002. Copyright 2002 by Elsevier.)

identifying preoperatively, the small subset of patients for whom renal artery revascularization makes sense.

G. L. Moneta, MD

Reconstruction for Renal Artery Aneurysm: Operative Techniques and Long-term Results
Pfeiffer T, Reiher L, Grabitz K, et al (Univ Hosp, Heinrich-Heine-Univ, Düsseldorf, Germany)
J Vasc Surg 37:293-300, 2003   9–8

Background.—There is ongoing debate over the indications for surgical reconstruction of renal artery aneurysm (RAA). One institution's experience with an aggressive and liberal policy toward surgical repair of RAA is reported.

Methods.—The 21-year experience included 94 patients (57 women, 37 men; mean age, 51 years) undergoing surgical reconstruction of RAA. The

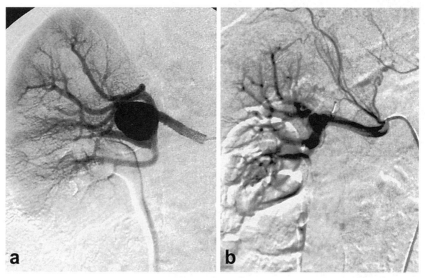

FIGURE 1.—Preoperative (A) and postoperative (B) angiography in 53-year-old woman with fibromuscular dysplasia that involved both kidneys and an aneurysm at the hilus of the right kidney. Saphenous vein bypass grafting had to be performed on the right side, and the patient became less hypertensive. Medication could be reduced from triple-drug to single-drug therapy. (Reprinted by permission of the publisher from Pfeiffer T, Reiher L, Grabitz K, et al: Reconstruction for renal artery aneurysm: Operative techniques and long-term results. *J Vasc Surg* 37:293-300, 2003. Copyright 2003 by Elsevier.)

underlying diagnosis was fibromuscular dysplasia in 48 patients, atherosclerosis in 28, dissection in 7, aortic coarctation in 5, nonspecific arteritis in 3, and giant cell arteritis, Marfan's syndrome, and trauma in 1 each. Reconstruction was performed for aneurysms that measured 1 cm or larger in patients with hypertension or ipsilateral and contralateral stenosis; and in women of childbearing age. In the absence of other risk factors, repair was performed for RAAs of 2 cm or larger.

Results.—Most repairs consisted of saphenous vein graft interposition or aneurysm resection with tailoring (Fig 1). The morbidity rate was 17%, including 1 case each of early graft occlusion, partial renal artery thrombosis, and branch artery stenosis. Among patients undergoing elective RAA repair, the mortality rate was 0; 1 patient died of myocardial infarction after emergency surgery for a ruptured RAA. At a mean of 46 months' follow-up in 83 patients, the rate of renal artery patency without stenoses was 81%. Hypertension was cured or improved in 47% of the patients.

Conclusions.—For patients with RAAs of 1 to 2 cm or larger and additional risk factors, surgical repair is safe treatment. Reconstruction prevents RAA rupture while normalizing or improving hypertension in about half of the cases, but this outcome is unpredictable. In nearly all cases, RAA repair can be achieved by autogenous reconstruction.

▶ The authors have a very aggressive approach to repair of RAAs. They advocate repair for RAAs as small as 1 cm in diameter in the presence of hypertension. Their approach is probably too aggressive for the occasional renal artery surgeon. Repair of a 1-cm RAA is a major procedure for a lesion of unclear pathologic significance with virtually no chance of rupture and a real potential for postoperative morbidity.

G. L. Moneta, MD

Renal Autotransplantation for Vascular Disease: Late Outcome According to Etiology
Chiche L, Kieffer E, Sabatier J, et al (Pitié-Salpétrière Univ Hosp, Paris)
J Vasc Surg 37:353-361, 2003   9–9

Background.—For patients with aneurysms or complex occlusive lesions of the renal artery, renal autotransplantation (RAT) is a well-established alternative to percutaneous transluminal angioplasty in cases where catheter-based techniques are contraindicated. The results of 68 RAT procedures were analyzed, with focus on differences in outcome among etiologic groups.

Methods.—The 16-year experience included 68 RAT procedures in 57 patients. The diagnosis was fibromuscular dysplasia (FMD) in 30 patients, Takayasu's disease (TD) in 19, and atherosclerosis in 8. Most patients with FMD and all of those with atherosclerosis were managed by intra-abdominal exposure in a single-stage procedure. Patients with TD generally underwent thoracoabdominal exposure because of the need to repair associated lesions of the aorta and intestinal arteries. The superficial femoral artery was the main arterial autograft used; because of the diffuse nature of their disease, patients with atherosclerosis were managed with greater saphenous vein grafts. Venous implantation was usually performed on the inferior vena cava in right RAT procedures and on the common iliac vein in left RAT procedures (Fig 1).

Results.—In the FMD group, early segmental infarction occurred in 4 of 34 procedures. One patient required late segmental nephrectomy. In FMD patients, the actuarial survival rate was 96.2% at 5 years and 84.1% at 10 years, with secondary patency rates of 100% and 92%, respectively. Nearly all patients had normalization or improvement in hypertension, and half had improvement in renal function.

Among TD patients, there was 1 early death from multiple organ failure and 1 patient required nephrectomy. At 5 and 10 years, the actuarial survival rate was 94.7% and the secondary patency rate was 91.3%. Eighty-nine percent of the patients had improvement or normalization of hypertension, and all had improved kidney function. Five patients in the atherosclerosis group required early or late nephrectomy. The survival rate decreased from 54.7% at 5 years to 18.2% at 10 years, and the secondary patency rate decreased from 50.0% to 33.3%. One half of the patients had improvement or normalization of hypertension, and only one third had improvement in renal function.

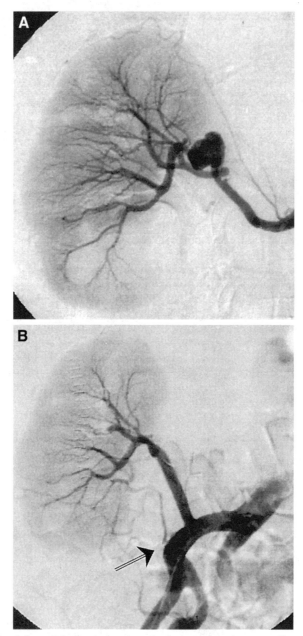

FIGURE 1.—A, Preoperative arteriogram shows dysplastic aneurysms in segmental branches of right renal artery. **B,** Follow-up arteriogram after RAT on common iliac artery, with indirect reimplantation of main artery with SFA autograft and direct reimplantation of lower polar artery (*arrow*). (Reprinted by permission of the publisher from Chiche L, Kieffer E, Sabatier J, et al: Renal autotransplantation for vascular disease: Late outcome according to etiology. *J Vasc Surg* 37:353-361, 2003. Copyright 2003 by Elseiver.)

Discussion.—The experience shows good outcomes of RAT in patients with an underlying diagnosis of FMD or TD. The results are not as good in patients with atherosclerosis.

▶ Two main points need emphasis here.

1. Autotransplantation for atherosclerotic renal artery disease does not work well. However, it is effective in patients with complex FMD not amenable to angioplasty, and in patients with TD, a condition that responds poorly to angioplasty.

2. The ureter can be left intact in virtually all cases of autotransposition, and arterial autographs seem to work well for nonatherosclerotic conditions. The authors frequently use the superficial femoral artery as an autograph in patients with FMD or TD. Replacement of the superficial femoral artery with a vein graft resulted in little trouble during late follow-up of these patients.

G. L. Moneta, MD

Ostial Renal Artery Stent Placement in Patients 75 Years of Age or Older
Bloch MJ, Trost DA, Whitmer J, et al (Cornell Univ, New York; Univ of Nevada, Reno)
Am J Hypertens 14:983-988, 2001   9–10

Background.—In patients with atherosclerotic renovascular disease, renal artery stent placement improves blood pressure (BP) and stabilizes renal function in some patients. However, information on outcomes in patients 75 years and older is limited.

Methods and Findings.—The prestent characteristics and clinical outcomes of patients aged 75 years and older undergoing renal artery stenting between 1992 and 1997 at one center were compared with those of the rest of the cohort. Of the 89 patients undergoing renal artery stent placement, 19 were 75 years or older. The elderly group were more likely to be women and current or former smokers, and they received a greater number of antihypertensive medications. The mean clinical follow-up was similar in both groups: 23.9 and 23.2 months. At most recent follow-up, 7 of the 19 elderly patients had died, compared with 5 of 70 patients younger than 75 years. The need for dialysis after intervention was comparable in the 2 groups. BP was improved in 74% of patients 75 years and older, stable in 21%, and worse in 5%. Renal function was improved in 26%, stable in 53%, and worse in 21%. Patients aged 75 years and older had a significant decline in systolic BP and a trend toward reduced diastolic BP and medications. The clinical outcomes of the elderly group did not differ significantly from those younger than 75 years.

Conclusions.—Mortality 2 years after renal artery stent placement is greater in patients with atherosclerotic renovascular disease aged 75 years and older than in those younger than 75 years. However, these elderly patients appear to derive comparable clincal benefits.

▶ One reason to treat hypertension is to lower death rates from cardiovascular causes. The reason to place a renal stent, other than to improve the appearance of the angiogram, is therefore to improve death rates from cardiovascular causes, an end point not analyzed in this paper. An additional reason to place a renal artery stent is to improve renal function. This did not happen in this study. In both groups of patients, those younger than 75 years and those 75 years or older, the need for dialysis after stent placement was high: 10% in those younger than 75 and 16% in those 75 or older. The only real conclusion possible is that patients with renal artery stents do poorly regardless of age. Whether the patients do better than they would have otherwise is unknown.

G. L. Moneta, MD

10 Leg Ischemia

Age at Onset of Smoking Is an Independent Risk Factor in Peripheral Artery Disease Development
Planas A, Clará A, Marrugat J, et al (Hospitalet de Llobregat, Barcelona; Hosp del Mar, Barcelona; Institut Municipal d'Investigació Mèdica, Barcelona; et al)
J Vasc Surg 35:506-509, 2002   10-1

Introduction.—Overwhelming evidence shows a causal role of cigarette smoking in cardiovascular disease. Data regarding the potential impact of age at smoking onset on cardiovascular disease are sparse. The association between age at smoking onset and the development of symptomatic peripheral arterial occlusive disease (PAOD) was examined.

Methods.—A population-based sample of 573 active or former male smokers (ages 55-74 years) was evaluated. Present or previous symptomatic PAOD was verified by noninvasive testing (history, physical examination, and ankle–brachial index). Differences in participants with and without PAOD and late versus early smoking onset were assessed.

Results.—Sixty-one research subjects (10.6%) had symptomatic PAOD. The prevalence of disease rose with an earlier starting age of smoking (15.6% if 16 years or younger vs 5.4% if older than 16 years). After controlling for confounding risk factors, including age and number of pack-years, men who started smoking at age 16 years or younger had a markedly higher risk of having PAOD develop (odds ratio, 2.19; 95% CI, 1.15-4.15; $P = .016$) compared with men who started smoking at a later age.

Conclusion.—A starting age for smoking of 16 years or younger more than doubles the risk of future symptomatic PAOD, regardless of the amount of exposure to cigarette smoking.

▶ The study underscores the importance of preventing smoking in young people. It is not just how much you smoke but when you start that puts you at risk for developing arterial disease. Age of onset of smoking, not just pack-years, should be part of the history and physical in patients with occlusive arterial disease.

G. L. Moneta, MD

The Impact of Walking Impairment, Cardiovascular Risk Factors, and Co-morbidity on Quality of Life in Patients With Intermittent Claudication

Breek JC, Hamming JF, De Vries J, et al (Martini Hosp, Groningen, The Netherlands; St Elisabeth Hosp, Tilburg, The Netherlands; Tilburg Univ, The Netherlands)

J Vasc Surg 36:94-99, 2002   10–2

Introduction.—The impact of intermittent claudication (IC) on quality of life (QOL) has been extensively evaluated, but the role of cardiovascular risk factors and the impact of concomitant disease on QOL are usually not included as variables in analysis of patients with IC. The relative impact of age, sex, degree of claudication, cardiovascular risk factors, comorbidity, and the presence of back, hip, or knee symptoms on QOL were examined in 200 consecutive patients with IC in a prospective observational trial.

Methods.—All patients were from a vascular outpatient department of a teaching hospital. QOL was evaluated with the use of a reduced version of the World Health Organization Quality of Life Assessment Instrument-100. This instrument examines 17 facets of QOL within 5 domains (physical and psychological health, level of independence, social relationships, and environment). Age, sex, degree of IC, risk factors, comorbidity (as recommended by the Society for Vascular Surgery/North American Chapter of the International Society for Cardiovascular Surgery [SVS/ISCVS]), and the presence of back, hip, or knee symptoms were assessed as possible predictors of QOL. Multiple regression analyses examined each of the QOL facets and domains as a dependent variable. A probability value of less than 0.05 was considered to be of statistical significance.

Results.—Male sex was predictive of better scores for energy and fatigue and sleep and rest facets; women had higher scores on the facet of negative feelings. The presence of back, hip, or knee symptoms had significant predictive value for many components of QOL. With more concomitant diseases, patients had lower scores on the domain of overall QOL and general health and the facet of energy and fatigue and demonstrated more dependence on medication and treatments. The intensity of IC, as expressed in the SVS/ISCVS classification, was a significant predictor of QOL on the domain of level of independence and its facets of mobility, activities of daily living, and working capacity and the facets of pain and discomfort, sexual activity, and transport.

Conclusion.—QOL in patients with IC is only partially determined by the severity of the limitation in walking. The significant impact of cardiovascular risk factors and comorbidity and the presence of back, hip, or knee symptoms on QOL need to be recognized and considered when deciding the treatment approach.

► We need to remember that IC is not the only thing impairing QOL in patients with arterial occlusive disease. No patient with claudication should be considered for revascularization without careful assessment of other comorbidities, such as joint pain, back pain, obesity, and cardiac and pulmonary disease, that may also limit ambulation.

G. L. Moneta, MD

The Ankle Brachial Index Is Associated With Leg Function and Physical Activity: The Walking and Leg Circulation Study
McDermott MM, Greenland P, Liu K, et al (Northwestern Univ, Chicago; Catholic Health Partners, Chicago; Natl Inst on Aging, Bethesda, Md; et al)
Ann Intern Med 136:873-883, 2002   10–3

Introduction.—Peripheral artery disease (PAD) is often asymptomatic and may be missed during the course of a physical examination. The ankle-brachial index (ABI) is a simple, noninvasive means of assessing for the presence of PAD, yet this test appears to be used rarely in patients without suspected PAD. A cross-sectional study tested the hypothesis that the ABI would be an independent marker of objectively measured impaired lower-extremity function.

Methods.—Participants were identified from 3 academic medical centers. From a total of 2662 consecutive vascular laboratory patients aged 55 years and older, 597 met eligibility requirements and agreed to take part in the study. From a total of 467 general medicine patients aged 55 years and older, 143 met eligibility requirements and consented to participate. Tests to measure ABI were usually performed before functional measures, which included accelerometer-measured physical activity over 7 days, a 6-minute walk, 4-meter walking velocity, and standing balance. The ABI for each leg was calculated by averaging pressures from the dorsalis pedis and posterior tibial arteries. Participants with an ABI of less than 0.90 were classified as having PAD.

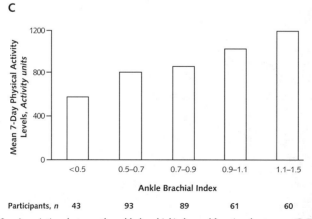

FIGURE 2.—Associations between the ankle-brachial index and functional outcomes. C, 7-day physical activity level, as measured by Caltrac accelerometer. (Courtesy of McDermott MM, Greenland P, Liu K, et al: The ankle brachial index is associated with leg function and physical activity: The walking and leg circulation study. *Ann Intern Med* 136:873-883, 2002.)

Results.—PAD was diagnosed in 447 vascular laboratory patients and 13 general medicine patients. The average ABI of participants with PAD was 0.65. Classic symptoms of intermittent claudication were present in 33%. A lower ABI was associated with lower accelerometer-measured activity over 7 days (Fig 2), a shorter distance walked in 6 minutes, poorer standing balance, slower walking velocity at usual and fastest pace, and a lower summary performance score. Among patients with mild to moderate PAD, these findings did not change substantially with regard to results of the 6-minute walk, 4-meter walk at fastest pace, and tandem stand. Associations between ABI and function were stronger than those between leg symptoms and function.

Conclusion.—The ABI can be used to identify PAD in relatively asymptomatic patients. Interventions to limit progression of PAD may prevent functional decline.

▶ I am a great fan of Dr McDermott's work. I have to say, however, the results of this study are not even a little surprising to vascular surgeons. This is a good example of your tax dollars being used to quantify the obvious for our more cerebral but less informed medical colleagues.

G. L. Moneta, MD

Exercise Rehabilitation Improves Functional Outcomes and Peripheral Circulation in Patients With Intermittent Claudication: A Randomized Controlled Trial
Gardner AW, Katzel LI, Sorkin JD, et al (Univ of Maryland, Baltimore; Maryland Veterans Affairs Health Care System, Baltimore)
J Am Geriatr Soc 49:755-762, 2001   10–4

Introduction.—The primary therapeutic goal for most patients with peripheral artery occlusive disease (PAOD) is the improvement of ambulatory function through exercise. Many studies have analyzed the effects of exercise rehabilitation on claudication distances. Other outcomes, such as perceived quality of life (QOL), are not frequently reported. The effects of a 6-month treadmill exercise program on ambulatory function, free-living daily physical activity, health-related QOL, and peripheral circulation were assessed in a prospective, randomized controlled study.

Methods.—The study included 61 patients with Fontaine stage II PAOD who were nonsmokers and who were randomly assigned to either an exercise rehabilitation group (n = 31) or to a usual-care, no-exercise control group (n = 30). Patients in the exercise group performed supervised, intermittent treadmill walking to near-maximum claudication pain 3 days per week. Benefits in free-living daily physical activity were reported by answers to questionnaires and confirmed by accelerometer monitoring.

Results.—Three patients from the exercise group and 6 from the control group withdrew from the trial. The 2 groups were comparable in baseline ambulatory function, peripheral hemodynamics, physical activity, health-related QOL, and self-reported ambulatory function. The mean compliance in the exercise group was 73%. Exercise rehabilitation increased the distance walked on the treadmill to the onset of claudication by 134% and to maximal claudication by 77%. The maximal calf blood flow increased by 30%. The walking economy and 6-minute walk distance were both increased by 12% in the exercise group. Exercisers walked greater distances, but the time-to-relief of claudication pain was unchanged. The increase in distance walked to onset of claudication was directly correlated with increases in free-living daily physical activity.

Conclusion.—A 6-month program of exercise rehabilitation significantly improved ambulatory function and peripheral circulation in older patients with PAOD and intermittent claudication. Exercise rehabilitation should be offered to older patients whose walking is limited by intermittent claudication.

▶ Exercise treatment of claudication can work. I have not, however, been all that impressed that it works all that well for most patients. Like any treatment, exercise must be prescribed judiciously. In this study, patients with significant comorbidities such as arthritis, poorly controlled diabetes, hypertension, significant coronary artery disease, or chronic obstructive pulmonary disease were excluded. My impression is that these comorbidities are present in the majority of patients we all see for intermittent claudication. Like surgery and catheter-based treatment for claudication, exercise is best prescribed selectively.

G. L. Moneta, MD

Exercise Training Reduces the Acute Inflammatory Response Associated With Claudication
Turton EPL, Coughlin PA, Kester RC, et al (St James's Univ Hosp, Leeds, England)
Eur J Vasc Endovasc Surg 23:309-316, 2002   10–5

Background.—Chronic inflammation is thought to be an important component in the pathogenesis of atherosclerosis. Markers of inflammation are elevated in patients who eventually have arterial disease and in patients with established atherosclerosis. Recent studies in patients with peripheral vascular disease (PVD) have shown that markers of inflammation rise when patients with PVD exercise to the point of maximum claudication pain. Concern exists that endothelial injury may be accelerated in patients with claudication because they are often instructed to perform regular walking exercise as part of therapy for PVD. The baseline markers of ischemia-reperfusion injury were assessed in patients with claudication and in control participants after short-term treadmill exercise, and the effect of a 3-month supervised exercise-training program on these markers was examined in the patients with claudication.

Methods.—Two groups, 1 comprising 46 patients with claudication and 1 comprising 22 age-matched control subjects, performed short-term treadmill exercise. Markers of ischemia-reperfusion injury, including neutrophil activation, degranulation, free radical damage, and antioxidants, were measured at rest and at 5, 30, and 60 minutes after exercise by flow cytometry, enzyme-linked immunosorbent assay, and chemiluminescence. The patients in the claudication group were then recruited into an intensive 3-month supervised exercise program. The same markers of ischemia-reperfusion injury were then reassessed at different time points at 3 and 6 months.

Results.—The markers of ischemia-reperfusion injury were similar in both groups at rest. Exercise had no effect on the control group; however, patients in the claudication group had significant neutrophil activation and degranulation with free radical damage immediately after exercise. This effect was diminished in a sequential manner after 3 months of exercise training.

Conclusions.—This study is the first to indicate that exercise training provides a benefit to patients with claudication not only in improved walking distance but also by decreasing the deleterious effects of ischemia-reperfusion injury that develop during claudication. Exercise training should be an essential component of the management of these patients.

▶ This group found that when claudicants were initially exercised, markers of endothelial cell activation and ischemia/reperfusion were released into the bloodstream. They proposed that such a repeated systemic inflammatory state could promote progression of atherosclerosis. While I view this as unlikely, proinflammatory and prothrombotic effects of vigorous exercise are well established. They subsequently measured the inflammatory response after chronic exercise training and found it resolved as claudication symptoms improved. This study brings us a little closer to understanding the underlying adaptation of skeletal muscle to chronic ischemia.

R. L. Geary, MD

Statin Use and Leg Functioning in Patients With and Without Lower-Extremity Peripheral Arterial Disease

McDermott MM, Guralnik JM, Greenland P, et al (Northwestern Univ, Chicago; Natl Inst on Aging, Bethesda, Md; Univ of California, San Diego; et al)
Circulation 107:757-761, 2003   10–6

Background.—In patients with atherosclerosis, statin drugs have numerous beneficial effects leading to reduction in the risk of cardiac and cerebrovascular events. By affecting lower-extremity arterial obstruction, these drugs might also influence functional status in patients with peripheral artery disease (PAD). The effects of statin drug treatment on leg function were assessed in PAD and non-PAD patients.

Methods.—The study included 392 patients with PAD, all having an ankle-brachial index (ABI) of less than 0.90, and 249 non-PAD patients, with ABI values of 0.90 to 1.50. Lower-extremity function was assessed by

6-minute walking distance and 4-meter walking speed. Together with performance on 5 trials of rising from a chair, the subjects' performance was ranked on an ordinal scale of 0 to 12.

Results.—Six-minute walking distance was 1276 feet in patients taking statin drugs versus 1218 feet in patients not taking statins ($P = .045$). Walking velocity was 0.93 mile/sec for statin-treated patients versus 0.89 mile/sec for untreated patients ($P = .008$); summary performance score was 10.2 versus 9.4, respectively ($P < .001$). All 3 performance measures were significantly better among statin-treated patients, with adjustment for age, sex, ABI, comorbid conditions, education, insurance status, cholesterol level, and other variables. Adjustment for C-reactive protein reduced the strength of these associations somewhat, but the effects of statin treatment on walking speed and performance score remained significant. The functional measures were unrelated to use of other medications, including aspirin, ACE inhibitors, vasodilator drugs, or β-blockers.

Conclusions.—With or without PAD, patients using statin drugs have better leg functional performance than statin nonusers. This is true even after adjustment for cholesterol levels and other confounding factors. Thus, statin drugs, in addition to their cholesterol-lowering properties, may have beneficial effects on functional status.

▶ Few drug classes have made so rapid an impact on a disease process as the statins on atherosclerosis. Introduced as lipid-lowering agents, a mountain of data has accumulated on pleiotrophic effects independent of lipid lowering, including anti-inflammatory, antioxidant, antithrombotic, and antiproliferative properties. These investigators found that statin use was associated with improved walking distance and speed in patients with reduced ABIs. This is consistent with the landmark 4S trial where long-term simvistatin use significantly reduced claudication. Curiously, in the present study, the benefit was not limited to persons with PAD, as those with normal ABIs had a similar improvement in walking distance. Even without these data, we should consider statins more often for our patients with PAD because the benefits are significant, while serious side effects are less common than many of us fear.

R. L. Geary, MD

The Influence of Hyperhomocysteinemia on Graft Patency After Infrainguinal Bypass Surgery in the Dutch BOA Study
de Borst GJ, for the Dutch BOA Study Group (Univ Med Ctr Utrecht, Nijmegen, The Netherlands; Univ Med Ctr St Radboud, Nijmegen, The Netherlands)
J Vasc Surg 36:336-340, 2002   10–7

Introduction.—Hyperhomocysteinemia (HHCA) has been confirmed as an independent risk factor for cardiovascular disease. It is not known whether HHCA contributes to graft failure after peripheral bypass surgery. The influence of HHCA on graft patency after infrainguinal bypass surgery was examined in the Dutch Bypass Oral Anticoagulants or Aspirin Study, a nested case-control investigation.

Methods.—One hundred fifty patients with graft occlusion were each matched with 2 randomly selected control subjects with patent grafts from the same investigation. Venous blood samples were obtained from case patients and control subjects to determine total plasma homocysteine levels.

Results.—The mean plasma homocysteine levels were 14.4 µmol/L and 14.9 µmol/L in case patients and control subjects, respectively. The resulting mean difference was –0.4 (95% CI, –1.8-0.9), and the odds ratio of HHCA was 0.81 (95% CI, 0.49-1.33). The adjustment for risk factors of graft occlusion did not alter these findings.

Conclusion.—High postoperative serum levels of homocysteine are not a risk factor for graft occlusion after infrainguinal bypass grafting.

▶ Patients with graft occlusion did not have higher homocysteine levels than patients with patent grafts. This may not be all that surprising. While elevated homocysteine levels are accepted as a risk factor for atherosclerosis, bypass graft failure within the first 6 postoperative months is not due to atherosclerosis. Further, it may have been harder to show a difference between the case and control groups in this study since both groups had mean homocysteine values near or above the upper limits of normal, again not surprising since both groups had already demonstrated a need for revascularization. The authors speculate that other factors may be more important in determining the fate of a bypass graft during the first postoperative year. This is probably true.

L. W. Kraiss, MD

Pre-operative Hand-held Doppler Run-off Score Can Be Used to Stratify Risk Prior to Infra-inguinal Bypass Surgery
Stewart AHR, Lucas A, Smith FCT, et al (Bristol Royal Infirmary, England)
Eur J Vasc Endovasc Surg 23:500-504, 2002   10–8

Background.—Adequacy of calf vessel run-off is an important factor when making the decision to perform an infrainguinal bypass. However, arteriography may be unreliable when there is underfilling of calf vessels distal to an arterial stenosis or occlusion. These vessels may not be clearly demonstrated with arteriography, resulting in an underestimation of calf vessel run-off. US may enable the detection of calf and pedal vessels not seen with arteriography, and pulse-generated run-off, dependent Doppler, and duplex US have all been advocated for use in the preoperative assessment of run-off. Another technique that may aid in this assessment is the use of a hand-held Doppler. The relationship of calf vessel run-off, assessed by means of hand-held Doppler, with graft patency and patient survival after infrainguinal graft surgery was assessed.

Methods.—Ankle Doppler auditory waveform characteristics were documented for 235 patients who underwent 258 infrainguinal bypass grafts. The patients had a median age of 71 years, and 67% were male. Doppler

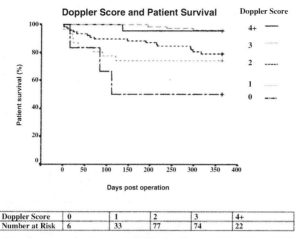

Doppler Score	0	1	2	3	4+
Number at Risk	6	33	77	74	22

FIGURE 1.—Doppler score and patient survival. (Reprinted by permission of the publisher from Stewart AHR, Lucas A, Smith FCT, et al: Pre-operative hand-held Doppler run-off score can be used to stratify risk prior to infra-inguinal bypass surgery. *Eur J Vasc Endovasc Surg* 23:500-504, 2002.)

signals from the anterior tibial, posterior tibial, and dorsalis pedis arteries were scored triphasic/biphasic (2), monophasic (1), or absent (0). A total Doppler run-off score (0-6) was calculated. After surgery, graft surveillance was accomplished with duplex US at 6, 12, 26, and 52 weeks. Graft and patient survival were assessed by using Cox regression analysis (Fig 1).

Results.—Doppler scoring was obtained for 82% of patients who subsequently underwent infrainguinal bypass grafting. Overall primary assisted graft patency at 1 year was 80%. With an increasing Doppler score from 0 to 6, primary assisted graft patency rose steadily from 50% to 100% (Fig 2).

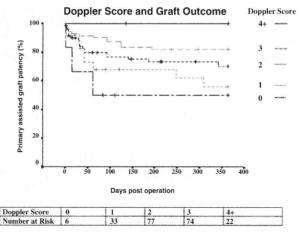

Doppler Score	0	1	2	3	4+
Number at Risk	6	33	77	74	22

FIGURE 2.—Doppler score and graft outcome. (Reprinted by permission of the publisher from Stewart AHR, Lucas A, Smith FCT, et al: Pre-operative hand-held Doppler run-off score can be used to stratify risk prior to infra-inguinal bypass surgery. *Eur J Vasc Endovasc Surg* 23:500-504, 2002.)

This rise was accompanied by a steady decline in patient mortality from 50% to 5%.

Conclusions.—In patients undergoing infrainguinal bypass surgery, simple scoring of run-off with hand-held Doppler signal characteristics of cruropedal vessels is predictive of graft patency and patient mortality in the first year after bypass surgery. This procedure may provide a method for stratifying operative risk for infrainguinal bypass surgery.

▶ Patients with good runoff do better than those with poor runoff. Internists aren't the only ones guilty of quantifying the obvious. (See also Abstract 10–3.)

G. L. Moneta, MD

Can Screening for Genetic Markers Improve Peripheral Artery Bypass Patency?

Kibbe MR, Hassett ALC, McSherry F, et al (Univ of Pittsburgh, Pa; Inst for Transfusion Medicine, Perry Point, Md; Veterans Affairs Cooperative Studies Coordinating Ctr, Boston; et al)

J Vasc Surg 36:1198-1206, 2002   10–9

Background.—Three genetic mutations have been associated with an increased risk of thromboembolic events: factor V Leiden R506Q, prothrombin G20210A, and methylenetetrahydrofolate reductase C677T (MTHFR) mutations. The effects of these 3 mutations on the patency of peripheral bypass procedures and preoperative and postoperative thromboembolic events were determined.

Methods.—The study group included 244 randomly selected participants in the Veterans Affairs Cooperative Study #362, all of whom were tested for factor V Leiden, prothrombin, or MTHFR mutations. Patients were randomly assigned to receive either aspirin or aspirin and warfarin therapy after undergoing a peripheral bypass procedure. The frequencies of preoperative and postoperative thromboembolic events and primary patency, assisted primary patency, and secondary patency rates were compared among carriers of the 3 mutations.

Results.—Fourteen patients (5.7%) were heterozygous for factor V Leiden mutation, 7 patients (2.9%) were heterozygous for the prothrombin mutation, and 108 patients (44.6%) and 15 patients (6.2%) were heterozygous and homozygous, respectively, for the MTHFR mutation. After surgery, patients who were homozygous for the MTHFR gene mutation had increased graft thrombosis (33.3%) compared with patients who were heterozygous for the MTHFR mutation (11.1%) and also had lower primary patency, assisted primary patency, and secondary patency than patients who were heterozygous for MTHFR. Patients who were heterozygous for the MTHFR mutation had fewer graft thromboses, fewer below-knee amputations, and higher primary patency, assisted primary patency, and secondary patency rates compared with wild-type control participants. Patients with factor V Leiden or prothrombin mutations undergoing peripheral bypass procedures were not at an increased risk for postoperative graft occlusion or thromboembolic events.

Conclusion.—Patients who were homozygous for the MTHFR mutation had lower graft patency rates compared with heterozygous patients, and there was a trend toward lower patency rates compared with wild-type control subjects. Preoperative screening for the MTHFR mutation may identify patients at an increased risk of graft thrombosis.

▶ The authors of this paper continue to glean important information from the Veterans Affairs Cooperative Study #362. These data, collected prospectively, suggest a correlation between heterozygous and homozygous point mutations for the methylenetetrahydrofolate reductase (MTHFR) gene and graft patency. This paper is truly a statistical tour de force, but there is no sense that the authors are trying to overstate or understate their findings. In the results section of the paper, the rationale for why certain end points could not reach statistical significance are lucidly explained. This paper, along with the known life-threatening complication associated with anticoagulant therapy, provides a compelling argument for routine screening for MTHFR in patients undergoing operative interventions. Similar data need to be collected and analyzed for patients undergoing catheter-based peripheral interventions. These data may, however, grossly underestimate the effects of genetic polymorphism on issues related to vascular graft patency because very few women were likely to have been included in this analysis.

M. T. Watkins, MD

Vein Versus Polytetrafluoroethylene in Above-Knee Femoropopliteal Bypass Grafting: Five-Year Results of a Randomized Controlled Trial

Klinkert P, Schepers A, Burger DHC, et al (Red Cross Hosp, The Hague, The Netherlands; Leiden Univ, The Netherlands)
J Vasc Surg 37:149-155, 2003   10–10

Background.—Controversy still exists whether to use polytetrafluoroethylene (PTFE) or vein for above-knee femoropopliteal bypass. Vein and PTFE grafts were prospectively compared for above-knee femoropopliteal bypasses in a randomized trial with 5-year follow-up.

Methods.—Of the 151 above-knee femoropopliteal bypasses performed between 1993 and 1996, 120 were done for severe claudication, 20 for rest pain, and 11 for ulceration. Patients were randomly assigned to undergo reversed saphenous venous bypass (75 procedures) or PTFE bypass (76 procedures).

Results.—The venous group had a significantly lower incidence of diabetes mellitus, but other risk factors and angiographic results were evenly distributed between the 2 groups. Venous bypasses required a significantly longer operating time than PTFE grafts. No perioperative deaths occurred, and none of the 7 superficial wound infections that developed led to reoperation or a loss of the bypass. Forty-two patients with an open bypass and 15

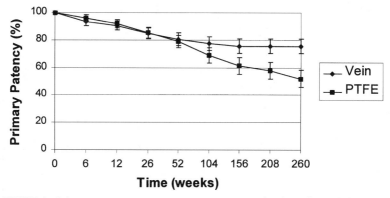

FIGURE 1.—Primary patency rates over time comparing vein with polytetrafluoroethylene in above-knee femoropopliteal bypass. *Error bars*, standard error of mean. (Reprinted by permission of the publisher from Klinkert P, Schepers A, Burger DHC, et al: Vein versus polytetrafluoroethylene in above-knee femoro-popliteal bypass grafting: Five-year results of a randomized controlled trial. *J Vasc Surg* 37:149-155, 2003. Copyright 2003 by Elsevier.)

with an occluded bypass died within 5 years. Primary patency rates at 5 years were 75.6% and 51.9%, respectively, for venous bypass and PTFE grafts (Fig 1). Venous grafts had a 79.7% secondary patency rate, whereas PTFE grafts had a 57.2% rate (Fig 2). Fourteen of the venous bypasses and 29 of the PTFE grafts failed. Comparing the failing cases, PTFE grafts required significantly more reinterventions than venous bypasses.

Conclusions.—At 2 years, PTFE grafts were an acceptable alternative to venous grafts; however, 5-year follow-up revealed a significant difference in primary and secondary patency rates between the 2 procedures favoring vein grafts. It appears that PTFE is acceptable for above-knee femoropoplit-

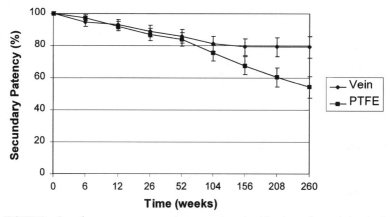

FIGURE 2.—Secondary patency rates over time comparing vein with polytetrafluoroethylene in above-knee femoropopliteal bypass. *Error bars*, standard error of mean. (Reprinted by permission of the publisher from Klinkert P, Schepers A, Burger DHC, et al: Vein versus polytetrafluoroethylene in above-knee femoro-popliteal bypass grafting: Five-year results of a randomized controlled trial. *J Vasc Surg* 37:149-155, 2003. Copyright 2003 by Elsevier.)

eal bypass in patients with short life expectancy or when vein is unavailable. All other patients are better treated with saphenous vein grafts.

▶ Vein works best. Concerns over "preserving the vein" are just excuses. No one has ever shown that choosing a relatively poor operation over a better one is ever a good idea. (See also comment on Abstract 10–13 for a slightly different view.)

G. L. Moneta, MD

Infrainguinal Bypass Conduit: Autogenous or Synthetic—A National Perspective
Merrell GA, Gusberg RJ (Yale School of Medicine, New Haven, Conn)
Vasc Endovasc Surg 36:247-254, 2002   10–11

Introduction.—Numerous studies have described the relative advantages and disadvantages of venous grafts (VGs) versus synthetic grafts (SGs) for infrainguinal bypass (IB). VGs appear to have superior patency rates, and many reports have documented their superiority over SGs when used in the infrapopliteal position. Two data sets were analyzed to define and explain practice patterns of graft usage in the United States.

Methods.—The first data set was Medicare part B billing data for patients in 49 states (excluding Alaska) who received an IB in 3 specific calendar years (1995 through 1997). Procedures were defined by 9 CPT billing codes. For the second data set, hospitals with more than 150 beds in 6 geographically diverse states (California, Colorado, Connecticut, Iowa, Minnesota, and Mississippi) were asked for volume statistics on the same CPT codes. The first data set included 254,677 procedures; the second included 1063 procedures performed at 27 institutions. The correlation between SG usage and smoking prevalence or diabetes prevalence was analyzed.

Results.—National data indicated that 41% of all infrainguinal grafts were synthetic, although geographic variation was considerable. Massachusetts had the lowest rate of SG use (27%) and Wyoming had the highest (80%). Nationwide, 60% of femoral popliteal grafts were synthetic; Oregon was lowest with 40% and Wyoming highest with 90%. The nationwide rate of synthetic infrapopliteal grafts was 14%, with a range of 4% (Montana) to 33% (Wyoming). The geographic variation in use of SGs showed no correlation with the prevalence of either diabetes mellitus or smoking. Analysis of data from the 27 hospitals surveyed indicated a significantly lower use of SGs for IB at teaching hospitals.

Conclusion.—Numerous series have confirmed the patency advantage of VGs over SGs for IB, but the use of SGs is substantial. Significant interstate and intrastate variations exist, however, and surgeons at teaching hospitals appear to use SGs less often than surgeons at nonteaching hospitals. Patient demographics do not appear to explain practice variations.

▶ I am amazed and disappointed at the high utilization of synthetic grafts for infrainguinal bypass. Shame on us. (See Abstract 10–10.)

G. L. Moneta, MD

A Decade of Experience With Dorsalis Pedis Artery Bypass: Analysis of Outcome in More Than 1000 Cases

Pomposelli FB, Kansal N, Hamdan AD, et al (Harvard Med School, Boston)
J Vasc Surg 37:307-315, 2003   10–12

Background.—An experience during the last decade with dorsalis pedis (DP) bypass for ischemic limb salvage in diabetic patients was reviewed. Outcomes of DP bypass were analyzed in terms of durability, limb salvage, and patient factors that may affect results.

Methods.—This retrospective analysis included 1032 DP bypass procedures in 865 patients from 1990 to 2000. These procedures accounted for 27.6% of the 3731 lower extremity arterial bypass procedures performed during that period. The majority of the patients (69%) were men, with a mean age of 66.8 years. Most of the patients (92%) had diabetes mellitus. All the procedures were performed for limb salvage and all but 2 were autogenous vein.

Results.—The mortality rate was 0.9% within 1 month of surgery. There were 42 graft failures (4.2%) within the first month, although 13 of these failures were successfully revised. In follow-up of 1 to 120 months (mean, 23.6 months), primary patency, secondary patency, limb salvage, and patient survival rates were 56.8%, 62.7%, 78.2%, and 48.6%, respectively, at

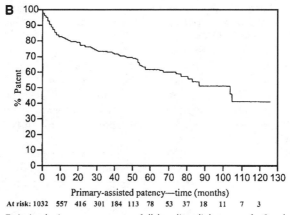

At risk: 1032 557 416 301 184 113 78 53 37 18 11 7 3

FIGURE 1.—B, Assisted primary patency rates of all dorsalis pedis bypass grafts. Standard error was less than 10% at all time intervals. (Reprinted by permission of the publisher from Pomposelli FB, Kansal N, Hamdan AD, et al: A decade of experience with dorsalis pedis artery bypass: Analysis of outcome in more than 1000 cases. *J Vasc Surg* 37:307-315, 2003. Copyright 2003 by Elsevier.)

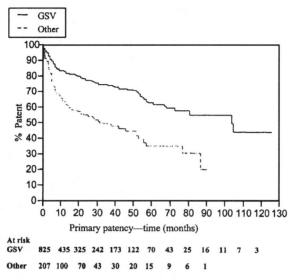

FIGURE 4.—Primary patency rate of greater saphenous vein (*GSV*) versus all other conduits. Difference is significant (*P* < .0001). Standard error was less than 10% at all time intervals. (Reprinted by permission of the publisher from Pomposelli FB, Kansal N, Hamdan AD, et al: A decade of experience with dorsalis pedis artery bypass: Analysis of outcome in more than 1000 cases. *J Vasc Surg* 37:307-315, 2003. Copyright 2003 by Elsevier.)

5 years and 37.7%, 41.7%, 57.7%, and 23.8%, respectively, at 10 years (Fig 1, B). Primary graft patency was worse in female patients (46.5% vs 61.6% in males at 5 years) but better in patients with diabetes (65.9% vs 56.3% for patients without diabetes mellitus at 4 years). Saphenous vein grafts had a secondary patency rate of 67.6%, better than all other conduits at 5 years (46.3%). Multivariate analysis indicated that a length of stay of more than 10 days and DP bypass for the surgical indication of previous graft occlusion were independent predictors of worse graft patency at 1 year. The use of saphenous vein as conduit was predictive of better patency (Fig 4).

Conclusions.—DP bypass is a durable procedure with a high likelihood of ischemic foot salvage over many years. These findings support the use of pedal arterial reconstruction for patients with diabetes mellitus with ischemic foot complications.

▶ This huge experience with pedal bypass with outstanding results confirms that the dorsal pedal artery is an excellent target for distal bypass. I agree with the authors that using the Doppler to mark the course of the dorsal pedal artery before making the incision, use of autogenous conduit, and the foot wound and its closure are the most important elements of a successful dorsal pedal bypass.

G. L. Moneta, MD

Bypass in the Absence of Ipsilateral Greater Saphenous Vein: Safety and Superiority of the Contralateral Greater Saphenous Vein

Chew DKW, Owens CD, Belkin M, et al (Harvard Med School, Boston)
J Vasc Surg 35:1085-1092, 2002   10–13

Introduction.—An absent or inadequate ipsilateral greater saphenous vein (IGSV) is not uncommon in patients requiring lower extremity infrainguinal revascularization. There is no consensus, however, on the optimal alternative conduit. Long-term results of different autogenous conduits utilized for infrainguinal bypass were retrospectively evaluated in 203 patients who underwent 226 reconstructions.

Methods.—All autogenous infrainguinal reconstructions were performed at a single institution between January 1990 and June 2000. The venous conduits used included contralateral GSV (CGSV), single-segment lesser saphenous vein, single-segment arm vein (SSAV), and autogenous composite vein (ACV). Outcome was determined by review of patient records, operative reports, vascular laboratory and angiographic reports, and telephone follow-up of patients with incomplete information. The median follow-up was 15 months (range, 0.1-106 months).

Results.—There were 128 men and 98 women with a mean age of 69 years. None had adequate IGSV, and many had significant risk factors including diabetes mellitus (51%) and coronary artery disease (70%). The predominant indication for surgery (93%) was limb salvage. In 59% of pa-

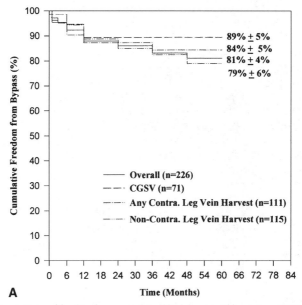

A

FIGURE 2.—A, Rates of freedom from contralateral limb bypass. *Abbreviation: CGSV,* Contralateral greater saphenous vein. (Reprinted by permission of the publisher from Chew DKW, Owens CD, Belkin M, et al: Bypass in the absence of ipsilateral greater saphenous vein: Safety and superiority of the contralateral greater saphenous vein. *J Vasc Surg* 35:1085-1092, 2002. Copyright 2002 by Elsevier.)

tients, there had been a previous failed lower limb bypass. All bypasses were completed with autogenous vein (ACV in 45%, CGSV in 31%, SSAV in 19%, and single-segment lesser saphenous vein in 5%). Bypasses in 84% of cases were performed to a tibial or pedal artery.

Thirty-day mortality was 1%. Overall postoperative morbidity was 24%; however, only 7% of patients experienced major morbidity. The rate of donor wound site complications was 6% and the 30-day rate of graft occlusion was 9%. The mean 5-year primary patency rates were significantly better for CGSV (61%) than for ACV (39%), but 5-year secondary patency rates were comparable in the CGSV (73%), SSAV (60%), and ACV (63%) groups. Five-year limb salvage rates were 81%, 81%, and 78%, respectively. Nine contralateral limbs were amputated at a mean of 36 months after bypass. The overall 5-year freedom from contralateral limb bypass was 81% (Fig 2).

Conclusion.—The alternative conduit of choice for most patients with inadequate IGSV is the CGSV, which offers desired length, superior performance, ease of harvest, and minimal risk to the donor limb. Long-term outcome of the contralateral limb does not appear to be compromised with this approach.

▶ The authors in this study from a center of excellence in lower extremity arterial reconstruction showed that in patients without significant ischemia, the use of the contralateral saphenous vein showed that these patients are unlikely to lose their limb as the result of the vein harvest, and they argue strongly against the concept of "saving the contralateral vein." It is interesting to note some clinical biases in their practice, including the frequent use of proximal superficial femoral, common femoral artery for inflow, where most of the outflow arteries were tibial or pedal vessels, which necessitates the need for a long conduit. Other centers that routinely avoid the use of the contralateral saphenous vein often have a large population of diabetic patients, where distal inflow sites and shorter vein grafts are more frequently possible, making alternative conduits more attractive. My personal opinion is that it is reasonable to use the contralateral saphenous vein in patients without significant contralateral ischemia. In patients being operated on for limb salvage indications, particularly those requiring redo procedures, it's unusual in my experience to find normal circulation in the opposite leg, especially in those patients who have diabetes mellitus. Moreover, while use of arm vein conduits is clearly more technically challenging than the use of the contralateral saphenous vein, even the most "arm-vein-averse" vascular surgeons rapidly become devotees the first time they have to amputate a contralateral limb because of an ischemic complication of vein harvest.

F. B. Pomposelli, Jr, MD

Long-term Results of Revised Infrainguinal Arterial Reconstructions

Darling RC III, Roddy SP, Chang BB, et al (Albany Med College, NY)
J Vasc Surg 35:773-778, 2002   10–14

Background.—Secondary interventions for continued patency of infrainguinal vein grafts are needed in as many as 20% of the patients. The need for these reconstructions raises concern about the continued patency of these revascularizations. The long-term patency of revised venous reconstructions was retrospectively investigated.

Methods.—Data on 3944 infrainguinal arterial reconstructions completed with vein as the conduit in the past 15 years were analyzed. Vein in situ was used in 2780 procedures, and excised vein in a single piece or spliced configuration was used in 1164. Duplex US scans were obtained at 3, 6, and 12 months in the first year and every 6 months thereafter.

Findings.—Nine percent of excised veins and 10% of in-situ reconstructions were revised: 6% of single-piece venous conduits and 14% of spliced venous reconstructions. At 5 years, the patency rates for revised and unrevised reconstructions were 67% and 78%, respectively ($P < .0001$). The patency rates for unrevised in situ bypass grafts were 81% versus 69% for revised in situ reconstruction ($P < .0001$) and 68% for unrevised excised veins versus 59% for revised excised vein ($P = NS$).

Conclusions.—The long-term patency rates of venous conduits that need revision are lower than those of unrevised grafts. An aggressive surveillance protocol is warranted for revised grafts to maximize long-term patency.

▶ The authors' conclusions parallel our experience in Oregon in some ways but not others. We found patency of revised grafts to be equal to that of nonrevised grafts. In this study, however, revised graft patency was diminished compared with nonrevised grafts. This may reflect different levels of aggressiveness in repairing all vein graft lesions and in performing repeat revisions. This paper once again emphasizes the fact that while the majority of revisions are performed in the first year, grafts requiring revision are identified in some cases many years postimplantation. It is my belief graft surveillance should continue as long as the graft remains patent and the patient remain a candidate for revision.

G. L. Moneta, MD

Tissue Loss, Early Primary Graft Occlusion, Female Gender, and a Prohibitive Failure Rate of Secondary Infrainguinal Arterial Reconstruction

Henke PK, Proctor MC, Zajkowski PJ, et al (Univ of Michigan, Ann Arbor)
J Vasc Surg 35:902-909, 2002   10–15

Background.—Primary autologous vein infrainguinal bypass has overall 5-year patency and limb salvage rates between 70% and 85%, regardless of whether the vein bypass was reversed, in situ, or in a nonreversed translocated configuration. Secondary infrainguinal bypasses generally have inferior long-term patency compared with primary bypass procedures. This is most often attributed to the severity of the arterial disease. Factors related to early and late graft failure in patients who underwent secondary infrainguinal arterial reconstructions were identified.

Methods.—A retrospective medical record review of 330 consecutive patients who underwent infrainguinal bypasses between 1992 and 2000 at a university hospital was performed. From this review, a series of 79 patients who had undergone either primary or secondary procedures before final bypasses became the subjects for this study. Data from these 44 men and 35 women were analyzed with life-table analysis, logistic regression, and descriptive statistics.

Results.—The mean age of the patients was 60 years. Secondary infrainguinal reconstructions were performed in patients who had undergone earlier ipsilateral bypasses once (35 patients) or twice (44 patients). Comorbidities included coronary artery disease (72%), tobacco use (77%), and diabetes mellitus (34%), but no patients had hemodialysis-dependent renal failure. Disabling claudication, with an average ankle brachial index of 0.48, had been the indication for the primary operation in 77% of the cases. A femoral–popliteal bypass was the primary procedure in 67%, and a prosthetic graft was used in 62%. The mean duration of patency of these earlier bypasses was 25 months. In 51% of the patients, the indication for the final bypass was rest pain or tissue loss, and the average ankle brachial index was 0.37. The most common procedure was a femoral–distal bypass with the use of an autologous vein (63%). The mean patency duration of the secondary bypass was 30 months. In 22 patients (28%), graft failure occurred within 30 days of the operation, and amputation was necessary in 86% of these patients. The presence of rest pain or tissue loss, when accompanied by a history of early prior graft thrombosis in women, correlated with inferior patency rates, recurrent graft failure, and a 94% amputation rate; in contrast, the amputation rate in men in a similar setting was 57%. Final patency was not associated with age, number of prior bypasses, conduit types, tobacco use, or diabetes.

Conclusions.—Secondary infrainguinal bypasses are associated with an increased rate of graft failure and significant limb loss, particularly in patients with a history of rest pain or tissue loss, female sex, and early prior graft failure. More appropriate initial procedures in carefully selected patients coupled with aggressive postoperative graft surveillance may improve these outcomes.

▶ Although the number of patients in this study is relatively small, the results are particularly sobering. While 77% of patients had claudication as an indication for their initial operation, 51% of patients had a limb-threatening indication for arterial reconstruction at the time of the final procedure. Patency at 60 months for patients with limb-threatening ischemia for these secondary/ tertiary reconstructions was only 31%, compared with 49% for patients operated on for intermittent claudication at the final operation. Even more sobering is that of the 42 patients who had graft occlusions over the course of the study, 30 required major limb amputation, including 10 of whom who had a final indication for surgery being claudication. These results emphasize many points that we all know, but occasionally ignore. First, claudication is best managed conservatively whenever possible. Second, the use of venous conduits is preferred over prosthetic conduits in most situations, including those done for claudication. And finally, and perhaps most importantly, *do it right the first time!*

F. B. Pomposelli, Jr, MD

Modifiable Patient Factors Are Associated With Reverse Vein Graft Occlusion in the Era of Duplex Scan Surveillance
Giswold ME, Landry GJ, Sexton GJ, et al (Oregon Health & Science Univ, Portland; Veterans Affairs Med Ctr, Portland, Ore)
J Vasc Surg 37:47-53, 2003   10–16

Background.—From 10% to 30% of infrainguinal bypass grafts occlude, with 10% of patients requiring amputation after reverse vein graft (RVG) occlusion. Factors that affect the outcome of infrainguinal bypass grafts include anatomic considerations, end-stage renal disease, hypercoagulable states, gender, choice of conduit, diabetes mellitus, and other potentially modifiable variables under the control of the patient and physician. The causes of RVG occlusion that are under patient and physician control were

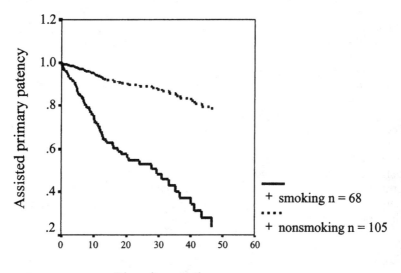

Time in months

FIGURE 1.—Adjusted assisted primary patency curve of RVGs comparing patients currently smoking (n = 68) with nonsmoking patients (n = 105). Curve was generated with Cox proportional hazard model. *P* < .001. (Reprinted by permission of the publisher from Giswold ME, Landry GJ, Sexton GJ, et al: Modifiable patient factors are associated with reverse vein graft occlusion in the era of duplex scan surveillance. *J Vasc Surg* 37:47-53, 2003. Copyright 2003 by Elsevier.)

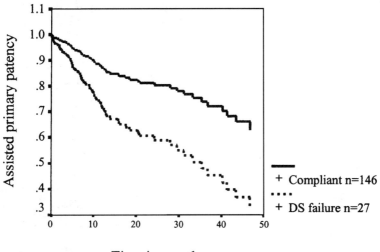

Time in months

FIGURE 2.—Adjusted assisted primary patency curve of RVGs comparing patients who fail early duplex scan surveillance (*DS*; n = 27) with compliant patients (n = 146). Curve was generated with Cox proportional hazard model. *P* = .006. (Reprinted by permission of the publisher from Giswold ME, Landry GJ, Sexton GJ, et al: Modifiable patient factors are associated with reverse vein graft occlusion in the era of duplex scan surveillance. *J Vasc Surg* 37:47-53, 2003. Copyright 2003 by Elsevier.)

assessed through an evaluation of patient characteristics and risk factors and duplex scan surveillance (DS) patterns.

Methods.—Six hundred seventy-four patients who underwent RVG between 1996 and 2000 were identified from prospectively maintained registries. The cases of 118 randomly selected patients whose grafts remained patent were compared with those of 55 patients whose grafts occluded. DS was performed every 3 months for the first year postoperatively, then every 6 months. The follow-up period extended a mean of 32.4 months. Having no DS within the first 3 months was termed early DS failure.

Results.—Occlusion occurred a mean of 13.4 months after surgery. Significantly lower assisted primary patency rates were noted for patients who were currently smoking than for nonsmokers, for patients on dialysis therapy versus those not on dialysis, for patients with early DS failure than for those with compliant DS, and for patients who had a known hypercoagulable state versus those who did not (Figs 1 and 2). Compliance with regular clinical visits and regular DS examinations for the duration of the follow-up period did not correlate with cigarette smoking, distance to drive to the institution, diabetes mellitus, previous ipsilateral bypass, gender, or age.

Conclusions.—The modifiable patient factors identified in this population were continued smoking and failure to participate in DS in the first 3 months postoperatively. Patients who continued to smoke and did not participate in follow-up evaluation had a higher likelihood of having occlusion of their graft.

▶ In the final analysis, it all seems so simple. Operate only when really necessary, get the patients to stop smoking, and follow the grafts with duplex. On the other hand, we all know what seems simple can be so difficult to achieve in real life.

G. L. Moneta, MD

Outcome of Catheter-Directed Thrombolysis for Lower Extremity Arterial Bypass Occlusion
Nehler MR, Mueller RJ, McLafferty RB, et al (Univ of Colorado, Denver; Southern Illinois Univ, Springfield; Colorado Prevention Ctr, Denver)
J Vasc Surg 37:72-78, 2003   10–17

Background.—Catheter-directed thrombolysis (CDT) is sometimes successful in opening an acutely occluded lower extremity arterial bypass (LEAB) graft and can reveal possible underlying lesions that can be addressed with either angioplasty or surgical revision. If reocclusion develops, CDT may be repeated under some circumstances. The long-term outcome of CDT used for the management of acute LEAB occlusion was evaluated.

Methods.—One hundred four patients had 109 acute LEAB occlusions treated with CDT by two practices between 1988 and 2001. Outcome measures included technical success, complications, secondary patency determination, and limb salvage. The number of secondary procedures required for residual lesions or failed CDT and the number of LEABs replaced or becoming infected were also noted.

Results.—Ninety-eight percent of the procedures were either completed or abandoned within 48 hours. In 77% of cases, CDT successfully restored patency. Of the 25 that failed CDT, 15 required surgical thrombectomy and revision, 4 were replaced, and 6 had no further revision procedures; 18 limbs were salvaged initially, and 7 were amputated. Three deaths occurred, and 14% of patients had bleeding complications requiring transfusion (7 required surgical evacuation/repair). Thirteen percent had other complications including compartment syndrome requiring fasciotomy, nonfatal myocardial infarction, and acute renal failure. A total of 2.9% of the patients having CDT died, and 6.7% had major amputations. With intention to treat analysis at 1 year, the secondary graft patency rate was 32%; at 3 years, 25%; and at 5 years, 19% (Fig 1). The 1-year secondary patency rates for LEABs with and without residual lesions where CDT was successful were 42% and 45%, respectively. Overall limb salvage rates were 73% at 1 year and 55% at 5 years, with 56% patient survival at 5 years. Recurrent interventions led to infection in 7 LEABs (8.3%) that had been salvaged with CDT, and 20 of the LEABs that were initially salvaged with CDT eventually required graft replacement, with 4 done immediately and 16 done after re-

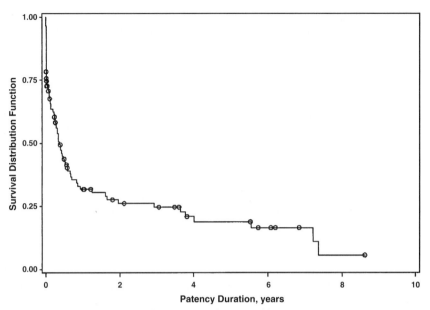

FIGURE 1.—Secondary patency for 109 LEABs after CDT. *Abbreviations: LEAB*, Lower extremity arterial bypass; *CDT*, catheter-directed thrombolysis. (Reprinted by permission of the publisher from Nehler MR, Mueller RJ, McLafferty RB, et al: Outcome of catheter-directed thrombolysis for lower extremity arterial bypass occlusion. *J Vasc Surg* 37:72-78, 2003. Copyright 2003 by Elsevier.)

current ischemic episodes. Two patients died while hospitalized for treatment of recurrent ischemia.

Conclusions.—The initial technical success for CDT as a treatment for acute LEAB occlusion was acceptable, but many cases eventually failed. Significant morbidity resulted from recurrent LEAB occlusion, leading to recurrent interventions, infection or replacement of the graft, and limb loss. CDT is reasonable treatment for acutely occluded LEAB grafts with liberal use of graft replacement for early and late failures in patients with favorable remaining autogenous conduit.

▶ CDT for occluded infrainguinal bypass grafts does not work well. In fact, it is really bad. Of course, placement of a new infrainguinal bypass for an occluded graft also has substantial problems. The take-home point is to avoid graft occlusion. You avoid graft occlusion by using autogenous grafts at all levels, including the above-knee popliteal (see Abstract 10–10), limiting the number of grafts by operating only for limb salvage or extreme claudication, and actively following up the patients with graft surveillance.

G. L. Moneta, MD

Vascular Training in the U.K.: Femorodistal Bypass, an Index Procedure?

Nasr MK, Taylor PJ, Horrocks M (Royal United Hosp, Bath, England)
Eur J Vasc Endovasc Surg 25:135-138, 2003   10–18

Introduction.—In the United Kingdom, the 3 index procedures for vascular surgical training are abdominal aortic aneurysm repair, carotid endarterectomy, and infrapopliteal bypass grafting. As more patients with critical limb ischemia have undergone primary treatment with percutaneous transluminal angioplasty (PTA), the number of primary bypass procedures has declined. The management of patients with critical limb ischemia was analyzed to assess the appropriateness of femorodistal bypass as a vascular index procedure.

Methods.—The analysis included a total of 608 limbs of 526 patients with chronic, critical ischemia admitted to a vascular surgery unit from 1994 through 1999. By policy, active revascularization was pursued if possible. Bypass surgery was reserved mainly for patients who were not candidates for PTA or in whom PTA had failed.

Results.—Either PTA, bypass surgery, or both were attempted in 86% of the limbs. Fourteen percent of the revascularized limbs underwent crural procedures. Of these 71 limbs, 34 underwent PTA as a sole treatment whereas 37 underwent femorodistal bypass grafting, alone or in combination with PTA. Diabetic patients were more likely to undergo PTA (Fig 2). Of

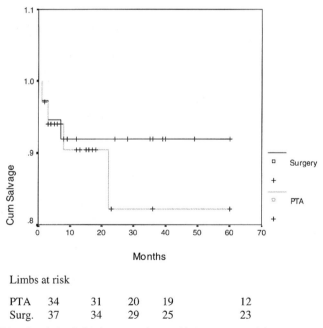

Limbs at risk

PTA	34	31	20	19	12
Surg.	37	34	29	25	23

FIGURE 2.—Cumulative limb salvage rates for crural lesions. (Reprinted from Nasr MK, Taylor PJ, Horrocks M: Vascular training in the U.K.: Femorodistal bypass, an index procedure? *Eur J Vasc Endovasc Surg* 25:135-138, 2003. Copyright 2003 by permission of the publisher.)

453 limbs with aortoiliac or femoropopliteal lesions, 304 were treated with PTA alone, 125 with surgery alone, and 24 with a combination of PTA and surgery.

Conclusions.—At a vascular surgery unit with an aggressive revascularization policy, only a small percentage of critically ischemic limbs are treated with primary femorodistal bypass. For these patients, including those with distal lesions, PTA has emerged as the first-line therapy and often the only treatment for critical limb ischemia. This practice pattern questions the relevance of considering femorodistal bypass as an index procedure for vascular surgical training.

▶ I think many would disagree that PTA is the initial procedure of choice for critical limb ischemia. This paper to me represents a particular practice pattern and nothing more.

G. L. Moneta, MD

Improved Patency of Infrainguinal Polytetrafluoroethylene Bypass Grafts Using a Distal Taylor Vein Patch

Yeung KK, Mills JL Sr, Hughes JD, et al (Univ of Arizona, Tucson)
Am J Surg 182:578-583, 2001   10–19

Introduction.—Graft patency and limb salvage rates for infrainguinal polytetrafluoroethylene (PTFE) bypass grafts with the use of distal anastomotic Taylor vein patch were examined in patients who did not have suitable vein conduit.

Methods.—Forty-four patients who underwent inguinal 6-mm PTFE leg bypasses with distal Taylor vein patches between January 1996 and August 2000 were reviewed retrospectively. All inpatient, outpatient, and vascular laboratory records were reviewed for data concerning patient demographics, preoperative risk factors, operative indications, inflow and outflow sites, postoperative management, and perioperative and postoperative complications. Eighty percent of patients received postoperative oral anticoagulation. Patient and graft status were updated during regular clinical examinations and serial graft duplex scanning.

Results.—Indications for surgery in 76% of patients were pain at rest, nonhealing ulcer, or gangrene. Forty-three percent of patients had undergone a prior ipsilateral leg bypass. Distal anastomotic sites were below-knee popliteal and tibial-peroneal arteries in 29% and 67%, respectively. The primary patency rates (SE <10%) for 1 month, 1 year, and 2 years were 86%, 71%, and 71%, respectively; limb salvage rates were 95%, 75%, and 66%, respectively; mortality rates were 5%, 20%, and 20%, respectively.

Conclusion.—These early results with PTFE and distal Taylor vein patch are promising and substantially superior to earlier reports of PTFE without anastomotic modification. Further long-term follow-up is needed to ascertain the 3- and 5-year durability of these reconstructions.

▶ This retrospective study from a center with a long interest in lower extremity arterial reconstruction and whom I know is committed to the use of vein whenever possible, lends further credence to the concept of applying some adjunctive measure to improve patency in prosthetic grafts in the lower extremity. The authors' early and midterm results are certainly compelling and suggest that the Taylor patch can improve patency. Unfortunately, this is a retrospective study, as are most of the other studies investigating these adjunctive techniques. The patency of grafts is dependent on many factors, and in the absence of a well-conducted, multicenter, controlled trial, I think it is unlikely that the question of whether vein patches and cuffs really improve prosthetic graft patency will ever be answered. I think the time has come to perform such a study. Like the authors, I prefer the use of the Taylor patch for infrapopliteal prosthetic arterial reconstructions on the infrequent occasion when I do them.

F. B. Pomposelli, Jr, MD

Graft Patency Is Not the Only Clinical Predictor of Success After Exclusion and Bypass of Popliteal Artery Aneurysms

Jones WT III, Hagino RT, Chiou AC, et al (Wilford Hall Med Ctr, Lackland Air Force Base, Tex)

J Vasc Surg 37:392-398, 2003   10–20

Background.—Surgical management of popliteal artery aneurysm (PAA) is undertaken with the goal of isolating the aneurysm, thereby preventing distal embolization and achieving revascularization. Three methods of PAA exclusion were evaluated with respect to long-term outcomes.

Methods.—Thirty patients (1 woman and 29 men; mean age, 76 years) had 41 reconstructions for PAA. Three methods of reconstruction were used—type 1: proximal and distal aneurysm ligation with short segment isolation (Fig 1); type 2: proximal and distal ligation with long segment isolation (Fig 2); and type 3: single ligature alone (Fig 3). The long-term outcomes were evaluated, with a mean follow-up of 46 months (range, 11-123 months).

Results.—Of the 38 procedures in which the method of PAA exclusion was clearly documented, 20 were type 1 exclusions, 10 were type 2, and 8 were type 3. Three patients were lost to follow-up, and 2 patients lost their limbs within 2 months of surgery because of extensive wound complications. Of the remaining 36 limbs, most aneurysms were occluded on follow-up, with only 2 patent PAAs. The mean maximum diameter of the excluded PAA decreased from 2.4 to 2.0 cm during the course of follow-up, with two thirds of the excluded aneurysms decreasing from 2.5 to 1.7 cm.

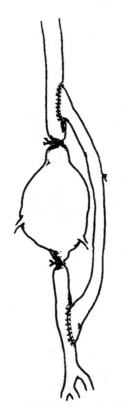

FIGURE 1.—Type 1 exclusion: proximal and distal ligation with short segment isolation. (Reprinted by permission of the publisher from Jones WT III, Hagino RT, Chiou AC, et al: Graft patency is not the only clinical predictor of success after exclusion and bypass of popliteal artery aneurysms. *J Vasc Surg* 37:392-398, 2003. Copyright 2003 by Elsevier.)

One third of the aneurysms were greatly enlarged when evaluated, with one fourth of these causing new compressive symptoms, such as local pain and tenderness. The method of PAA exclusion was significantly correlated with the late size of the excluded PAA. Type 1 was superior to both type 2 and type 3 exclusions in reducing aneurysm diameters. Final aneurysm size was a function of the presence or absence of visible arterial branches feeding the excluded aneurysm sac. The final PAA diameter did not correlate with either native arterial or vein graft enlargement. At 5 years, the graft primary patency rate was 86%, and the assisted primary patency was 92%. The limb salvage rate after 2 years was 89%.

Conclusions.—In general, the PAA exclusions produced aneurysm thrombosis and reduced size, but aneurysms enlarged in a third of patients, with several enlarging as much as 50% and producing compressive symptoms. Enlargement of the vein graft did not influence patency adversely. A

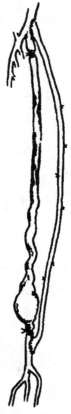

FIGURE 2.—Type 2 exclusion: proximal and distal ligation with long segment isolation. (Reprinted by permission of the publisher from Jones WT III, Hagino RT, Chiou AC, et al: Graft patency is not the only clinical predictor of success after exclusion and bypass of popliteal artery aneurysms. *J Vasc Surg* 37:392-398, 2003. Copyright 2003 by Elsevier.)

short bypass graft with proximal and distal ligation of the aneurysm produced the best overall results.

▶ This study seems to answer a question that I would think would be self-evident to most vascular surgeons. Proper isolation exclusion of a PAA requires a ligature both proximal and distal to the aneurysm sac. The anatomic variability of PAAs is such that the so-called type 1 exclusion cannot always be performed. However, there is really no reason why aneurysms cannot be ligated both proximally and distally. It should be no surprise to any vascular surgeon that even with proximal and distal ligatures, PAAs may still occasionally enlarge due to the phenomenon that is analogous to type 2 endoleak in aortic aneurysms treated with stent grafts. Continued surveillance of these patients

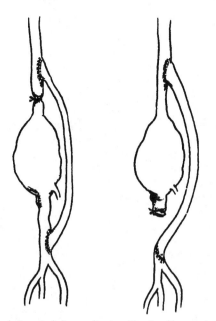

FIGURE 3.—Type 3 exclusion: single ligature ligation. (Reprinted by permission of the publisher from Jones WT III, Hagino RT, Chiou AC, et al: Graft patency is not the only clinical predictor of success after exclusion and bypass of popliteal artery aneurysms. *J Vasc Surg* 37:392-398, 2003. Copyright 2003 by Elsevier.)

even after aneurysm ligation is therefore critical, not only to assess grafts for patency, but also for continued aneurysm enlargement.

F. B. Pomposelli, Jr, MD

A Randomised, Double Blind, Placebo-controlled Study to Determine the Efficacy of Immune Modulation Therapy in the Treatment of Patients Suffering From Peripheral Arterial Occlusive Disease With Intermittent Claudication

McGrath C, Robb R, Lucas AJ, et al (Bristol Royal Infirmary, England; Ninewells Hosp and Med School, Dundee, Scotland)

Eur J Vasc Endovasc Surg 23:381-387, 2002   10–21

Background.—Current treatment for intermittent claudication includes risk factor modification, exercise therapy, balloon angioplasty, medication, and surgery. Immune modulation therapy (IMT) is a new therapeutic approach to treatment of claudication. IMT involves the administration of autologous blood components after their ex vivo exposure to thermal and oxidative stress. While several studies have indicated that IMT may be helpful in relieving symptoms of claudication, the exact mechanism of therapy is unclear. The effect of IMT on claudication distances was investigated.

Methods.—This double-blind placebo-controlled trial randomly assigned 85 patients with disabling intermittent claudication stratified for short- and long-distance intermittent claudication. For IMT, 10 mL of citrated autologous blood was administered by IM injection after exposure to ultraviolet light, oxidation, and a temperature of 42.5°C. Patients received 2, 3, or 4 courses, depending on their response, with each course consisting of 6 injections in 3 weeks, followed by 3 weeks of rest. The main outcome measure was the number of patients who had a greater than 50% increase in initial claudication distance in each group. Secondary outcome measures included percentage changes in initial claudication distance and change in quality of life.

Results.—At week 24, there were more responders in the IMT group (65%) than in the placebo group (41%). In the subgroup of short-distance claudicants, this difference was statistically significant (17/26 or 65%). The median increase in initial claudication distance was significantly greater in the IMT group (81%) than in the placebo group (44%). Quality of life measurements paralleled these results.

Conclusion.—Immune modulation therapy may be effective treatment for patients with short-distance intermittent claudication.

▶ IMT consists of exposing 10 mL of a patient's blood to UV light, ozone, and heat, then returning the blood to the patient via an IM injection. At first, this sounds akin to chelation therapy. It's not clear that anyone really knows what the biological response is to IMT except that, in this study, claudicants had a sustained trend toward improved walking distance and quality of life. The sponsor of the study, Vasogen, manufactures the all-in-one device that "treats" the patient's blood sample before reinjection. While intriguing and at least in this case, subjected to rigorous scientific scrutiny, IMT is not yet ready for prime time treatment of claudication. This study needs to be replicated, and a more complete biological characterization of the host response to IMT is necessary.

L. W. Kraiss, MD

Naked Plasmid DNA Encoding Fibroblast Growth Factor Type 1 for the Treatment of End-Stage Unreconstructible Lower Extremity Ischemia: Preliminary Results of a Phase I Trial
Comerota AJ, Throm RC, Miller KA, et al (Temple Univ, Philadelphia; Gencell, Aventis Pharma, Bridgewater, NJ; Hennepin County Med Ctr, Minneapolis; et al)
J Vasc Surg 35:930-936, 2002   10–22

Background.—Therapeutic angiogenesis is a new treatment strategy designed to improve collateral blood vessel formation by stimulation of neovascularization through expression of angiogenic growth factors. This study evaluated the safety and tolerance of increasing single and repeated (2) doses of IM naked plasmid DNA encoding for fibroblast growth factor (FGF) type

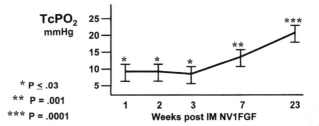

FIGURE 2.—Foot transcutaneous oximetry (*TcPO₂*) (millimeters of mercury; mean) after IM fibroblast growth factor type 1 (*NV1FGF*) (change from baseline). (Reprinted by permission of the publisher from Comerota AJ, Throm RC, Miller KA, et al: Naked plasmid DNA encoding fibroblast growth factor type 1 for the treatment of end-stage unreconstructible lower extremity ischemia: Preliminary results of a phase I trial. *J Vasc Surg* 35:930-936, 2002. Copyright 2002 by Elsevier.)

1 (NV1FGF) administered to patients with unreconstructible end-stage peripheral arterial occlusive disease.

Methods.—Intramuscular NV1FGF was administered to 51 patients with critical limb ischemia and unreconstructible peripheral arterial occlusive disease. Increasing single and repeated doses of NV1FGF were injected into the ischemic thigh and calf. Arteriography was performed before treatment and was repeated 12 weeks after treatment. Side effects and serious adverse events were monitored. Measurements of plasma and urine levels were performed to evaluate the distribution of NV1FGF plasmid. Serum FGF-1 was measured as an analysis of gene expression at the protein level. Transcutaneous oxygen pressure, ankle brachial index, toe brachial index, pain assessment by visual analogue scale, and ulcer healing were also assessed. The safety results presented here apply to 51 patients, and clinical outcomes are presented for the first 15 patients who completed the 6-month follow-up study.

Results.—The NV1FGF was well tolerated by all patients. There were 66 serious adverse events, but none were considered to be related to NV1FGF. Four patients had adverse events that may have been related to the study treatment, including pain, injection site pain, peripheral edema, myasthenia, and paresthesia. There were no laboratory adverse events related to

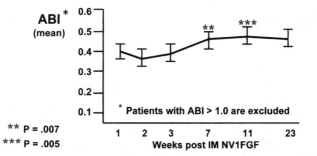

FIGURE 3.—Mean ankle-brachial index (*ABI*) after IM fibroblast growth factor type 1 (*NV1FGF*). (Reprinted by permission of the publisher from Comerota AJ, Throm RC, Miller KA, et al: Naked plasmid DNA encoding fibroblast growth factor type 1 for the treatment of end-stage unreconstructible lower extremity ischemia: Preliminary results of a phase I trial. *J Vasc Surg* 35:930-936, 2002. Copyright 2002 by Elsevier.)

NV1FGF. Biodistribution of plasmid was limited and transient in plasma and absent in urine, and there was no increase in FGF-1 serum level. Compared with pretreatment values, there were significant reductions in pain and aggregate ulcer size and an increase in transcutaneous oxygen pressure (Fig 2). A significant increase in ankle-brachial index was also observed (Fig 3).

Conclusion.—NV1FGF was well tolerated in patients with unreconstructible peripheral arterial occlusive disease. NV1FGF may be effective for the treatment of end-stage limb ischemia. Further investigation of NV1FGF is needed in a placebo-controlled, double-blind clinical trial.

▶ This ambitious clinical trial was designed to test the safety of a gene therapy for FGF in patients with unreconstructible occlusive peripheral vascular disease. Sixty-six severe adverse events occurred in this critically ill patient population. The paper is essentially descriptive because there are no controls. I suspect the adverse events were more characteristic of the kinds of problems akin to patients with end-stage limb ischemia rather than a systemic effect of the therapy, but there's no way to prove it. Given our knowledge of the natural history of end-stage occlusive peripheral vascular disease, it's probably unethical to recruit a control patient population for such a study. The results are encouraging (decreased pain, increased tissue oxygen, increased ankle-brachial index), but the lack of a dose-response curve casts doubt on the efficacy of the plasmid delivery system (naked plasmid DNA administered IM).

M. T. Watkins, MD

Influence of Lipoprotein(a) on Restenosis After Femoropopliteal Percutaneous Transluminal Angioplasty in Type 2 Diabetic Patients
Maca TH, Ahmadi R, Derfler K, et al (Univ of Vienna)
Diabetic Med 19:300-306, 2002   10–23

Background.—Diabetes increases the risk of early cardiovascular events. Elevated levels of lipoprotein(a) (Lp[a]) may worsen the prognosis of patients with diabetes and vascular disease. The rate of restenosis after percutaneous transluminal angioplasty (PTA) is increased in patients with type 2 diabetes. This study is the first to compare the rates of recurrent stenosis after femoropopliteal PTA in diabetic and nondiabetic patients with respect to Lp(a) levels.

Methods.—The clinical course and risk profile were prospectively followed in 132 patients (54 with type 2 diabetes and 78 nondiabetic patients) with peripheral arterial occlusive disease (PAD) after PTA. Clinical examination, oscillometry, ankle-brachial blood pressure index, and the toe systolic blood pressure index were assessed during follow-up. Duplex sonography and reangiography were also used to verify suspected restenosis or reocclusion of angioplasty sites.

Results.—Patients with type 2 diabetes had a lower median Lp(a) than patients without diabetes (9 vs 15 mg/dL). Recurrence within 1 year after PTA occurred in 25 (46%) diabetic and 30 (38%) nondiabetic patients. Patients with type 2 diabetes with 1 year of patency had a median Lp(a) of 7, compared with a median Lp(a) of 11 mg/dL in nondiabetic patients. However, 12 months after angioplasty, Lp(a) correlated negatively with the ankle-brachial index in both diabetic and nondiabetic patients. The probability of recurrence after PTA increased continuously with higher levels of Lp(a) in each subgroup of patients.

Conclusion.—These findings indicate that Lp(a) is generally lower in patients with peripheral arterial occlusive disease and type 2 diabetes than in nondiabetic patients. The increased risk for restenosis with rising levels of Lp(a) is set at a lower Lp(a) in patients with diabetes.

▶ Most surgeons and other interventionalists have focused on anatomy and medical comorbidities rather than potential serum markers as predictors of recurrence after intervention. In this study, Maca et al have reviewed a number of serum markers in diabetics and nondiabetics undergoing femoropopliteal PTA to identify a potential serum marker for recurrence, with specific reference to Lp(a).

The authors conclude that while diabetic patients have a baseline lower level of Lp(a), they tend to be more sensitive to even mild elevations of this serum constituent in terms of the response to arterial intervention. They further recommend that Lp(a) data be separated for diabetic and nondiabetic patients in forthcoming studies. Unfortunately, until the cause of this lipoprotein effect on disease recurrence can be clearly elucidated, the real benefits of this knowledge cannot be realized.

D. G. Clair, MD

Does Subintimal Angioplasty Have a Role in the Treatment of Severe Lower Extremity Ischemia?
Lipsitz EC, Ohki T, Veith FJ, et al (Albert Einstein College of Medicine, Bronx, NY)
J Vasc Surg 37:386-391, 2003   10–24

Background.—Subintimal angioplasty (SIA) has been proposed for the treatment of long lower extremity arterial occlusions; however, this technique has not gained wide acceptance despite promising results in a number of small centers in Europe. There are no reports of positive results with SIA in the North American literature. The role of SIA in a group of patients with severe lower extremity arterial occlusive disease was evaluated.

Methods.—During a 2.5-year period, 39 patients with arterial occlusions (median length, 8 cm) were treated with SIA on an intention-to-treat basis. Gangrene was present in 25 patients, 5 patients had rest pain, and 9 had disabling claudication. There were 24 superficial femoral, 2 superficial femoral–popliteal, 4 popliteal, 2 popliteal-tibial, 5 tibial, and 2 external iliac artery lesions. With the use of fluoroscopic guidance via a prograde common femoral artery puncture or a contralateral common femoral artery puncture,

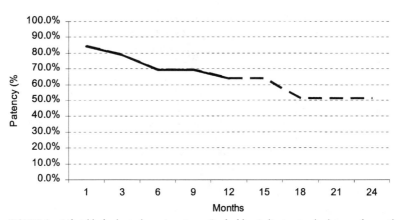

FIGURE 2.—Life-table for hemodynamic patency. *Dashed line* indicates standard error of more than 10%. Details of analysis are available in Table 1 (online only). (Reprinted by permission of the publisher from Lipsitz EC, Ohki T, Veith FJ, et al: Does subintimal angioplasty have a role in the treatment of severe lower extremity ischemia? *J Vasc Surg* 37:386-391, 2003. Copyright 2003 by Elsevier.)

a subintimal dissection plane was created across the occlusion with a standard guidewire and catheter. The arterial lumen was reentered distal to the occlusion. The recanalized segment was then dilated. All the patients were followed up with arterial duplex scan.

Results.—The SIA procedure was technically successful in 34 of 39 patients (87%). The 5 failures resulted from an inability to reenter the patent lumen distally, and these 5 patients underwent successful bypasses. In the 34 technically successful procedures, pain was resolved completely in 14 of 14 patients, and areas of gangrene healed in 21 of 25 patients. The cumulative patency rate in patients in whom SIA was successful was 74% ± 10% at 12 months (Fig 2). The mean increase in ankle-brachial index after SIA was 0.34. Two distal embolic events occurred, both of which were successfully treated with surgical or catheter-directed techniques. Three patients underwent subsequent bypass, and the remaining 5 patients are asymptomatic at last report.

Conclusions.—SIA is a feasible and effective approach in certain patients with lower extremity artery occlusions and threatened limbs. These findings are supportive of a greater role for SIA in the treatment of lower extremity arterial occlusive disease.

▶ This article suggests SIA has a role in the treatment of occlusive disease. It neither defines this role well nor clarifies well the patient population for whom SIA might be used as primary therapy. Hopefully, as more experience with this technique is gained, definition of the population benefiting the most can be identified.

D. G. Clair, MD

Intravascular Gamma Radiation for In-Stent Restenosis in Saphenous-Vein Bypass Grafts

Waksman R, Ajani AE, White RL, et al (Washington Hosp Center, DC; Oschner Clinic, New Orleans, La; Scripps Clinic, San Diego, Calif)
N Engl J Med 346:1194-1199, 2002   10–25

Background.—The effects of intravascular gamma radiation in patients with in-stent restenosis of coronary saphenous vein bypass grafts were examined.

Methods.—A total of 120 patients were enrolled between August 1998 and August 2000. The patients were assigned to 1 of 2 groups: 60 to the ^{192}Ir group and 60 to the placebo group. Angiographic and intravascular US studies were performed before revascularization of the saphenous vein graft to determine the length of the lesion and the size of the vessel. The prescribed dose of radiation was 14 to 15 Gy in vessels 2.5 to 4.0 mm in diameter and 18 Gy in vessels greater than 4.0 mm in diameter.

Results.—All patients tolerated the radiation treatment. Between the 2 groups, there were no significant differences in in-hospital complications. At 6 months, angiography was performed in 85% of the ^{192}Ir group and 89% of the placebo group. The rate of restenosis in the stented segment in the ^{192}Ir group was 65% lower (21% vs 44%) than in the placebo group ($P = .005$). At 12 months' clinical follow-up, data were obtained for all patients. The risk of a major cardiac event was significantly lower in the ^{192}Ir group than in the placebo group ($P < .001$). Event-free survival over a 24-month period is shown in Fig 2.

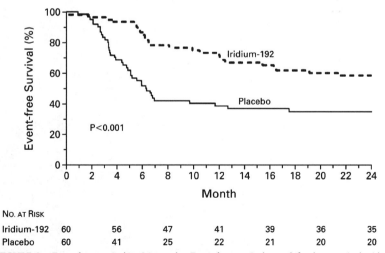

FIGURE 2.—Event-free survival at 24 months. Event-free survival was defined as survival without Q-wave myocardial infarction or revascularization of the target vessel. Data were available for 79 of 120 patients at 24 months. (Reprinted by permission of *The New England Journal of Medicine* from Waksman R, Ajani AE, White RL, et al: Intravascular gamma radiation for in-stent restenosis in saphenous-vein bypass grafts. *N Engl J Med* 346:1194-1199, 2002. Copyright 2002, Massachusetts Medical Society. All rights reserved.)

Conclusions.—Intravascular gamma radiation reduces the risk of in-stent restenosis in saphenous-vein grafts for a 12-month period.

▶ Peripheral vein grafts have high rates of restenosis when treated with interventional therapies for disease. While this study does not address directly the effect of radiation therapy for peripheral vein grafts, it clearly offers a potential therapy that might be of benefit in this patient population and poses the potential for a peripheral trial of radiation therapy to treat vein grafts after interventional therapy.

D. G. Clair, MD

11 Hemoaccess and Upper Extremity Vascular

Prospective Validation of an Algorithm to Maximize Native Arterio-venous Fistulae for Chronic Hemodialysis Access

Huber TS, Ozaki CK, Flynn TC, et al (Univ of Florida, Gainesville)

J Vasc Surg 36:452-459, 2002   11–1

Introduction.—The National Kidney Foundation Dialysis Outcome Quality Initiative Clinical Practice guidelines recommend increasing the placement of native arteriovenous fistulas (AVFs). The target goal is 50% of all new permanent hemodialysis accesses; however, only 17% of all initial permanent hemodialysis access procedures in Medicare patients between 1996 and 1997 were native AVFs. An algorithm to maximize native AVF procedures for hemodialysis access was prospectively evaluated in an academic, tertiary care medical center.

Methods.—All adults referred for permanent upper extremity dialysis access between April 1999 and May 2001 underwent Doppler arterial pressures and waveforms and duplex imaging of the basilic, cephalic, and central veins. The optimal configuration for an AVF was ascertained (criteria: vein greater than 3 mm, no arterial inflow stenosis, no venous outflow stenosis), based on the noninvasive procedures and unilateral arteriography and venography to verify the choice. Permanent hemodialysis access was based on imaging studies. Remedial imaging or an intervention was performed if the AVF did not mature. Outcome measures were the impact of the noninvasive and invasive imaging, perioperative morbidity and mortality, incidence of successful AVF, time to cannulation, and predictors of AVF failure.

Results.—One hundred thirty-nine access procedures were performed in 131 patients (mean age, 53 years). Of these, 49% were actively undergoing dialysis and 26% had a prior permanent access. Sixty percent had diabetes. Noninvasive imaging revealed that 83% of patients were candidates for AVF (mean, 2.7 possible configurations). Invasive imaging was abnormal in 38% and affected the surgical plan in 19%. Abnormalities included significant forearm arterial disease in 30%, significant central vein stenosis in 8%, and inflow stenosis in 5%. An AVF was ultimately performed in 90% (brachio-basilic in 39%, brachiocephalic in 36%, radiocephalic in 22%, and radio-basilic in 3%). In patients who underwent AVF procedures, the 30-day mortality rate was 1%, the complication rate was 20% (wound, 10%; hand ischemia, 8%), and 24% required a remedial procedure. The AVF matured adequately for cannulation in 84% and was suitable for cannulation within a mean of 3.4 months. On the basis of intention to treat, an AVF sufficient for cannulation was achieved in 71%. Female gender and radiocephalic configuration were independent predictors of failure of the fistula to mature.

Conclusion.—When this aggressive algorithm is used, the construction of a native AVF is possible in most patients referred for new hemodialysis access.

▶ Noninvasive imaging to assess the arterial and venous anatomy of the upper extremity should be the standard of care for planning dialysis access. Such studies result in performance of a higher proportion of autogenous dialysis access. Whereas most use noninvasive tests as definitive information, the authors of this paper follow their noninvasive tests with contrast studies of the arteries and veins. Nineteen percent of the time, the contrast studies changed the operative plan that had been based on the noninvasive studies. More information is usually better. We don't know, however, whether the addition of contrast studies results in a higher proportion of eventually usable autogenous fistulas.

G. L. Moneta, MD

Prediction of Wrist Arteriovenous Fistula Maturation With Preoperative Vein Mapping With Ultrasonography

Mendes RR, Farber MA, Marston WA, et al (Univ of North Carolina, Chapel Hill)
J Vasc Surg 36:460-463, 2002   11–2

Background.—Several studies have shown that arteriovenous fistulas have the highest primary and secondary patency rates when compared with prosthetic access. There are few clinical pathways used to predict the success of fistula maturation for arteriovenous fistula construction. Whether the preoperative minimal cephalic vein size in the forearm is predictive of successful wrist fistula maturation to a functional hemodialysis access was investigated.

Methods.—A consecutive series of 44 patients was evaluated before surgery with US scan imaging to map the entire cephalic vein in preparation for the construction of an arteriovenous fistula at the wrist. Measurements of the vein diameter were obtained from US scan images at 8 representative sites. Patients were monitored clinically to determine the maturation of the fistula in terms of it being able to provide a functional hemodialysis access. The smallest diameter of the cephalic vein was then used for the preoperative prediction of fistula maturation.

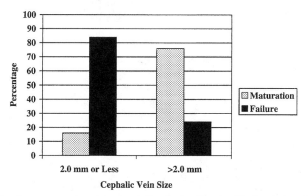

FIGURE 2.—Outcome rates for minimal cephalic vein size. (Reprinted by permission of the publisher from Mendes RR, Farber MA, Marston WA, et al: Prediction of wrist arteriovenous fistula maturation with preoperative vein mapping with ultrasonography. *J Vasc Surg* 36:460-463, 2002. Copyright 2002 by Elsevier.)

Results.—The success rate for maturation of the arteriovenous fistula was 50% (22 procedures). Cephalic veins with a minimal diameter of 2 mm or less were used for anastomosis in 19 patients (43%), and 3 of these procedures (16%) led to a functional access site. The other 25 patients (57%) had minimal cephalic vein diameters greater than 2 mm, and successful maturation of the fistula creations was accomplished in 19 of these patients (76%). The rate of successful fistula maturation was significantly higher in patients with a preoperative minimal cephalic vein size greater than 2 mm (Fig 2).

Conclusions.—A procedure other than wrist fistula should be considered to optimize dialysis access in patients with a minimal cephalic vein size of 2 mm or less.

▶ The authors have focused on only a tiny component of what needs to be done to evaluate a patient before placement of an autogenous dialysis access. The conclusion is obvious: little veins don't do as well as big ones. The article by Huber et al (see Abstract 11–1) is more inclusive.

G. L. Moneta, MD

Factors Predictive of Failure of Brescia-Cimino Arteriovenous Fistulas
Zeebregts C, van den Dungen J, Bolt A, et al (Univ Hosp Groningen, The Netherlands)
Eur J Surg 168:29-36, 2002   11–3

Introduction.—Patient-related factors predictive of failure of Brescia-Cimino fistulas were retrospectively examined to improve patient selection and perioperative management.

Methods.—Between January 1995 through December 1999, 153 fistulas were created in 150 consecutive patients. The mean age of 95 males and 55 females was 56 years (range, 17-80 years). The primary outcome measures were patency rates determined by the Kaplan-Meier method and the possible predictive value of 20 different variables evaluated by the Cox proportional hazards model.

Results.—Primary patency was 70% at 3 months. Predictors of failure identified by univariate analysis that had a hazard ratio (HR) greater than 2.5 for failure were initiation of dialysis before creation of the fistula (HR, 2.79; $P < .01$), moderate or poor quality of the artery (HR, 2.54; $P < .01$) or vein (HR, 3.55; $P < .001$), and postoperative use of acenocoumarol instead of acetylsalicylic acid (HR, 3.14, $P < .01$) (Fig 2). Seven distinct factors were significantly correlated with the predictive factors identified by univariate analysis and may have had an indirect influence on fistula failure: these included sex, age, diabetes mellitus, cause of end-stage renal disease, preoperative systolic blood pressure, preoperative serum urea concentration, and side of the fistula.

Conclusion.—The major determinates for a successfully created Brescia-Cimino fistula were creation of the fistula before initiation of dialysis, use of acenocoumarol, and good quality of both the artery and the vein. Timely creation of arteriovenous fistulas in patients with end-stage renal disease and accurate preoperative assessment to establish the quality of the vessels are essential for success.

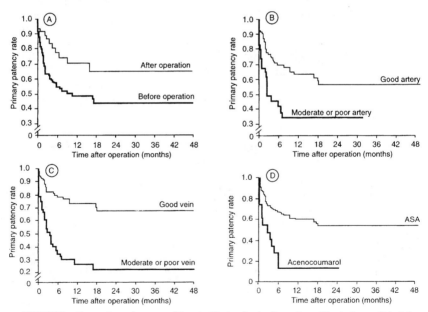

FIGURE 2.—Comparison of patency of Brescia-Cimino fistulas for patients (**A**) who began dialysis before operation compared with those who started after creation of the fistula; (**B**) who had good compared with moderate or poor quality arteries; (**C**) who had good compared with moderate or poor quality veins; and (**D**) who were given acetylsalicylic acid compared with those given acenocoumarol postoperatively. (Courtesy of Zeebregts C, van den Dungen J, Bolt A, et al: Factors predictive of failure of Brescia-Cimino arteriovenous fistulas. *Eur J Surg* 168:29-36, 2002. Copyright 2002 Elsevier Science Inc.)

▶ The importance of a good artery and vein for long-term patency of a Cimino fistula is obvious. However, when the fistula is created after dialysis begins, access patency is considerably worse. Part of this relates to placement of central venous catheters to initiate dialysis. The results of Cimino fistula placement after dialysis begins appear sufficiently poor to obviate the otherwise improved patency of an autogenous dialysis access. One wonders whether autogenous access is worth the effect in patients who require dialysis via central catheters before placement of a permanent access.

G. L. Moneta, MD

Transposed Saphenous Vein Arteriovenous Fistula Revisited: New Technology for an Old Idea
Illig KA, Orloff M, Lyden SP, et al (Univ of Rochester, NY)
Cardiovasc Surg 10:212-215, 2002   11–4

Background.—The greater saphenous vein can be used for dialysis access as a thigh saphenofemoral loop. The procedure is infrequently performed, in part because of the morbidity of vein harvesting and the risk of a groin infection. The use of endoscopic vein harvesting was evaluated for making lower extremity arteriovenous fistula (AVF) for dialysis access.

Methods.—The greater saphenous vein is harvested from the groin to as far distally as possible through several small incisions. The vein, still attached at the saphenofemoral junction, is brought to the surface after dissection is complete and is distended with saline solution containing heparin and papaverine. An inflow site is then obtained at the common or superficial femoral artery. The vein is laid in a gentle curve on the anterior thigh and the position marked. The vein is then tunneled superficially with the use of a sheath and trocar tunneler. After heparinization, the proximal anastomosis is constructed in the conventional manner.

Results.—This procedure has been used on 4 patients since December 1999. The procedure was technically successful in 3 patients; however, in the fourth patient, the vein was of extremely poor quality and failed in the postanesthetic unit. All 4 veins were thought to be of poor quality and fragile. No major wound complications occurred, but 1 patient had a small to moderate thigh hematoma. All patients were discharged on the second postoperative day. The 3 successful TSV-AVFs matured and were used for access. In 2 patients, the fistulas remained patent for 6 and 12 months but then thrombosed. The remaining patient had a functioning fistula 13 months after implantation. Thigh access was satisfactory, and no late infections or unusual bleeding episodes occurred at the time of writing.

Conclusions.—The use of the saphenous vein for AV access is not new. The transposed thigh saphenous vein AVF procedure described in this article using the endoscopic vein harvest may reduce wound complications and has theoretical advantages of using an autologous conduit and a native venous anastomosis.

▶ Transposed thigh saphenous vein AVFs are generally constructed with a loop configuration with the arteriovenous anastomosis in the groin. An alternative technique is to construct a "straight" fistula, similar to a basilic vein transposition, with the arteriovenous anastomosis placed on the distal superficial femoral artery and the saphenous vein transposed anteriorly on the thigh. In such cases, preoperative documentation of a relatively thin-walled distal superficial femoral artery is suggested.

G. L. Moneta, MD

Salvage of Immature Forearm Fistulas for Haemodialysis by Interventional Radiology
Turmel-Rodrigues L, Mouton A, Birmelé B, et al (Clinique St-Gatien, France; Clinique de l'Archette, Olivet, France; Centre Hospitalier Universitaire, Tours, France; et al)
Nephrol Dial Transplant 16:2365-2371, 2001   11–5

Background.—DOQI guidelines encourage the use of the native fistulas in hemodialysed patients. A recent publication in Europe confirmed the long-term superiority of forearm fistulas over upper arm fistulas and any type of native fistula over any type of graft. However, more attempts to create native fistulas will inevitably lead to more native fistulas that fail to mature. The value of endovascular techniques for the salvage of fistulas that fail to mature was investigated.

Methods.—Catheter-based techniques were used to treat 52 dysfunctional and 17 thrombosed immature forearm fistulas over a period of 6 years. The patients had a mean age of 63 years (range, 22-86 years) and the mean age of the fistulas was 10.25 weeks. Angiography was performed by puncture of the brachial artery, but dilation of underlying stenoses was performed after cannulation of the fistula, whenever possible, with a balloon never smaller than 5 mm. In the thrombosed fistulas, significant clots were removed by manual catheter-directed aspiration.

Results.—An underlying stenosis was diagnosed in all 69 patients, with half of these stenoses located in the anastomotic area. The initial success rate was 97%. Dilation-induced rupture occurred in 9 patients (13%). Stents were needed in only 2 patients. The rate of significant complications was 2.8%, with these complications consisting of bacteremia and pseudoaneurysm. The secondary patency rate at 1 year was 79%.

Conclusions.—Delayed maturation of native fistulas should systematically be investigated by clinical examinations and US or angiographic evaluation because an underlying stenosis will be diagnosed in almost all cases. Most cases can be treated with a catheter-based technique with a success rate of 97%. However, early recurrence of stenoses is possible, so re-evaluation must be performed after salvage of the fistula.

▶ I don't share the authors' "evangelic" position regarding the use of catheter-based procedures for salvaging fistulas that fail to mature. The article, however, has at least 1 interesting observation. All fistulas in this study that failed to mature were associated with a stenosis that was usually at or near the arteriovenous anastomosis.

G. L. Moneta, MD

Restoration of Thrombosed Brescia-Cimino Dialysis Fistulas by Using Percutaneous Transluminal Angioplasty

Liang H-L, Pan H-B, Chung H-M, et al (Natl Yang-Ming Univ, Kaohsiung, Taiwan)
Radiology 223:339-344, 2002   11–6

Introduction.—Thrombosed arteriovenous fistulas (AVFs) may be treated within 24 hours of thrombosis with angioplasty. Success has also been reported with occlusions of 24 to 72 hours. Described is the experience with a percutaneous technique for management of thrombosed Brescia-Cimino AVFs.

Methods.—Forty patients with 42 thrombosed AVFs underwent percutaneous treatment. Thrombosis developed within 24 hours before attempted angioplasty in 5 fistulas, between 24 and 72 hours in 27, and longer than 72 hours in 10 fistulas treated with angioplasty. Thrombosed fistulas were approached in a retrograde fashion, followed by direct balloon dilation with the use of 5- to 8-mm balloon catheters. If retrograde catheterization failed to cross the arterial anastomosis, an antegrade puncture directly into the thrombosed drainage vein close to the anastomosis was performed via US guidance as an aid to catheterization of the arterial inflow. Thrombolytic therapy with infusion of urokinase directly into the thrombus was undertaken in selected patients with visible thrombi that had compromised blood flow in the partially restored vascular access. Postintervention primary and secondary patency was determined, and patency rates between patients with and without urokinase infusion were compared.

Results.—Anatomical success was accomplished in 39 of 42 fistulas (93%), with clinical patency in 38 (90%). Rates of postintervention primary and secondary patency (including initial technical failure) at 6, 12, and 18 months were 81% and 84%, 70% and 80%, and 63% and 80%, respectively. There was no difference in patency between patients with and without urokinase infusion ($P = .912$). Three patients died of unrelated causes at 1, 2, and 5 months after their procedures. No major complications occurred.

Conclusion.—High anatomical success and excellent clinical patency is possible in the salvage of thrombosed AVFs. To optimize the outcomes in patients receiving hemodialysis, percutaneous restoration of AVFs should be attempted before recreation of a new dialysis access.

▶ The previous paper from France (see Abstract 11–5) addressed catheter-based techniques to salvage Cimino fistulas that failed to mature. In this paper from Taiwan, mature fistulas that thrombosed were treated with catheter-based techniques. Patency could be restored in 90% of cases. Seventy percent required no further intervention and remained patent at 18 months. Whereas the French data were a bit of crowing over not all that much, the Chinese appear to have a little more to be proud of. Restoration of patency with a resulting functioning fistula in 70% of cases at 18 months is excellent.

G. L. Moneta, MD

Using Pullback Pressure Measurements to Identify Venous Stenoses Persisting After Successful Angioplasty in Failing Hemodialysis Grafts
Funaki B, Kim R, Lorenz J, et al (Univ of Chicago; Racine Radiologist Group, Wis)
AJR 178:1161-1165, 2002   11–7

Introduction.—Angiographically, inconspicuous stenoses in patients with synthetic hemodialysis grafts may be ascribed to patient positioning, graft type, lesion configuration, or a combination of these factors. Anastomotic stenosis may be masked by superimposition of adjacent outflow veins, especially in the upper arm and thigh. Pressure measurement has been recommended by the Dialysis Outcomes Quality Initiative to prolong graft patency and overall access life. Data are scarce concerning the use of pressure measurements at the time of angiography to assess the hemodynamic significance of venous stenoses. Pullback pressure measurements were used to assess venous stenoses persisting after angioplasty of failing hemodialysis grafts.

Methods.—Thirty-two patients with elevated venous pressures at dialysis underwent 50 angioplasty procedures. Grafts were initially assessed via digital subtraction angiography. Angiography was performed for all stenoses measuring greater than 50% on angiography. Pullback measurements were obtained from the superior vena cava to the graft in successful cases (residual stenosis, <30%) to identify hemodynamically significant stenoses (>10 mm Hg). Lesions were treated with repeated angiography.

Results.—Hemodynamically significant stenoses with a gradient range of 10 to 27 mm Hg (mean, 16 mm Hg) were identified in 9 procedures (18%). All gradients were located at sites of prior angioplasty. Repeated angioplasty of these stenoses performed with larger angioplasty balloons decreased the gradients to below 3 mm Hg in 6 stenoses and to 5 mm Hg in 3 stenoses. The primary patency rate was 89% (8 of 9 stenoses) in this subgroup at 1 and 2 months and 56% (5 of 9 stenoses) at 6 months. Life table analysis showed that the primary patency of the entire population was 84% at 1 month, 66% at 2 months, and 47% at 6 months. The mean time between interventions was 6 months. The thrombosis rate was 0.32 per year.

Conclusion.—Angiographically subtle, hemodynamically significant stenoses are observed in about 1 of 5 failing dialysis grafts. These lesions may be identified via pullback pressure measurements. These measurements are a useful adjunct to angiography in assessing the hemodynamic results of angioplasty in patients with failing hemodialysis grafts.

▶ One should optimize what one does. If you are going to dilate a lesion, use whatever is necessary to ensure you get the best hemodynamic result possible.

G. L. Moneta, MD

Prospective, Randomized Evaluation of a Cuffed Expanded Polytetrafluoroethylene Graft for Hemodialysis Vascular Access
Sorom AJ, Hughes CB, McCarthy JT, et al (Mayo Clinic, Rochester, Minn)
Surgery 132:135-140, 2002   11–8

Background.—A cuffed expanded polytetrafluoroethylene (ePTFE) hemodialysis graft was compared with noncuffed, standard ePTFE grafts in terms of patency and blood flow rates achieved during dialysis.

Methods.—Forty-eight patients required new permanent hemodialysis vascular access and were randomly allocated to receive either the cuffed ePTFE graft or a standard, uncuffed ePTFE graft. All of the patients in the cuffed group and 91% of those in the standard group were at high risk of graft failure on the basis of age over 65 years, history of diabetes, or history of graft failure.

Results.—Overall primary graft patency was similar in the 2 groups, whereas secondary graft patency was significantly increased in the cuffed group. The cuffed group had graft patency rates of 64% at 12 months and 58% at 24 months, whereas the standard group had rates of 32% and 21%, respectively (Fig 2). The average time to failure or completion of the study was 426 days for the cuffed group and 219 days for the standard group.

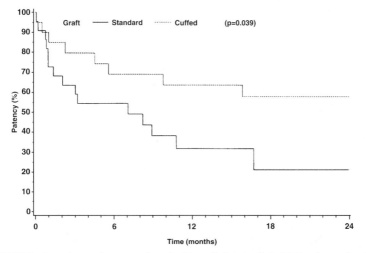

FIGURE 2.—Secondary graft patency of standard (uncuffed) and cuffed ePTFE grafts as a function of time after placement. A significantly larger number of cuffed grafts were patent at 24 months (P = .039). (Reprinted by permission of the publisher from Sorom AJ, Hughes CB, McCarthy JT, et al: Prospective, randomized evaluation of a cuffed expanded polytetrafluoroethylene graft for hemodialysis vascular access. *Surgery* 132:135-140, 2002. Copyright 2002 by Elsevier.)

None of the cuffed grafts failed because of venous outflow stenosis. At 3 months the average flow rates did not differ statistically between the 2 groups, but at 12 months the flow was 623 mL/min for the cuffed group and 253 mL/min for the standard group; flow declined to 531 mL/min for the cuffed group and 121 mL/min for the standard group at 24 months.

Conclusions.—Overall patency was improved and hemodialysis blood flow rates were increased with the use of the cuffed ePTFE graft for hemodialysis when they were compared with a standard graft. With no cuffed grafts failed secondary to venous anastomotic stenosis, improved hemodynamic profiles resulted in a decreased incidence of graft failure for these patients.

▶ There is a steady trickle of papers on "cuffed" PTFE grafts for dialysis access. This one suggests such grafts may offer some improvement over standard PTFE without distal cuffs. The study is reasonably well done. The evaluation was blinded, and the patients appear at high risk for failure, perhaps explaining the below-standard results for noncuffed PTFE grafts. There is enough here to merit a multicenter study of cuffed grafts in patients who truly require prosthetic dialysis access.

G. L. Moneta, MD

Evaluation of 4-mm to 7-mm Versus 6-mm Prosthetic Brachial-Antecubital Forearm Loop Access for Hemodialysis: Results of a Randomized Multicenter Clinical Trial

Dammers R, Planken RN, Pouls KPM, et al (Univ Hosp Maastricht, The Netherlands; Medisch Spectrum Twente, Enschede, The Netherlands; Albert Schweitzer Hosp, Dordrecht, The Netherlands)
J Vasc Surg 37:143-148, 2003   11–9

Background.—Thrombosis of a vascular access graft is common in hemodialysis patients with prosthetic arteriovenous fistulas. Some researchers have used tapered 4- to 7-mm grafts in an effort to reduce shear stress–induced intimal hyperplasia. However, results with these tapered stents have been contradictory. The patency rates of 4- to 7-mm tapered prosthetic grafts were prospectively compared with those of standard 6-mm prosthetic grafts during brachial-antecubital forearm loop access for hemodialysis.

Methods.—One hundred nine patients (40 men and 69 women; mean age, about 64 years) who required vascular access for hemodialysis were studied. Patients were randomly assigned to receive either a 6-mm (n = 57) or a 4- to 7-mm tapering (n = 52) polytetrafluoroethylene brachial-antecubital forearm loop access. At 1, 6, and 12 months after surgery, duplex US was used to measure blood flow, peak systolic velocity, and stenosis (>50%). Primary, assisted primary, and secondary patency rates were compared between the groups.

Results.—At 1 year, the 6-mm prostheses and the 4- to 7-mm prostheses did not differ significantly in primary patency rates (43% vs 46%, respectively; Fig 1), assisted primary patency rates (58% vs 62%), and secondary

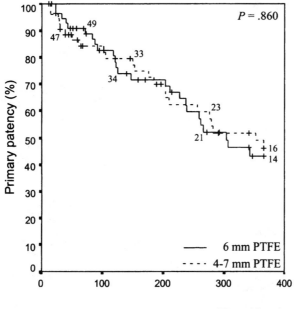

Time (days)

FIGURE 1.—Primary patency rates. Patency rate is shown in percentages, and survival time in days. Number of patients is presented in graph. *P* values are calculated with log-rank test. *Abbreviation: PTFE,* Polytetrafluoroethylene. (Reprinted by permission of the publisher from Dammers R, Planken RN, Pouls KPM, et al: Evaluation of 4-mm to 7-mm versus 6-mm prosthetic brachial-antecubital forearm loop access for hemodialysis: Results of a randomized multicenter clinical trial. *J Vasc Surg* 37:143-148, 2003. Copyright 2003 by Elsevier.)

patency rates (91% vs 87%). The 2 groups also had a comparable incidence of thrombotic occlusion (0.88 vs 0.74 per patient-year, respectively). The mean graft flow in the 6-mm and the 4- to 7-mm groups was also similar at 1 month (1415 vs 1416 mL/min), 6 months (1319 vs 1345 mL/min), and 12 months (1265 vs 1595 mL/min). Peak systolic velocities were also similar between the 2 groups in all parts of the grafts. At 1 year, the incidence of stenosis was also similar in the 6-mm and the 4- to 7-mm groups (20% vs 27%).

Conclusion.—No differences in patency rates, the incidence of thrombotic occlusion, blood flow, peak systolic velocity, or the incidence of stenosis were detected between standard 6-mm and tapered 4- to 7-mm prosthetic brachial-antecubital forearm loop access grafts.

▶ Tapered 4- to 7-mm PTFE dialysis access grafts were no better than 6-mm PTFE grafts with regard to patency, development of stenoses, and ischemic symptoms. On the other hand, they were no worse either. Provided there are no cost differences, graft choice is basically surgeon preference.

G. L. Moneta, MD

Early Result of Arteriovenous Graft With Deep Forearm Veins as an Outflow in Hemodialysis Patients

Won T, Min SK, Jang JW, et al (Ewha Women's Univ, Seoul, Korea)

Ann Vasc Surg 16:501-504, 2002   11–10

Introduction.—The result of arteriovenous (A-V) grafting with the deep forearm veins as an outflow system in patients with hemodialysis was examined.

Methods.—Between June 1999 and July 2001, 27 A-V grafts were constructed in 26 patients (mean age, 56.7 years; range, 34-78 years) by using expanded polytetrafluoroethylene with deep forearm veins. Patients were followed up until failure of the graft, first intervention (ie, thrombolysis, angioplasty, or surgical revision), or death.

Results.—The median follow-up was 17.3 months (range, 1-72 months). The failure rate during follow-up was 26% (7 fistulas). The patency at 3 months was 93%; at 12 months, it was 80%. No significant differences were observed in patency rates between men and women or between patients with diabetes versus those without diabetes. Excluding graft thrombosis, 5 patients experienced graft-related complications, including operative wound dehiscence in 2 patients, graft infection in 1, a seroma in 1, and mild hypoperfusion of the hand in 1.

Conclusion.—The early patency rate of A-V grafts that use a deep forearm veins as a venous outflow site is very good. This technique may be recommended for vascular access in patients with exhausted superficial veins.

▶ The deep forearm veins referred to in this paper are the paired brachial veins accompanying the brachial artery. I have been using these veins for years as an alternative for venous outflow when other antecubital veins are unsatisfactory. They work quite well, although they are somewhat thin and connected by venous bridges. Even when small, they seem to support a prosthetic fistula at least for several months. When patients return for revision, the veins beyond the old venous anastomosis are enlarged. A disadvantage is that exposure for revision usually requires a "T" type of incision perpendicular to the original horizontal antecubital fossa incision.

G. L. Moneta, MD

Does Surgical Intervention Significantly Prolong the Patency of Failed Angioaccess Grafts Previously Treated With Percutaneous Techniques?

Alexander J, Hood D, Rowe V, et al (Huntington Mem Hosp, Los Angeles; Univ of Southern California, Los Angeles)

Ann Vasc Surg 16:197-200, 2002   11–11

Introduction.—Several contemporary management strategies have attempted to combine both surgical and percutaneous approaches to optimize survival of thrombosed access grafts. The efficacy of surgical intervention for patients who have failed catheter-based therapy of prosthetic arterio-venous graft occlusion was prospectively investigated.

Methods.—During a 2-year period, 101 surgical procedures in 71 patients (ages 31-92 years; mean age, 67 years) were performed on failed bridge fistulas. All patients had previously undergone percutaneous thrombolysis and dilatation (range, 1-5 procedures). Survival curves for the bridge fistulas after surgical interventions were plotted, with the Kaplan-Meier method. Differences in times-to-first failure between types of grafts and interventions were analyzed.

Results.—The primary patency rates of the angioaccess grafts after operative revision were 43%, 24%, and 12% at 30, 60, and 90 days, respectively. Survival rate was not affected by patient sex, use of anticoagulation, or the number of prior interventions. Neither the anatomical location of the graft nor the type of surgical procedure affected fistula patency. Five patients died within 30 days of surgery.

Conclusion.—Surgical intervention did not significantly prolong the patency of angioaccess grafts that previously failed percutaneous interventions. The routine use of such intervention is not recommended.

▶ The answer to the question posed is "No." It is clear no matter what method is used to restore patency of thrombosed prosthetic dialysis access grafts, 2 and certainly 3 failures of the same access strongly predict another failure in very short order. If feasible, once an access has failed 3 times, it is probably best to let it go and place a new access.

G. L. Moneta, MD

Safety and Efficacy of Femoral-based Hemodialysis Access Grafts
Tashjian DB, Lipkowitz GS, Madden RL, et al (Tufts Univ, Springfield, Mass)
J Vasc Surg 35:691-693, 2002   11–12

Background.—Early experience with hemodialysis access in the groin was discouraging because of a high rate of infection and associated major limb amputation. However, the development of polytetrafluoroethylene (PTFE) for prosthetic subcutaneous hemodialysis access and improvements in surgical techniques and dialysis care have resulted in renewed attention to the groin as a valuable hemodialysis access site. The experience at 1 institution was reviewed to assess safety and viability of angioaccess grafts in the groin in a hemodialysis patient population.

Methods.—A retrospective review was conducted of all groin hemodialysis access grafts performed between June 1990 and February 1998. The grafts were PTFE loop grafts placed from the common or superficial femoral artery to the saphenous–common femoral vein junction or directly to the common femoral vein. The choice of the specific type of graft was made by the individual surgeon and included grafts ranging from 6 mm to 8 mm. Demographic information, complications, and subsequent treatment were recorded. Life-table analysis was used to analyze graft patency and infection rates.

Results.—Data were obtained for 73 graft insertions. There were 52 episodes of thrombosis in 26 grafts. The primary patency rate was 71% at 1 year, and the secondary patency rate was 83% at 1 year. The incidence of infection was 22%.

Conclusions.—The incidence of infection and thrombosis in this series of femoral-based hemodialysis grafts was comparable with the rates reported in the literature for upper extremity PTFE angioaccess grafts. While not a first choice, femoral artery–based hemodialysis access would appear to be a viable option in patients in whom it is not possible to construct arteriovenous fistulas in the upper extremity.

▶ The authors provide surprisingly little information about how patients were selected for operation or, perhaps more important, excluded from placement of a groin arteriovenous access. The secondary patency of 83% at 1 year is admirable. This, however, was associated with an infection rate of 22%. These procedures should be avoided in obese patients and those with poor personal hygiene.

G. L. Moneta, MD

Using a Cutting Balloon to Treat Resistant High-Grade Dialysis Graft Stenosis

Ryan JM, Dumbleton SA, Smith TP (Duke Univ, Durham, NC)
AJR 180:1072-1074, 2003   11–13

Background.—Treatment of dialysis graft stenoses generally involves balloon angioplasty or surgical revision of the graft. In this case, salvage of a dialysis graft was successfully accomplished using the cutting balloon for a resistant venous anastomotic stricture.

> *Case Report.*—Man, 68, had diminished dialysis flow rates and elevated venous pressures in his 15-month-old polytetrafluoroethylene forearm loop graft and underwent fistulography and central venography (Fig 1). The stenosis at the venous anastomosis exceeded 90%. Balloon angioplasty was unsuccessful with a persistent resisant stenosis exceeding 70%. A 4- × 10-mm cutting balloon was placed across the resistant stenosis over a 0.014-inch guidewire. Initial inflation was to 6 atm, then to 10 atm; 2 further overlapping inflations were performed. After angioplasty balloon exchange, a second conventional angioplasty was performed. The stenosis diminished to less than 30% and the patient's hemodynamic dialysis parameters improved markedly.

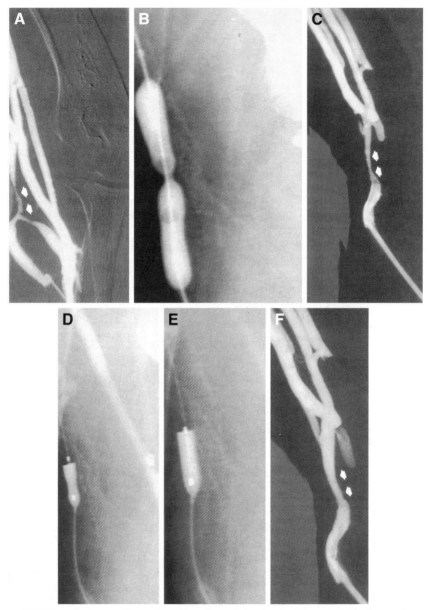

FIGURE 1.—A 68-year-old man with polytetrafluoroethylene forearm loop graft. **A,** Fistulogram shows high-grade stenosis (*arrows*) at venous anastomotic region. **B,** Radiograph of balloon angioplasty with 7 × 40 mm high-pressure balloon reveals tight resistant stricture at venous anastomosis. **C,** Fistulogram obtained after angioplasty shows 70% residual stenosis (*arrows*). **D,** Radiograph taken during initial inflation of cutting balloon (Interventional Technologies, San Diego, CA) at 6 atm reveals waist on balloon indicating area of stricture. **E,** Radiograph of cutting balloon in same position as in **D,** at 10 atm of inflation, shows that waist has resolved. **F,** Fistulogram obtained after second conventional angioplasty with 7 × 40 mm high-pressure balloon shows that residual stenosis (*arrows*) is markedly improved at 30%. (Courtesy of Ryan JM, Dumbleton SA, Smith TP: Using a cutting balloon to treat resistant high-grade dialysis graft stenosis. *AJR* 180:1072-1074, 2003. Reprinted with permission from the *American Journal of Roentgenology.*)

Conclusions.—This case demonstrates that the cutting balloon can be effective in treating resistant, highly stenotic lesions in dialysis grafts.

▶ I think using a cutting balloon on an arterial prosthetic anastomosis is unwise. Surgeons, however, have routinely cut across the suture lines of venous anastomoses of dialysis grafts to perform patch angioplasty for outflow anastomotic strictures. It therefore appears that using a cutting balloon on an anastomotic stricture at the venous end of a prosthetic dialysis graft may be okay. I don't have any idea if the results will be durable, but I doubt the technique will lead to pseudoaneurysms at the venous end of a prosthetic dialysis graft.

G. L. Moneta, MD

Distal Revascularization–Interval Ligation: A Durable and Effective Treatment for Ischemic Steal Syndrome After Hemodialysis Access

Knox RC, Berman SS, Hughes JD, et al (Univ of Arizona, Tucson)
J Vasc Surg 36:250-256, 2002   11–14

Background.—The treatment of hemodialysis access–induced steal syndrome is challenging. The distal revascularization–interval ligation (DRIL) procedure provided promising early results, but this procedure has not been widely accepted because of concerns about its complexity and long-term efficacy. The efficacy and durability of the DRIL procedure in relieving hand ischemia and in maintaining access patency were evaluated in the setting of hemodialysis access–induced ischemia (Fig 3).

Methods.—This retrospective review evaluated all patients who underwent the DRIL procedure for access-induced ischemia. Data compiled for this review included demographic information, data regarding access and bypass patency, limb salvage, and patient survival. Arteriovenous access and brachial artery bypass patency rates were determined with life-table methods.

Results.—From 1995 to 2001, a total of 55 DRIL procedures were performed in 52 patients (35 women and 17 men; mean age, 60.8 years). Indications for surgery were ischemic pain in 27 patients, tissue loss in 20 patients, loss of neurologic function in 4 patients, and pain on hemodialysis in 1 patient. Most of the patients (92%) had diabetes. The mean interval from access placement to DRIL was 7.4 months (range, 1-84 months). The mean follow-up interval was 16 months (range, 1-67 months). The brachial artery bypass primary patency rate was 80% at 4 years, and the arteriovenous access primary patency rate was 83% at 1 year. Substantial or complete relief of ischemic hand symptoms was obtained in 47 of 52 patients, and 15 of 20 patients' digital ischemic lesions have healed completely.

Conclusions.—DRIL is a durable and effective procedure that reliably provides persistent relief of hand ischemia and continued access patency in patients with hemodialysis access–induced ischemic steal syndrome.

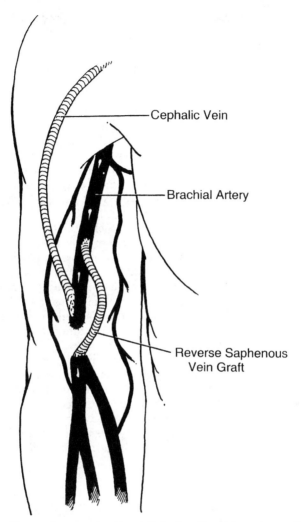

Cephalic Vein

Brachial Artery

Reverse Saphenous
Vein Graft

FIGURE 3.—Diagram of upper arm brachiocephalic fistula and brachial artery bypass with interval brachial artery ligation. In this case, brachial artery was divided below origin of fistula and distal anastomosis of vein bypass graft was performed end-to-end to distal brachial artery. (Reprinted by permission of the publisher from Knox RC, Berman SS, Hughes JD, et al: Distal revascularization–interval ligation: A durable and effective treatment for ischemic steal syndrome after hemodialysis access. *J Vasc Surg* 36:250-256, 2002. Copyright 2002 by Elsevier.)

▶ All surgeons performing dialysis access should be aware of this procedure. It is most useful in patients whose digital photoplethysmography waveforms improve dramatically with compression of the fistula. We have not found it as useful in patients with digital gangrene, likely because underlying distal occlusive disease contributes more to the gangrene than the steal phenomenon. (See Abstract 11–13.)

G. L. Moneta, MD

Relationship of Hemodialysis Access to Finger Gangrene in Patients With End-Stage Renal Disease

Yeager RA, Moneta GL, Edwards JM, et al (Portland Veterans Affairs Med Ctr, Ore; Oregon Health Sciences Univ, Portland)
J Vasc Surg 36:245-249, 2002   11–15

Background.—Finger gangrene resulting from upper extremity arterial occlusive disease is a relatively infrequent clinical problem. Little is known of the etiology, natural history, prognosis, and appropriate management of this disease. There are concerns regarding the etiology of finger gangrene in patients with end-stage renal disease (ESRD) with respect to the relationship of finger gangrene to an upper extremity hemodialysis access arteriovenous (AV) fistula or shunt. A comprehensive review of patients on hemodialysis with ESRD with finger gangrene is presented.

Methods.—Twenty-three patients with ESRD with finger gangrene were identified from a computerized vascular registry. The mean age of these patients at the start of dialysis was 53 years. The presence of an ipsilateral AV fistula in these patients was verified, and then they were compared with a group of patients with ESRD without finger gangrene. Management consisted of arteriography, selective AV fistula management, and finger amputation. Multivariate analysis was used to determine the risk factors associated with finger gangrene, and repeat finger amputation. Survival rates were determined with life-table analysis.

Results.—Of the 23 patients with ESRD and finger gangrene, 48% (11 patients) had a functional ipsilateral AV fistula. Arteriography consistently showed diffuse atherosclerosis involving the radial, ulnar, palmar, and digital arteries, precluding attempts at distal arterial bypass. In 52% of patients, repeat finger amputations were necessary (Fig 2). Bilateral finger gangrene developed in 61% of patients. The rate of patient survival after the onset of finger gangrene was 27% at 2 years (Fig 3). Starting dialysis at younger than

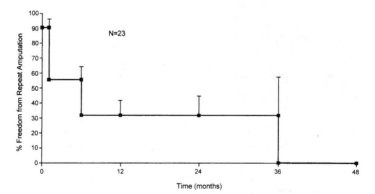

FIGURE 2.—Life table shows rate of freedom from repeat finger amputation. (Reprinted by permission of the publisher from Yeager RA, Moneta GL, Edwards JM, et al: Relationship of hemodialysis access to finger gangrene in patients with end-stage renal disease. *J Vasc Surg* 36:245-249, 2002. Copyright 2002 by Elsevier.)

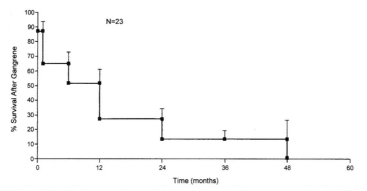

FIGURE 3.—Life table shows patient survival rate after onset of finger gangrene. (Reprinted by permission of the publisher from Yeager RA, Moneta GL, Edwards JM, et al: Relationship of hemodialysis access to finger gangrene in patients with end-stage renal disease. *J Vasc Surg* 36:245-249, 2002. Copyright 2002 by Elsevier.)

55 years of age, diabetes, coronary artery disease, and lower extremity arterial occlusive disease were significantly associated with finger gangrene.

Conclusions.—There is a high risk for development of finger gangrene in young diabetic patients with diffuse vascular disease and ESRD on chronic hemodialysis. Finger gangrene results from distal atherosclerosis and is not primarily related to dialysis access.

▶ Symptomatic steal syndrome is a well-recognized complication of AV dialysis shunts. It appears that when finger gangrene develops in dialysis patients, it is not the shunt but the underlying distal occlusive disease that is most to blame. However, when finger gangrene occurs ipsilateral to a dialysis access, it would still seem prudent to ligate the access or consider a DRIL (distal revascularization interval ligation) procedure. Distal bypass is not likely possible given the distal occlusive disease in these patients.

G. L. Moneta, MD

Race-Specific Association of Lipoprotein(a) With Vascular Access Interventions in Hemodialysis Patients: The CHOICE Study

Astor BC, for the CHOICE Study (Johns Hopkins Univ, Baltimore, Md; et al)
Kidney Int 61:1115-1123, 2002   11–16

Background.—Elevated serum levels of lipoprotein(a) (Lp[a]) and low molecular weight apolipoprotein(a) (apo[a]) isoforms are associated with atherothrombotic disease in the general population and in patients with kidney failure. Some studies have suggested that Lp(a) may be more atherothrombotic in whites than in blacks. However, data on the relationship of Lp(a) and apo(a) isoform size to hemodialysis vascular access complications are limited, particularly among black patients. This prospective study was conducted to evaluate the relationship of Lp(a) and apo(a) size with hemodialysis vascular access complications among a cohort of white and black patients initiating chronic hemodialysis.

Methods.—The intervention-free survival of the first arteriovenous access was analyzed in 215 white and 112 black incident hemodialysis patients participating in the CHOICE Study, a national multicenter prospective cohort study.

Results.—The black patients had higher median levels of Lp(a) protein than white patients (81.0 vs 37.5 nmol/L), and these levels were inversely correlated with apo(a) isoform size. The incidence rate of access interventions was much higher in synthetic grafts than in native fistulae (0.95 vs 0.49 interventions/access year) and in patients with kidney failure primarily resulting from diabetes mellitus versus other causes (0.90 vs 0.60 interventions/access year).

However, the incidence rate of access interventions did not differ by race. Black patients in the highest race-specific Lp(a) quartile (more than 145 nmol/L) had a significantly higher incidence rate than other black patients, while no association was found in white patients. This association in blacks remained after adjustment for access type and other characteristics. There was no association with apo(a) isoform size in either race.

Conclusion.—Elevated lipoprotein(a) may be a risk factor for venous access complications in black patients receiving hemodialysis.

▶ It is always interesting when a well-done study produces unexpected data. Elevated Lp(a) is a risk factor for atherosclerotic events. But, despite overall higher levels in black patients, the adverse atheroembolic effects of elevated Lp(a) appear to be more of a problem in white than black patients. Yet in this study, dialysis access failure was associated with high Lp(a) levels in black but not white patients. There is no apparent explanation for this association. To me, the data suggest the presence of an unknown race-specific factor acting in synergy with Lp(a).

G. L. Moneta, MD

Increased Expression of TGF-β1 and IGF-I in Inflammatory Stenotic Lesions of Hemodialysis Fistulas

Stracke S, Konner K, Köstlin I, et al (Univ of Ulm, Germany; Univ of Cologne, Germany)
Kidney Int 61:1011-1019, 2002   11–17

Background.—Hemodialysis fistula dysfunction caused by stenotic lesions is the most frequent cause of hospitalization for hemodialysis patients. The involvement of TGF-β1 and IGF-I in the pathogenesis of stenosis and subsequent thrombosis of primary arteriovenous fistulas was investigated.

Methods.—At the time of surgical revision, 15 occluded or severely narrowed vein segments of primary arteriovenous (AV) fistulas, 29 control vein segments from mostly predialysis patients, and 15 control saphenous vein segments from nonrenal patients were obtained. The tissue specimens were snap frozen in cold isopentane and stored at $-70°C$ until processed for immunohistochemistry. The serum levels of TGF-β1 and free IGF-I were determined with a commercially available enzyme-linked immunosorbent assay and with IRMA, respectively.

Results.—Pronounced intimal thickening was observed adjacent to the site of anastomosis. TGF-β1 expression was found to be significantly higher in the luminal (neo)intima, the medial layer, and the vasa vasorum of the stenosed vessels, compared with nonstenosed uremic vessels and with nonuremic control vessels; IGF-I expression was found to be significantly higher in the endothelium, the (neo)intima, and the medial layer of the stenosed vessels, compared with both types of control vessels. Among the groups, there was no statistically significant difference concerning serum levels of TGF-β1 or IGF-I, and no correlation could be observed between serum levels and the intensity of the local growth factor expression.

Conclusion.—Neointimal thickening of primary AV fistulas appears to be a local inflammatory process upregulating both TGF-β1 and IGF-I. Therapeutic strategies should be designed to prevent proatherogenic processes in AV fistulas and to improve shunt patency by blocking the signal for matrix production while leaving other activities such as TGF-β1 untouched.

▶ The authors suggest that stenotic AV fistulas are a model for accelerated atherosclerosis. I disagree. The lesion in a stenotic AV fistula doesn't look anything like an atherosclerotic plaque. While elevated levels of growth factors are found in the stenotic lesions of AV fistulas and in atherosclerosis, the only logical conclusion is that these growth factors are important in both atherosclerosis and neointimal hyperplasia.

G. L. Moneta, MD

Endoscopic Thoracic Sympathicotomy for Raynaud's Phenomenon
Matsumoto Y, Ueyama T, Endo M, et al (Natl Kanazawa Hosp, Japan)
J Vasc Surg 36:57-61, 2002   11–18

Introduction.—The efficacy of endoscopic thoracic sympathicotomy (ETS) for Raynaud's phenomenon and its applicability were examined.

Methods.—Of 502 consecutive patients who underwent ETS between December 1992 and August 2001, 28 were treated for Raynaud's phenomenon. Indications for ETS in patients with Raynaud's phenomenon included severe chronic symptoms or nonhealing digital ulceration refractory to intensive medical therapy. A self-assessment questionnaire was mailed to all patients after surgery to ascertain the immediate and long-term results. Data were recorded from initial and long-term follow-up examinations.

Results.—The 28 patients with Raynaud's phenomenon underwent 54 ETS procedures. No operative mortality occurred, and conversion to an open procedure was not needed in any patient. Initial resolution or improvement of symptoms was accomplished in 26 of 28 patients (92.9%). Symptoms recurred in 23 patients (82.1%). No recurrent digital ulcerations were observed during a median follow-up of 62.5 months. During follow-up, 25 patients (89.3%) reported overall improvement in the frequency and severity of symptoms.

Conclusion.—The recurrence rate was 82%, yet ETS provided a high rate of initial relief, promoted healing of digital ulcers, and demonstrated potential for diminishing the severity of refractory symptoms.

▶ Sympathectomy has been largely abandoned for treatment of Raynaud's syndrome. Patients improve initially, but recurrence is nearly universal within 1 to 2 years. The authors' experience with endovascular sympathectomy is really no different than that of open sympathectomy, and there is no reason it should be different. It makes no sense to perform a basically ineffective procedure just because it can be performed with an endoscope.

G. L. Moneta, MD

Endoscopic Transthoracic Sympathectomy for Upper Limb Hyperhidrosis: Limited Sympathectomy Does Not Reduce Postoperative Compensatory Sweating

Lesèche G, Castier Y, Thabut G, et al (Hôpital Beaujon, Clichy, France)
J Vasc Surg 37:124-128, 2003   11–19

Background.—Compensatory sweating (CS) is the most common complication of thoracodorsal sympathectomy. It is also the most common symptom reported by patients who are dissatisfied with the surgery. Limited or selective sympathectomy may limit CS. An alternate theory postulates that patients who have preexisting hyperhidrosis with more widespread pathologic sweating are at greater risk for developing CS. Whether there is a relationship between the extent of sympathectomy was investigated, along with the occurrence and severity of CS after endoscopic transthoracic sympathectomy for patients with upper limb hyperhidrosis.

Methods.—One hundred thirty-four patients (99 female and 35 male; mean age, 27.8 years) underwent 268 sympathectomies. Eighty-four patients had palmar sweating, 7 axillary sweating, and 43 a combination. None of the patients had responded to conservative treatment. All patients had single-stage bilateral endoscopic transthoracic sympathectomy under general anesthesia. In the 84 patients with palmar hyperhidrosis, 8 had T1-T2 resection, 4, T1-T3 resection; 8, T2-T3 resection; and 64, T2-T4 resection. In 43 patients with axillary and palmar hyperhidrosis, 8 had T1-T5 resection and 35 had T2-T5 resection. T3-T5 sympathectomy was performed in 7 patients who had isolated axillary hyperhidrosis. Follow-up extended for a mean of 44.3 months and included 98.5% of patients.

Results.—CS developed 2 to 7 months after sympathectomy in 95 patients (about 72%) and affected the back, chest, abdomen, or buttocks/thighs. Four patients thought their condition was disabling, 21 that it was embarrassing in a hot environment, and 70 that it was minor and intermittent. Overall, in 19% of cases, CS was classified as severe. The only variable linked to an increased occurrence of CS was age. Four patients who had limited sympathectomy for palmar hydrosis had temporary relief/recurrence after 2, 6, 9, and 45 months, respectively. Extending the thoracoscopic sympathectomy to T5 produced successful early and late outcomes for 3 of these 4 patients.

Conclusions.—The extent of sympathectomy did not influence the occurrence of CS. A positive family history of hyperhidrosis was similarly unconnected with either the incidence or the severity of CS. Limited sympathectomy did not produce a decrease in the magnitude of CS in these patients.

▶ This study emphasizes that CS after thoracic sympathectomy for hyperhidrosis is very common, some of it is severe, and there is not much a surgeon can do about it. Since limiting sympathectomy to T2 or T2 and T3 doesn't reduce CS, and including T4 with sympathectomy may improve the effectiveness of the procedure, there seems little role for a limited sympathectomy in the treatment of hyperhidrosis.

G. L. Moneta, MD

12 Carotid and Cerebrovascular Disease

Alcohol Consumption and Risk of Ischemic Stroke: The Framingham Study
Djoussé L, Ellison RC, Beiser A, et al (Boston Univ)
Stroke 33:907-912, 2002   12–1

Background.—The correlation between alcohol intake and ischemic stroke (IS) is still debated. Data from the Framingham Study were analyzed to further investigate this association.

Methods and Findings.—During three 10-year follow-up periods, 196 men and 245 women participating in the Framingham Study had IS. Participants were categorized as never drinkers (group 1); drinkers of 0.1 to 11 g/d of ethanol (group 2), of 12 to 23 g/d (group 3), of 24 g/d or more (group 4); and former drinkers of 0.1 to 11 g/d (group 5) and 12 g/d or more (group 6). Among men, the crude incidence rates of IS were 6.5 per 1000 person-years for group 1, 5.9 for group 2, 4.9 for group 3, 5.0 for group 4, 6.7 for group 5, and 17.8 for group 6. For women, the corresponding incidences were 5.9, 4.1, 4.1, 4.3, 8.3, and 7.1 per 1000 person-years. In a multivariate Cox regression analysis, current alcohol intake was not significantly associated with IS in either sex compared with never drinkers. Formerly drinking 12 g/d or more carried a 2.4 times greater risk of IS among men but not among women. When data were stratified by age, alcohol consumption correlated with a lower risk of IS among 60- to 69-year-olds. Only wine consumption was associated with a reduced risk of IS.

Conclusion.—There appears to be no overall significant correlation between total alcohol consumption and IS. However, alcohol intake may have a protective effect among persons aged 60 to 69 years.

▶ Epidemiologic studies do not agree on the relation between alcohol consumption and ischemic stroke. The results vary from no effect to increased risk to what is termed a "J" or "U" effect with decreasing risk in moderate drinkers only. This study therefore adds very little to previous data. It is somewhat encouraging that light to moderate drinkers at least do not appear to be at increased risk of stroke. Overall, it appears that one should not consider a beer on a warm day or wine with dinner to be a major component of your stroke prevention program.

G. L. Moneta, MD

Major Carotid Plaque Surface Irregularities Correlate With Neurologic Symptoms

Rapp JH, and the Assessment of Carotid Stenosis by Comparison With Endarterectomy Plaque Trial (ACSCEPT) Investigators (San Francisco Dept of Veterans Affairs Med Ctr; et al)

J Vasc Surg 35:741-747, 2002   12–2

Background.—Carotid plaque surface irregularities have been associated with the risk of stroke. Initial neurologic symptoms in patients were correlated with high-resolution MRI studies of ipsilateral plaque surface invaginations and ledges, lumen shape, and location of the plaque bulk producing the stenosis.

Methods.—The study included 83 men and 17 women (ages 45-81 years) undergoing surgery. Forty-five patients had had a transient ischemic attack (TIA) or stroke, and 55 had no symptoms. Fifty patients underwent angiography. Carotid plaques removed en bloc were placed in gadolinium-doped saline for imaging. Surface irregularities were classified as a ledge or ulcer and were measured.

Findings.—The average maximal stenosis was 81.5%. Surface contour irregularities were seen on 80 plaques. Of these, 35 (43.8%) were classified as having major surface contour irregularities, and 45 as minor irregularities. Major surface irregularity was associated significantly with TIA or stroke. Irregular plaques were also detected on angiograms, but sizes were underestimated. Circular lumens were seen on 28% of the plaques, elliptical lumens on 50%, and crescentic or multilobular lumens on 22%. Maximal stenosis occurred in the internal carotid artery in 82 plaques, in the bifurcation in 17, and in the common carotid artery in 1.

Conclusions.—Submillimeter resolution of the carotid plaques with MRI showed that surface irregularities were common. However, only the presence of major irregularities were associated with TIA or stroke. Neither lumen shape nor plaque location appeared to predict stroke risk, but these features may influence imaging accuracy for determining degree of stenosis.

▶ The fact that plaque irregularity correlates with previously symptomatic plaque confirms that plaque and not just the degree of stenosis is important in the pathophysiology of carotid artery disease. This was suggested years ago by the North American Symptomatic Carotid Endarterectomy Trial investigators, who felt that ulceration increased the risk of stroke in patients with significant carotid artery stenosis. The information presented in the current study is nice but not very clinically useful. The identification of asymptomatic plaques with the propensity to produce symptoms is the real goal of this sort of research. Hopefully, the eventual identification of asymptomatic plaques with the proclivity to produce symptoms will allow a decrease in the number of carotid endarterectomies performed for asymptomatic disease.

G. L. Moneta, MD

Carotid Artery Intima-Media Thickness in Children With Type 1 Diabetes
Järvisalo MJ, Putto-Laurila A, Jartti L, et al (Univ of Turku, Finland; Univ of Tampere, Finland)
Diabetes 51:493-498, 2002   12–3

Background.—Postmortem studies of adolescents have demonstrated an association between diabetes and atherosclerosis. Increased subclinical atherosclerosis and its risk factors in children with type 1 diabetes were investigated.

Methods.—Eighty-five children (mean age, 11 years) were studied. Fifty had type 1 diabetes, with a mean duration of 4.4 years, and 35 were healthy. The 2 groups were matched for age, sex, and body size. Carotid intima-media thickness (IMT) was measured by high-resolution US. Susceptibility of low-density lipoprotein (LDL) to oxidation was evaluated by measuring the formation of conjugated dienes induced by Cu^{2+} in subgroups of 21 children with diabetes and 21 healthy children.

Findings.—The mean carotid IMT was increased in the children with diabetes; the values were 0.47 and 0.42 mm in the diabetic and control groups, respectively. The 2 groups had similar total cholesterol and LDL cholesterol concentrations, but the children with diabetes had an increased rate of LDL diene formation. This suggested an increase in in vitro LDL oxidizability. Independent correlates for IMT in a multivariate model were diabetic state, LDL cholesterol, and systolic blood pressure. In the patients with diabetes, LDL oxidizability was significantly associated with the mean IMT. This relationship persisted after adjustment for LDL cholesterol concentration.

Conclusion.—Type 1 diabetes is an independent risk factor for increased carotid IMT in children. Increased oxidative modification of LDL may be associated with early structural atherosclerotic vascular changes in children with diabetes.

▶ Foam cell formation, the precursor of the atherosclerotic plaque, may be increased by oxidative modification of LDL. The reason for increased risk of atherosclerosis in diabetic patients has never been clarified. This study indicates that increased LDL oxidation in diabetes may lead to early atherosclerotic changes. The idea is these early changes then progress to clinically significant lesions over time. Of course, we still need to identify what leads to this progression in patients with diabetes who do not have additional atherosclerotic risk factors.

G. L. Moneta, MD

Regular Aerobic Exercise and the Age-Related Increase in Carotid Artery Intima-Media Thickness in Healthy Men

Tanaka H, Seals DR, Monahan KD, et al (Univ of Colorado, Boulder; Univ of Colorado, Denver)

J Appl Physiol 92:1458-1464, 2002   12–4

Background.—Stroke is the third leading cause of death in the United States. There is an exponential increase in stroke with advancing age, doubling in each successive decade after age 55 years. Several studies have demonstrated that carotid artery intima-media thickness (IMT), which is an independent risk factor for stroke, increases with advancing age in sedentary persons and thus is presumed to contribute to the age-associated increase in stroke incidence. Regular aerobic exercise is generally associated with a lower incidence of stroke, particularly in middle-age and older adults. The mechanisms of this protective effect are not fully understood, but it is possible that regular aerobic exercise acts to attenuate the age-related increase in carotid IMT. This potential association in both cross-sectional and intervention approaches was explored.

Methods.—In the cross-sectional phase, 137 healthy sedentary and endurance-trained men (aged 18-77 years) were studied. In the interventional phase of this study, 18 healthy sedentary men (mean age, 54 ± 2 years) were studied before and after 3 months of endurance training.

Results.—In the cross-sectional phase, carotid IMT and the IMT-to-lumen ratio was progressively higher with age in both the sedentary and endurance-trained groups. There were no significant differences in measures of carotid IMT between the endurance-trained and sedentary men at any age. Carotid systolic blood pressure increased progressively with age and was related to carotid IMT. In the second phase, there were no changes in carotid IMT, IMT/lumen ratio, or carotid systolic blood pressure in the 18 previously sedentary men after 3 months of endurance training.

Conclusion.—This exploration of the possible association of regular aerobic exercise and reversal of the age-associated increase in carotid IMT did not support the hypothesis that regular aerobic exercise exerts a protective effect against stroke by attenuating the age-related increase in carotid IMT.

▶ Noninvasive assessment of atherosclerotic risk is a hot topic. The present study and others have correlated carotid artery IMT with risk of ischemic events such as stroke. Given that regular exercise is known to reduce the risk of stroke, the authors ask whether exercise would also reduce carotid IMT. The flaw here is that a small change in IMT of the common carotid artery does not directly contribute to strokes (in contrast to a large complicated plaque in the bulb). I am not surprised that exercising patients with basically normal carotid arteries for only 3 months had no impact on IMT.

R. L. Geary, MD

Fish Consumption and Risk of Stroke in Men
He K, Rimm EB, Merchant A, et al (Harvard School of Public Health, Boston)
JAMA 288:3130-3136, 2002   12–5

Background.—The risk of ischemic stroke may be reduced and the risk of hemorrhagic stroke increased with the consumption of fish. Long-chain omega-3 polyunsaturated fatty acids (PUFAs), which inhibit platelet aggregation and are almost exclusively found in marine sources, may play an important role in this effect. Few studies have distinguished between risk factors for ischemic and hemorrhagic stroke. The relationship between fish intake and the risk of stroke was investigated in the Health Professional Follow-up Study, which consisted of a large cohort of men who completed dietary evaluations periodically during a 12-year period.

Methods.—The relationship linking fish consumption and PUFAs with risk of stroke in men was evaluated in 43,671 men aged 40 to 75 years. Participants completed a detailed semiquantitative food frequency questionnaire. None had evidence of cardiovascular disease at baseline. Assessments were carried out in 1986, 1990, and 1994, seeking the relative risk (RR) of stroke by subtype based on the cumulative average fish consumption or long-chain omega-3 PUFA intake.

Results.—The likelihood of smoking and being overweight was less in men with high fish consumption, but these men were more likely to have a history of hypertension and hypercholesterolemia, to be physically active, and to use aspirin or multivitamin supplements, requiring adjustments in the statistical analyses. Stroke developed in 608 participants, with 377 ischemic strokes, 106 hemorrhagic strokes, and the remainder unclassified. Compared with men who consumed fish less than once a month, the risk of ischemic stroke was significantly reduced among men who ate fish 1 to 3 times monthly, with no further benefit with greater levels of consumption. No significant association was noted between fish intake and the risk of hemorrhagic stroke. The RR of ischemic stroke was significantly less in men in relation to long-chain omega-3 PUFA intake except in the highest intake category compared with the lowest one. Hemorrhagic stroke risk and PUFA intake showed no corresponding relationship. Nineteen fish oil users had strokes, with 12 being of the ischemic variety and 7 unknown. The intake of α-linoleic acid and the risk of stroke were also not linked statistically. Comparing men who ate fish less than once a month and those who ate fish at least once a month, the multivariate RRs were 0.72 for total stroke, 0.56 for ischemic stroke, and 1.36 for hemorrhagic stroke. Neither aspirin nor vitamin E intake modified the risk of ischemic stroke, with too few cases of hemorrhagic stroke to analyze statistically.

Conclusions.—The risk of ischemic stroke among men who ate fish at least once a month was 40% lower than among men who ate fish less often. No relationship was found between fish consumption or long-chain omega-3 PUFA intake and the risk of hemorrhagic stroke.

▶ PUFAs, including eicosapentaenoic acid and docosahexaenoic acid, are almost exclusively derived from marine sources and are known to inhibit platelet aggregation. The authors conclude a 40% lower risk of ischemic stroke in men who consumed fish more than once per month compared with those who consumed fish less often. The results from these very large prospective epidemiological studies (43,671 men in this cohort) have a shortfall in relying on the potential inaccuracies of voluntary completion of survey materials. Nonetheless, the results are quite compelling. Certainly, this proposed prophylactic intervention of eating more fish has little risk. We should all make way to the sashimi (raw fish) counters! (See Abstract 1–9.)

R. M. Fujitani, MD

Risk of Arterial Thrombosis in Relation to Oral Contraceptives (RATIO) Study: Oral Contraceptives and the Risk of Ischemic Stroke

Kemmeren JM, Tanis BC, van den Bosch MAAJ, et al (Univ Med Centre Utrecht, The Netherlands; Leiden Univ, The Netherlands)
Stroke 33:1202-1208, 2002   12–6

Background.—Some evidence indicates third-generation oral contraceptives (OCs; ie, those containing the progestogens desogestrel or gestodene) may increase a woman's risk of venous thrombosis compared with earlier types of OCs. In a multicenter, population-based, case–control study, several types of OCs were examined for their risk of causing ischemic strokes.

Methods.—The medical records of 9 Dutch centers were reviewed to identify all women 19 to 49 years old who had first ischemic strokes between January 1990 and October 1995. Case patients were matched with control subjects without vascular disease from the same geographic region. Analyses were stratified by age, area of residence, and year of the stroke. All research subjects completed a questionnaire about their use of OCs and their risk factors for an ischemic stroke.

Results.—In all, 203 of 295 eligible case patients (69%) participated, as did 925 of 1259 eligible control subjects (73%). The majority of patients (93%) were white. After adjustment was made for stratification factors, subjects using any type of OC had twice the risk of having an ischemic stroke (odds ratio [OR], 2.3) compared with women who did not use OCs. The risk increased with age (Table 3). The risk also varied with the type of OCs: women who used first-generation OCs had an OR of 1.7, users of low-dose second-generation OCs (containing levonorgestrel) had an OR of 2.4, and users of third-generation OCs had a risk of 2.0. The risk of having an ischemic stroke did not differ significantly between women using second-generation OCs and those using third-generation OCs (OR, 1.0).

TABLE 3.—Odds Ratios (95% CI) for Women With First Ischemic Strokes in Relation to Oral Contraceptive Use (All Types) by Age Categories

| | Current OC Use/Noncurrent OC Use | | |
| | Stroke Patients | Control Women | |
Age Category	(*n*=203)	(*n*=925)†	OR (95% CI)*
18-29 y, n (%)	30/7 (81)	145/42 (78)	1.3 (0.5-3.3)
30-39 y, n (%)	31/21 (60)	123/184 (40)	2.3 (1.2-4.3)
40-49 y, n (%)	41/73 (36)	80/342 (19)	2.6 (1.6-4.2)

Note: Values are number (percentage using an OC) of individuals.
*Adjusted for stratification factors (area of residence and calendar year).
†Nine control women were left out of the analysis: OC use was unknown in 7 women, and 2 women used hormone replacement therapy.
Abbreviation: OC, Oral contraceptives.
(Courtesy of Kemmeren JM, Tanis BC, van den Bosch MAAJ, et al: Risk of arterial thrombosis in relation to oral contraceptives (RATIO) study: Oral contraceptives and the risk of ischemic stroke. *Stroke* 33:1202-1208, 2002.)

Conclusion.—The use of any type of OC increases the risk of having an ischemic stroke. However, the risk of having an ischemic stroke is no higher with third-generation OCs than with second-generation OCs.

▶ Third-generation OCs with a different form of progesterone are less androgenic and tend to increase HDL cholesterol. It was hoped they would therefore reduce the risk of arterial thrombosis. It appears these changes have made no difference with regard to stroke risk. We are where we were: The use of any OC agent increases the risk of stroke.

G. L. Moneta, MD

Risk Factors for Progression of Aortic Atheroma in Stroke and Transient Ischemic Attack Patients

Sen S, Oppenheimer SM, Lima J, et al (Johns Hopkins Univ, Baltimore, Md; Seton Hall Univ, Edison, NJ; New York Univ)
Stroke 33:930-935, 2002   12–7

Background.—Aortic atheromas of 4 mm or greater are an independent risk factor for new and recurrent strokes. There is no definitive treatment. This lack of therapeutic options is partly because of the unknown natural history of aortic atheromas in patients with strokes. However, it appears there may be regression and progression of aortic atheromas. This evidence of regression suggests that aortic atheromas may be treatable. Associations between stroke vascular risk factors and the risk of aortic atheroma progression were investigated in patients with cerebrovascular disease.

Methods.—A group of patients (57 with strokes and 21 with transient ischemic attacks) underwent multiplanar transesophageal echocardiograms within 1 month of symptom onset and again at 9 months. Stroke risk factors, the use of anticoagulant, antiplatelet, and hypolipidemic drugs, and the clinical and etiologic subtypes of strokes were recorded and compared in pa-

TABLE 4.—Stroke Subtypes According to TOAST Criteria

TOAST Subtype	Progression $(n=29), n$ (%)	No Progression $(n=49), n$ (%)	P (χ^2 Test)
Cardioembolic	0	5 (10)	0.08
Large-artery atherosclerosis	6 (21)	1 (2)	0.005
Small-artery occlusion	11 (38)	19 (39)	0.9
Other	4 (14)	11 (22)	0.8
TIA	8 (28)	13 (26)	0.9

Abbreviations: TOAST, Trial of Org 10172 in Acute Stroke Treatment; TIA, transient ischemic attack.
(Courtesy of Sen S, Oppenheimer SM, Lima J, et al: Risk factors for progression of aortic atheroma in stroke and transient ischemic attack patients. *Stroke* 33:930-935, 2002.)

tients and stratified for the presence or absence of aortic atheroma progression.

Results.—Of these 78 patients, the aortic atheroma in 29 patients (37%) progressed. In 32 patients (41%), it remained unchanged, and in 17 patients (22%), the atheroma regressed. Progression was most pronounced at the aortic arch, followed by the ascending segment. Among the patients in whom the aortic atheroma was unchanged over 9 months, nearly two thirds of these patients had no evidence of atheromas on baseline transesophageal echocardiograms. The only factors significantly correlated with progression were the homocysteine level ($\geq$14.0 μmol/L), the presence of a total anterior cerebral infarct, and large-artery atherosclerosis (Table 4).

Conclusions.—Elevated levels of homocysteine are associated with progression of aortic atheromas. Homocysteine levels should be assessed in patients with aortic atheromas who have also had strokes or transient ischemic attacks.

▶ Progression of aortic atheroma is common—37% in this article focusing on patients with cerebral symptoms presumably secondary to an aortic atheroma. Previous research has suggested statins may induce regression of aortic atheromas in hyperlipidemic patients. The current study suggests that decreasing homocysteine levels may also be of value in patients with aortic atheromas. Overall, it is clear from this study, and others like it, that aggressive medical management of symptomatic vascular disease in the future will consist of multidrug therapy. My guess is that while antiplatelet agents, statins, and β-blockers will be part of this management, warfarin will not.

G. L. Moneta, MD

High-Risk Carotid Endarterectomy: Fact or Fiction

Gasparis AP, Ricotta L, Cuadra SA, et al (SUNY Stony Brook Univ Hosp, NY; Winthrop Univ Hosp, Mineola, NY)
J Vasc Surg 37:40-46, 2003   12–8

Background.—Carotid angioplasty/stenting has been proposed for use with patients who are considered to be at high risk for carotid endarterectomy (CEA). The experience with a contemporary series of CEAs was reviewed retrospectively to identify patients who met the published criteria for high risk and to assess their outcome.

Methods.—Seven hundred eighty-eight consecutive cases were reviewed from June 1996 to June 2001. Two hundred twenty-eight patients were classified as high risk according to anatomic or physiologic criteria. The anatomic factors leading to a designation of high-risk patient were contralateral occlusion, lesion above C_2, the need for digastric division, reoperation, and neck radiation. The high-risk comorbid conditions identified were an age of 80 years or older, New York Heart Association class III/IV angina, Canadian class III/IV heart failure, myocardial infarct within 6 months, steroid-dependent or oxygen-dependent pulmonary disease, and a creatinine level of 3 or greater.

Results.—Thirty-eight percent of patients in a normal-risk group had surgery for symptomatic carotid disease, whereas 43% of those in the high-risk group had this indication. For 58% of patients, CEA was performed based only on the results of noninvasive carotid duplex scanning; 30% had MR angiography, and 12% had cerebral angiography. Of the 228 high-risk patients (29% of the sample), 28% had an anatomic risk factor, 63% had a physiologic risk factor, and 9% had both. Eighty-six percent of the normal-risk group had a patch, as did 84% of the high-risk group. General anesthesia and shunt placement were used in most of the patients in both groups. For the entire group, the 30-day risk of stroke and death was 1.1%; this rate was 1.3% for the high-risk group and 1.1% in the normal-risk group. Four patients (0.7%) in the normal-risk group and 2 (0.9%) in the high-risk group had postoperative strokes, and 5 patients (0.9%) in the normal-risk group (3 of whom died) and 2 (0.9%) in the high-risk group had myocardial infarctions. No statistically significant differences in event rates were noted between the 2 groups.

Conclusions.—Twenty-nine percent of the cases reviewed constituted high-risk patients, yet no evidence indicated that this designation influenced the results after CEA. No increased complication rate or risk for stroke or death was noted in the high-risk group in comparison with the normal-risk patients. Thus, any high-risk group that exists is small and limited to patients who are undergoing reoperation or who have a radiated neck, which occurred in 4% of the cases reviewed. With this possible exception, carotid angioplasty/stenting should be restricted to randomized clinical trials, while CEA is continued for all other cases.

▶ I agree with Gasparis et al that patients truly at high risk for CEA are uncommon. Whereas everything is a bit in the eye of the beholder, the sudden large numbers of patients considered high risk suggests that some of us are blinded by enthusiasm, are perhaps true visionaries, or have interests other than the patient's best interest.

G. L. Moneta, MD

Long-term Outcome After Angioplasty for Symptomatic Extracranial Carotid Stenosis in Poor Surgical Candidates

Fox DJ Jr, Moran CJ, Cross DT III, et al (Washington Univ, St Louis)
Stroke 33:2877-2880, 2002   12–9

Background.—Some patients with symptomatic carotid stenosis may not be good candidates for surgery because of age, anatomic factors, prior neck irradiation, previous surgery, or poor medical condition. Long-term outcomes after angioplasty were reported in a series of patients with high-grade carotid stenosis who were poor surgical candidates, and these data were compared with historical control data from the North American Symptomatic Carotid Endarterectomy Trial (NASCET).

Methods.—Forty-two consecutive patients considered poor candidates for surgery with greater than 70% carotid stenosis and ipsilateral ischemic symptoms within 120 days of undergoing angioplasty were identified. Baseline epidemiologic stroke risk factors were obtained from a review of the patients' medical records. Follow-up was from clinic records and by telephone.

Results.—The baseline epidemiologic stroke risk factors for these patients were similar to those of medically treated patients in NASCET. However, angioplasty patients tended to have higher degrees of stenosis or occlusion (45% with greater than 90% stenosis vs 24% in NASCET) and more frequent contralateral stenosis or occlusion (30% vs 9%) than patients in NASCET. Three patients had procedure-related strokes. One other patient had a central retinal occlusion 48 hours after angioplasty. There were no further ipsilateral strokes during a mean follow-up period of 1.7 years. Three patients were lost to follow-up. The cumulative risk for stroke among the angioplasty patients was 9.5% compared with 26% at 2 years for medically treated NASCET patients.

Conclusions.—The data from this pilot study suggest that there is a beneficial effect of angioplasty for patients with high-grade symptomatic carotid stenosis who are not good candidates for surgery.

▶ Comparing the incidence of ipsilateral stroke (26%) in the medically treated patients in the NASCET trial with that of the patients treated in this trial (9.5%), the authors conclude that angioplasty provides a reasonable alternative for high-risk patients. The patients presented here, however, have been retrospectively reviewed not only for the preoperative symptoms, but also for postoperative events, as opposed to the NASCET trial. Also, the patients are a very different group as many of these patients would have been excluded from the NASCET trial. Additionally, the perioperative stroke rate is higher than the perioperative stroke rate achieved with surgical intervention in the NASCET trial. It is unclear that the presented data justify the conclusion that stenting may provide a better long-term outcome for these patients.

D. G. Clair, MD

Initial Experience With Cerebral Protection Devices to Prevent Embolization During Carotid Artery Stenting

Ohki T, Veith FJ, Grenell S, et al (Albert Einstein College of Medicine, Bronx, NY)
J Vasc Surg 36:1175-1185, 2002   12–10

Background.—The initial results with carotid artery stenting (CAS) performed with cerebral protection devices for treatment of carotid bifurcation stenosis were reported.

Methods.—A total of 31 patients with carotid artery stenosis underwent treatment with CAS in conjunction with either the PercuSurge GuardWire (Medtronic, Minneapolis, Minn), the Cordis Angioguard filter (Cordis, Warren, NJ), or the ArteriA Parodi Anti-embolization catheter (ArteriA, San Francisco, Calif). Preoperative neurologic symptoms were present in 58% of patients, and the mean stenosis was 85% ± 12%. Data were prospectively analyzed on an intent-to-treat basis. Patients underwent preoperative and postoperative evaluation by a protocol neurologist.

Results.—The overall technical success rate was 97% (30 of 31 patients). One patient had a severely stenosed and tortuous lesion that could not be crossed with a guidewire. CAS had a good angiographic result in the remaining 30 patients, with residual stenosis of less than 10%. The protection devices were well tolerated by all patients, and there were no intraprocedural neurologic complications. Macroscopic embolic particles were recovered from each patient. There were no deaths, but one patient had a major stroke immediately after CAS, for a combined 30-day stroke/death rate of 3%. During a mean of 17 months, one patient experienced subacute occlusion of the stent that did not result in a stroke. Three patients had duplex scan–proved in-stent restenosis, and 2 patients underwent treatment with repeat percutaneous transluminal angioplasty. There were no cases of stroke during follow-up.

Conclusions.—CAS with cerebral protection devices can be performed safely, and the rate of technical success is high. The neurologic complication rate was low. Tight lesions and tortuous anatomy may make the use of distal protection devices difficult.

▶ The authors conclude protected CAS is an acceptable alternative for high-risk surgical candidates. While this study does report experience at a single institution with different devices, the series is a small sample overall and there is obviously a significant amount of initial operator experience with these devices. The need for ancillary devices for lesion traversal is much higher than has been reported in other series reporting experience with these devices. This series does, however, reinforce the potential benefit of interventional means of treating carotid artery disease in the high-risk surgical patient.

D. G. Clair, MD

Response to Intra-arterial and Combined Intravenous and Intra-arterial Thrombolytic Therapy in Patients With Distal Internal Carotid Artery Occlusion

Zaidat OO, Suarez JI, Santillan C, et al (Case Western Reserve Univ/Univ Hosps of Cleveland, Ohio)
Stroke 33:1821-1827, 2002   12–11

Introduction.—There are only a few reported cases addressing the outcome and results of thrombolytic therapy in angiographically confirmed acute distal internal carotid artery (ICA) occlusion. The clinical features, angiographic findings, and response to treatment with thrombolytic therapy were examined in patients with ischemic strokes caused by acute occlusion of the distal ICA.

Methods.—A retrospective case series from a prospectively collected stroke database for patients with acute ICA occlusion seen within 6 hours of stroke onset was assessed to determine safety, feasibility, and the response to thrombolytic therapy. Demographics, clinical features, stroke mechanisms, severity, imaging findings, type of thrombolysis, treatment responses, mortality, and long-term outcomes with the use of a modified Rankin Scale and Barthel Index were noted. Short-term outcomes were evaluated with the use of the National Institutes of Health Stroke Scale (NIHSS). Acute thrombolytic therapy was given with recombinant tissue plasminogen activator or urokinase intra-arterially only or in combination with IV administration.

Results.—Eighteen patients with acute ischemic strokes and ipsilateral occlusion of the distal ICA treated with thrombolysis were evaluated. The time to treatment was the strongest predictor of a response to thrombolytic therapy ($P < .001$). The therapeutic response correlated well with the severity of the initial clinical deficit, as determined by the NIHSS ($P < .001$). No difference was found in the recanalization rate, symptomatic hemorrhage, or NIHSS score for IV/intra-arterial (IA) therapy compared with IA therapy alone ($P =$ NS). Complete angiographic recanalization was achieved in 80% of patients who received combination IV/IA thrombolysis and in 62% of those who received IA therapy alone ($P =$ NS). Patients with distal occlusions extending to the middle and anterior cerebral arteries were least likely to respond to thrombolytic therapy. Symptomatic intracerebral hemorrhaging was observed in 20% of patients receiving IV/IA therapy and in 15% of those who received IA alone ($P =$ NS). At 24 hours, the NIHSS score fell by 3 points in the IA group and by 4 points in the IV/IA group ($P =$ NS). Mild disability with independence was seen in 77% of survivors at a 3-month follow-up. The mortality rate was 50%, despite thrombolysis.

Conclusion.—The mortality rate of acute stroke with distal ICA occlusion was 50% despite the use of thrombolytic therapy. Thrombolytic therapy with the use of a combination of IV and IA routes or with the use of the IA-only route provides equal outcomes in patients with occlusion of the distal ICA. Shorter intervals between stroke onset and treatment seem to be associated with a higher rate of recanalization and an improved outcome.

▶ The authors conclude there may be a trend toward improved efficacy with IV/IA therapy compared with IA alone; however, patients with simple IV therapy who had a good clinical response have not been included in the study as they did not have evaluation of the area of arterial occlusion. While this study may offer the possibility that IV/IA therapy is better than IA therapy or for that matter IV therapy alone, there clearly are not any strong statements that can be made because of the limited sample size.

D. G. Clair, MD

High Rate of Recanalization of Middle Cerebral Artery Occlusion During 2-MHz Transcranial Color-Coded Doppler Continuous Monitoring Without Thrombolytic Drug
Cintas P, Le Traon AP, Larrue V (Univ of Toulouse, France)
Stroke 33:626-628, 2002   12–12

Introduction.—Experimental evidence suggests that US may accelerate thrombolysis. Reported are findings on early recanalization during transcranial color-coded Doppler (TCCD) continuous monitoring in 6 consecutive patients with acute strokes resulting from middle cerebral artery (MCA) occlusion.

Methods.—All patients underwent continuous TCCD monitoring through a temporal bone window with a 2-MHz transducer. The diagnosis of MCA occlusion was made with the use of both color-coded imaging and pulse-wave Doppler US. Patients did not receive recombinant tissue plasminogen activator (rtPA). The clinical severity of the stroke was assessed at baseline, 2 hours, and 24 hours with the use of the National Institutes of Health Stroke Scale.

Results.—The mean patient age was 54.3 years. IV aspirin, 250 mg, was administered in all patients as part of the initial therapy. The mean time from symptom onset to initiation of TCCD monitoring was 210 minutes. Recanalization of the initially occluded MCA was observed during monitoring in 5 patients (83%). The mean time to initiation of recanalization was 17.2 minutes. Complete recanalization at 24 hours occurred in 1 patient. The mean National Institutes of Health Stroke Scale score in the 5 patients who had recanalization during monitoring was 21.2 at baseline, 19.2 at 2 hours, and 15.6 at 24 hours ($P = .1$).

Conclusion.—In this small series of consecutive patients with acute MCA occlusion who were not treated with rtPA, a high incidence of recanalization was observed during continuous exposure to low-intensity 2-MHz US. These findings suggest that US may have a role in thrombolysis.

▶ Therapeutic US is a new concept in patients with acute stroke. I think it is too early to start using continuous transcranial Doppler monitoring in patients with MCA stroke. Low-intensity US in the range used for transcranial Doppler studies can enhance plasminogen activator–induced thrombolysis. This makes US an interesting, and potentially safer, alternative to lytic therapy for acute MCA stroke.

G. L. Moneta, MD

Clinical Utility of Quantitative Cerebral Blood Flow Measurements During Internal Carotid Artery Test Occlusions
Marshall RS, Lazar RM, Young WL, et al (Columbia College of Physicians and Surgeons, New York; Univ of California, San Francisco)
Neurosurgery 50:996-1005, 2002   12–13

Background.—Occlusion of the internal carotid artery (ICA) may cause no symptoms or may lead to a devastating hemispheric stroke, but sometimes the ICA, however, must be deliberately occluded in the course of treatment. How well a patient will tolerate permanent ICA occlusion (PCO) is evaluated by balloon test occlusion (BTO) of the ICA. Predicting the status of the brain during BTO has relied on various electrophysiologic and cerebral blood flow (CBF) measures, but no standard criteria currently exist. An assessment was undertaken of patients who underwent BTO and then PCO to determine whether a specific quantitative CBF threshold exists during BTO that predicts stroke outcomes after PCO.

Methods.—ICA BTO was carried out in 33 patients who had clinical indications for PCO, then PCO was performed as appropriate. Standard neurologic examinations, sustained-attention testing, and quantitative CBF evaluations were carried out during BTO; in addition, 2 scalp scintillation detectors recorded washout data after xenon-133 was injected through a port at the tip of the occluding balloon. The follow-up period extended for a mean of 34 months. Data were analyzed with the use of statistical methods.

Results.—None of the patients experienced adverse neurologic events in response to the BTO alone. Two patients died: 1 of cancer and 1 of sepsis; 7 strokes occurred, all of which were ipsilateral to the occluded ICA with 5 occurring within 18 hours of PCO—1 at 2 months and 1 at 1 year. Minor hemiparesis and good recovery accompanied all but 1 stroke. Eight patients had extracranial–intracranial (EC-IC) bypass after BTO; only 1 of these patients had a stroke, and that patient had a nonfunctioning bypass. For the prediction of a stroke after PCO, standard clinical testing had a positive predictive value of 33% and a negative predictive value of 70%. In addition, CBF values less than 30 mL/100 g/min had a positive predictive value of 42% and a negative predictive value of 100%. The cumulative life-table rates of ipsilateral strokes for patients with CBF values less than 30 mL/100 g/min were 25% at 30 days and 50% at 1 year (Fig 1). Thus, patients with CBF values less than 30 mL/100 g/min had a significantly greater risk than did those whose CBF values were 30 mL/100 g/min or greater. Sustained-attention testing showed a positive predictive value of 25% and a negative predictive value of 90% for predicting strokes after PCO.

Conclusions.—Variables found to be predictive of the success or failure of BTO included CBF values less than 30 mL/100 g/min, particularly when

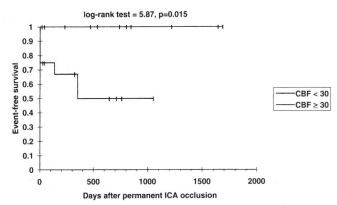

FIGURE 1.—Event-free survival plots of strokes occurring among patients after PCO. These Kaplan-Meier curves demonstrate that patients with CBF values of more than 30 mL/100 g/min during BTO experienced no ipsilateral strokes in the 34-month follow-up period, whereas patients with CBF values of less than 30 mL/100 g/min exhibited a 50% cumulative risk of strokes in the first year. *Abbreviations: CBF*, Cerebral blood flow; *ICA*, internal carotid artery; *PCO*, permanent ICA occlusion; *BTO*, balloon test occlusion. (Courtesy of Marshall RS, Lazar RM, Young WL, et al: Clinical utility of quantitative cerebral blood flow measurements during internal carotid artery test occlusions. *Neurosurgery* 50:996-1005, 2002.)

measured during induced hypotension while BTO was performed. The specificity of low CBF values may be increased if sustained-attention testing during BTO is also undertaken. A suggested protocol would be a 30-minute BTO, with 15 minutes of normotension and 15 minutes of hypotension to 60% to 70% mean systemic arterial pressure. If a patient's CBF value declines below 30 mL/100 g/min, an EC-IC bypass is recommended, as well as retesting before PCO.

▶ ICA BTO protocols with only clinical neurologic signs for predicting success or failure of PCO have been shown not to predict stroke outcomes well, exhibiting low negative and positive predictive values. Other adjunctive evaluations have been proposed to enhance the sensitivity of BTO procedures. Previous studies have proposed a CBF value of less than 30 mL/100 g per minute as a BTO failure criterion. In this series, the authors describe an intracarotid ^{133}Xe injection technique to measure real-time CBF measurements. With a less than 30 mL/100 g per minute threshold, under both normotensive and induced hypotensive mean arterial pressures, patients requiring EC-IC bypass may be identified before permanent ICA ligation. While these authors propose a reasonable algorithm to predict ipsilateral cerebral ischemia, we have yet to fully understand the adaptability of the collateral circulation of the brain and its affect on neurologic outcomes.

R. M. Fujitani, MD

Assessment of Cerebrovascular Reserve Capacity in Asymptomatic and Symptomatic Hemodynamically Significant Carotid Stenoses and Occlusions

Orosz L, Fülesdi B, Hoksbergen A, et al (Univ of Debrecen, Hungary; Academic Med Ctr, Amsterdam)
Surg Neurol 57:333-339, 2002   12–14

Background.—Cerebrovascular reactivity measurements may be a useful tool for selecting patients with carotid stenoses and occlusions who are at increased risk of a hemodynamic stroke. Cerebral vasoreactivity was compared among patients with asymptomatic stenosis, asymptomatic occlusion, symptomatic stenosis, and symptomatic occlusion of the internal carotid artery.

Methods.—A total of 62 patients with asymptomatic and symptomatic internal carotid artery stenoses and occlusions underwent transcranial Doppler–acetazolamide tests. Absolute velocities of the middle cerebral arteries (MCAV), percent increases of the MCAV at different time points of the test, and the maximal percent increase after administration of acetazolamide were compared on the affected and nonaffected sides. Asymmetry indices were compared among the groups of obstructive lesions of varying severity.

Results.—The resting MCAV was similar on both sides in all groups. In the symptomatic groups, a significant side-difference of the MCAV values after acetazolamide was observed. The difference in cerebrovascular reserve capacity (CRC) between the affected and nonaffected side was statistically significant only in the symptomatic groups. The asymmetry index of the CRC was close to 1 in the asymptomatic stenosis group only; in all other groups, this index indicated a significant hemispheric vasoreactivity asymmetry.

Conclusions.—CRC is compromised in patients with hemodynamically significant carotid lesions. Studies are needed to clarify whether the clinical efficiency of carotid endarterectomy and extra-intracranial bypass may be improved by selecting patients on the basis of hemodynamic criteria.

▶ Interesting, but is it clinically practical? In this study, cerebrovascular reactivity and reserve capacity measurements with transcranial Doppler-acetazolamide testing was found only to be significantly decreased in symptomatic patients. The clinical application of this apparently cumbersome study is still questionable since there is no proven correlation to improvements in clinical outcomes. It would not seem to change the management algorithm of a patient with a symptomatic, hemodynamically significant stenosis—he or she would still undergo an elective carotid endarterectomy.

R. M. Fujitani, MD

Control of Emboli in Patients With Recurrent or Crescendo Transient Ischaemic Attacks Using Preoperative Transcranial Doppler-Directed Dextran Therapy

Lennard NS, Vijayasekar C, Tiivas C, et al (Coventry and Warwickshire Univ Hosps, England)
Br J Surg 90:166-170, 2003   12–15

Background.—The risk of stroke is highest after the first transient ischemic attack (TIA), with 4% to 8% of all strokes occurring in the first month after TIA. An aggressive approach with urgent carotid endarterectomy has been advocated for patients with recurrent or crescendo TIAs, although published results are variable. The efficacy of IV Dextran 40 at controlling symptoms and emboli before elective carotid endarterectomy was assessed in patients with recurrent or crescendo TIAs.

Methods.—Nineteen patients were recruited for this prospective pilot study. All of these patients had greater than 70% internal carotid artery stenosis, 2 or more symptomatic episodes within 30 days, and microemboli detected on transcranial Doppler US. Dextran 40 was initiated at 20 mL/h and increased in 20-mL/h increments until symptoms and emboli were controlled. Patients then underwent carotid surgery.

Results.—Dextran 40 controlled the symptoms and emboli in all the patients. One patient with both unstable angina and crescendo TIAs died of myocardial infarction while awaiting urgent surgery. Of the 18 patients who underwent surgery, 1 patient had a nondisabling stroke on the third postoperative day.

Conclusions.—Transcranial Doppler US–directed Dextran 40 provides safe and effective control of symptoms and emboli in high-risk patients before elective carotid endarterectomy.

▶ Fifteen of the 18 patients in this study had their symptoms controlled with 20 ml/h infusions of Dextran 40. This suggests the source of recurrent TIA is platelet aggregates. A combination of Dextran and clopidogrel in patients with multiple TIAs and a negative CT scan for hemorrhage seems reasonable as long as surgery is performed promptly. I agree with the authors that a middle-of-the-night carotid operation is very seldom indicated.

G. L. Moneta, MD

Risk of Stroke, Transient Ischemic Attack, and Vessel Occlusion Before Endarterectomy in Patients With Symptomatic Severe Carotid Stenosis

Blaser T, Hofmann K, Buerger T, et al (Univ of Magdeburg, Germany)
Stroke 33:1057-1062, 2002   12–16

Introduction.—Delaying endarterectomy after an ischemic vascular event may expose patients to an increased stroke risk. A prospective follow-up of consecutive patients scheduled for carotid endarterectomy examined the hypothesis that rapid progression of a severe symptomatic stenosis toward occlusion is a prominent cause of disabling stroke.

Methods.—The study group comprised 143 patients (105 men and 38 women; mean age, 66 years). All had symptomatic severe carotid artery stenosis and had experienced an ischemic vascular event in the ipsilateral anterior circulation. Data obtained at admission included medical history, neurologic status, extracranial and transcranial Doppler/duplex sonography, CT/MRI, ECG, and routine laboratory examination. Patients were re-evaluated before surgery and at recurrence of an ischemic event. The end point of follow-up (median duration, 19 days) was carotid endarterectomy, recurrent ipsilateral ischemia, or carotid occlusion.

Results.—Carotid endarterectomy was performed in 120 patients, 15 had an ipsilateral recurrent ischemic event (including 8 disabling strokes and 4 cases of carotid occlusion), and 8 had asymptomatic carotid occlusion. The only independent predictor for disabling stroke (odds ratio [OR], 9.7) was an exhausted cerebrovascular reactivity as determined by transcranial Doppler examination of the middle cerebral artery ipsilateral to the stenosis. The stroke rate in patients with this finding was 27% per month versus 5.2% in patients with normal reactivity. Twelve patients exhibited progression of stenosis toward occlusion, an event associated with decreased poststenotic peak systolic velocity (OR, 0.75), poststenotic arterial narrowing (OR, 22.7), and very severe stenosis (OR, 13.6). In the absence of hemodynamic compromise, occlusion was not associated with increased stroke risk.

Conclusion.—After an ischemic vascular event, patients with recently symptomatic high-grade carotid artery stenosis and ipsilateral hemodynamic compromise are at high risk for early disabling stroke. An assessment of hemodynamic status might identify those in whom endarterectomy should not be delayed.

▶ The timing of carotid endarterectomy after an ischemic or neurologic event, particularly a stroke, is a clinical problem that tests the judgment of even the most experienced vascular surgeon. This interesting study identifies exhausted cerebrovascular reactivity, as determined by the transcranial Doppler test after inhalation of carbon dioxide or hyperventilation, as a significant independent predictor of stroke following the initial event. Reduced blood flow in the internal carotid artery just distal to a critically stenotic lesion was an independent predictor for carotid artery occlusion but, interestingly, not for stroke, except in those patients with exhausted cerebrovascular reactivity. The data are quite compelling; however, I am concerned by the fact that many units, including our own, do not incorporate transcranial Doppler measurements into their routine evaluation of patients with carotid artery disease. For those of us making these decisions without the availability of transcranial Doppler analysis or physiologic testing of cerebrovascular reactivity, a prudent course would seem to suggest erring on the side of operating early on most patients with small strokes and good recovery, and then all patients with transient ischemic symptoms if possible.

F. B. Pomposelli, Jr, MD

Carotid Artery Closure for Endarterectomy Does Not Influence Results of Angioplasty-Stenting for Restenosis

Hobson RW II, Lal BK, Chakhtoura EY, et al (Univ of Medicine and Dentistry of New Jersey, Newark; St Michael's Med Ctr, Newark, NJ)

J Vasc Surg 35:435-438, 2002   12–17

Background.—Symptomatic or asymptomatic carotid restenosis occurs rarely after carotid endarterectomy (CEA) for extracranial carotid occlusive disease, but intervention for this complication is reported by some to carry an increased risk of postoperative neurologic events and cranial nerve palsies. Carotid angioplasty and stenting (CAS) has been proposed as an alternative to surgical management for recurrent carotid stenosis. However, the need for guidewire placement and balloon dilatation at the site of a previous arterial suture line represents potential drawbacks. A series of CAS procedures performed to treat high-grade restenosis after prior CEA was evaluated.

Methods.—Fifty-four CAS procedures (54 patients; 28 men and 26 women; mean age, 69 years) were performed for restenosis after previous CEA. Nineteen patients had symptoms and 35 did not. These procedures were undertaken from 6 to 62 months after the CEA (mean, 16 months), and follow-up extended for 1 to 48 months (mean, 18 months). The severity of

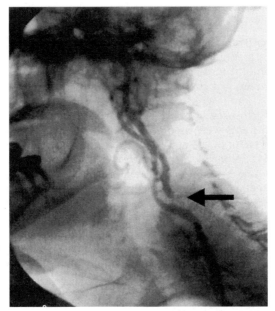

FIGURE 1.—Selective lateral carotid angiogram results show high-grade restenotic lesion in proximal internal carotid artery (*arrow*) near apex of polyethylene terephthalate (Dacron) patch angioplasty used in this patient. (Reprinted by permission of the publisher from Hobson RW II, Lal BK, Chakhtoura EY, et al: Carotid artery closure for endarterectomy does not influence results of angioplasty-stenting for restenosis. *J Vasc Surg* 35:435-438, 2002. Copyright 2002 by Elsevier.)

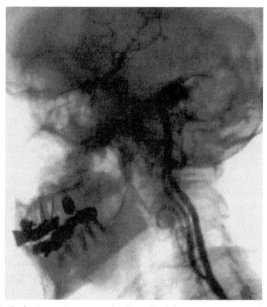

FIGURE 3.—Final selective angiogram results showed satisfactory post-stent result. (Reprinted by permission of the publisher from Hobson RW II, Lal BK, Chakhtoura EY, et al: Carotid artery closure for endarterectomy does not influence results of angioplasty-stenting for restenosis. *J Vasc Surg* 35:435-438, 2002. Copyright 2002 by Elsevier.)

the stenosis was evaluated with the use of digital angiography in the lateral, anteroposterior, and oblique planes (Fig 1); the mean severity of the restenosis was 84%, and the mean residual stenosis after CAS was 8%.

Results.—Fifteen percent of the closures were classified as primary, 9% were classified as autologous patch angioplasty, and 76% were classified as synthetic patch closures. All CAS procedures were successful (Fig 3). Self-expanding Wallstents were used in 91% of the procedures, self-expanding nickel–titanium stents were used in 7.5%, and a balloon expandable stent was used in 1.5%. None of the patients experienced contrast extravasation, arterial disruption, or subintimal dissection. None of the residual stenosis after CAS exceeded 15%. One patient had a stroke; this individual had a prior CEA and polyethylene terephthalate (Dacron) patch closure.

Conclusions.—CAS provided a safe and effective alternative to repeated CEA procedures and was not linked to excessive numbers of serious complications. Care is required in passing the guidewire across the stenosis, suture line, or patch angioplasty: 1 patient required retraction and replacement of the guidewire. Whether primary closure or patch angioplasty was used to obtain closure of the original arteriotomy had no impact on the incidence of complications.

▶ The authors periprocedure results are reported for CAS for recurrent carotid stenosis. Initial results do not appear to be influenced by the method of original closure of the endarterectomy site. The results are excellent and were obtained with the use of protection devices in only 2 of the patients. Since therapy was for recurrent stenosis, a more definitive evaluation will require long-term analysis of in-stent restenosis and the development of symptoms after carotid artery stenting for recurrent stenosis.

G. L. Moneta, MD

Hospital and Surgeon Determinants of Carotid Endarterectomy Outcomes
Feasby TE, Quan H, Ghali WA (Univ of Calgary, Alta, Canada)
Arch Neurol 59:1877-1881, 2002   12–18

Background.—Hospital and physician factors that may affect outcome after carotid endarterectomy (CEA) include volume of cases, teaching status, and participation in randomized controlled trials (RCTs) of CEA. A national data source for all CEAs performed in Canada was analyzed to determine whether there are relationships between hospital and surgeon characteristics and the rates of adverse events after CEA.

Methods.—All the CEAs performed in fiscal years 1994 through 1997 were included for a total of 14,368 patients. The specific characteristics analyzed were case volume, teaching status, and participation in RCTs of CEA for hospitals, and specialty and case volume for surgeons. Logistic regression analysis was performed to correlate adverse outcomes after CEA with these hospital and surgeon characteristics. Outcome measures were in-hospital stroke, death, or both.

Results.—Low hospital volume was predictive of significantly worse adjusted outcomes, with a rate of 5.1% when fewer than 150 patients had CEA and 4.0% when more than 150 patients had CEA. Participation in the 2 large North American CEA RCTs carried a significantly lower adjusted adverse outcome rate of 3.7% when compared with the 4.5% rate of other hospitals. Hospital teaching status did not influence outcome rate. General surgeons had a statistically significant worse outcome when compared with vascular surgeons, neurosurgeons, and thoracic surgeons combined. A strong inverse relationship was found between surgeon case volume and adverse events, especially when the surgeon had performed fewer than 15 procedures during the 4-year period covered. Low-volume surgeons at low-volume hospitals had an adverse outcome rate of 13.6%; low-volume surgeons at high-volume hospitals had an adverse outcome rate of 5.9%; high-volume surgeons at low-volume hospitals had an adverse outcome rate of 4.7%; and high-volume surgeons at high-volume hospitals had an adverse outcome rate of 3.9%. Participation in RCTs and surgeon volume proved to be independently significant characteristics on statistical analysis.

Conclusions.—Low hospital and surgeon case volumes had a significant negative impact on outcome after CEA. Participation in RCTs carried a positive influence, and patients having CEA performed by general surgeons had worse outcomes overall than those whose procedures were performed by specialists in thoracic, vascular, or neurologic disciplines. Thus, the best results for CEA were found at high-volume hospitals, with high-volume specialist surgeons and when the institution was involved in RCTs in CEA.

▶ Although I am generally somewhat skeptical of the conclusions drawn from data analyzed from large national databases, the results of this study support those of many other studies. Specifically, the result of CEA is most significantly affected by the experience of the operating surgeon. Low-volume surgeons have worse outcomes for CEA than high-volume surgeons, regardless of their specialty or in the type of hospital in which they practice. What is disconcerting in this study, as is in several trials from the United States, is that more than one third of the surgeons performing CEA in Canada did less than 1 procedure per year. Clearly, this is unacceptable. While the application of minimal volume standards for surgeons performing CEA is debatable, data from this study, as in many others, strongly suggest that surgeons who perform CEA very infrequently should probably stop doing so.

F. B. Pomposelli, Jr, MD

Distal Vertebral Artery Reconstruction: Long-term Outcome
Kieffer E, Praquin B, Chiche L, et al (Pitié-Salpêtrière Univ Hosp, Paris)
J Vasc Surg 36:549-554, 2002   12–19

Background.—Surgical reconstruction of the distal vertebral artery (DVA) has been performed for more than 20 years. Long-term outcomes in a total of 352 procedures in 323 patients are described.

Methods.—From December 1978 to July 2001, DVA reconstruction was performed in 323 patients (177 men, 148 women; mean age, 60 ± 12.9 years; range, 8-82 years). The preoperative cardiovascular status was normal in 147 patients (45.5%). The remaining patients had hypertension, coronary artery disease, or both. Nearly all the patients (94.3%) had symptoms of vertebrobasilar insufficiency. Bypass grafting (mostly saphenous vein grafts) was performed in 240 cases (68.2%). In 102 cases (29%), the DVA was transposed onto the internal carotid artery (ICA). Other techniques were used in 10 cases.

Results.—Seven deaths (2%) occurred and were all caused by strokes in the early postoperative period. Five nonfatal strokes (1.4%) occurred. Strokes were hemispheric in 7 cases and vertebrobasilar in 5 cases. There were 6 strokes (2.3%) in the subgroup of 264 isolated DVA reconstructions and 6 strokes (6.8%) in the subgroup of 88 cases that had combined ICA and DVA reconstruction. Temporary paralysis of the spinal accessory nerve occurred in 26 cases (7.4%). Intraoperative or early postoperative angiographic findings were available in 341 of 345 cases and showed that early postoperative occlusion occurred after 25 procedures (7.1%). Complete clinical follow-up was available for 313 of the surviving patients. The mean duration of follow-up was 99.5 ± 62.5 months. A total of 65 patients died during follow-up, but no deaths resulted from vertebrobasilar or hemispheric strokes. The cumulative Kaplan-Meier survival rate was $89.0\% \pm 3.9\%$ at 5 years and 75.4% ± 7.1% at 10 years. The significant vertebrobasilar symptom-free rate was 94.0% ± 3.5% at 5 years and 92.8% ± 3.8% at 10 years. The primary patency rate was 89.3% ± 3.6% at 5 years and 88.1% ± 4.0% at 10 years.

Conclusions.—Excellent long-term results can be obtained with reconstruction of the DVA. However, early postoperative occlusions occur in 7%. The subgroup of patients undergoing combined ICA and DVA reconstruction are at higher risk of postoperative stroke.

► This is an impressive series summarizing the results of DVA reconstruction for patients with vertebrobasilar ischemic symptoms over a 23-year span, with an average more than 8-year follow-up. Similar to carotid artery disease, however, we may predict that the development of refined endovascular neurointerventional techniques will change the future treatment algorithm of these patients presenting with focal vertebrobasilar lesions.

R. M. Fujitani, MD

Congenital Absence of the Internal Carotid Artery: Case Reports and Review of the Collateral Circulation

Given CA II, Huang-Hellinger F, Baker MD, et al (Wake Forest Univ, Winston-Salem, NC; Florida Hosp, Orlando)
AJNR Am J Neuroradiol 22:1953-1959, 2001   12–20

Introduction.—The absence of the internal carotid artery (ICA) is a rare finding. Reported are 4 new cases of congenital absence of the ICA.

Case 1.—Man, 56, was seen for transient right-sided weakness. Sonographic examination identified a diffuse narrowing of the left ICA, with a peak systolic velocity of 20 cm/s. The contralateral side was remarkable for mildly increased flow in the common carotid artery (CCA). MRI demonstrated attenuated flow within the petrous portion of the left ICA and collateral flow to the left hemisphere through the circle of Willis. Hypoplasia of the left carotid canal was detected on CT angiography, verifying a congenital small left ICA. His symptoms resolved spontaneously.

Case 2.—Girl, 6 years, had a single episode of slurred speech and headache. An MR angiogram revealed absence of flow-related signal intensity within the left supraclinoid ICA with collateral flow to the left anterior cerebral (ACA) and middle cerebral (MCA) arteries through a patent anterior communicating artery (ACOM). The absence of the carotid canal on a skull base CT scan verified agenesis of the left ICA.

Case 3.—Man, 62, was seen for transient ischemic attacks. Arteriogram showed a right CCA of diminished caliber that terminated in the external carotid artery. No remnant of a cervical right ICA could be seen. The right ACA was supplied via a patent ACOM. The right

MCA was a continuation of the right supraclinoid ICA. The right carotid siphon received blood flow via an intercavernous collateral vessel that arose from the left ICA and coursed through the sella turcica. The intercavernous communication verified a congenitally absent right ICA.

Case 4.—Woman, 33, had sudden onset of left upper extremity weakness 10 days after a motor vehicle accident. Cerebral angiography demonstrated a focal dissection of the right cervical ICA. The left CCA terminated into the external carotid artery (ECA) with no detectable remnant of the ICA. Collateral flow to the left hemisphere was supplied across a patent ACOM and through a patent posterior communicating artery. Head CT showed a diminutive left carotid canal, verifying the diagnosis of left ICA aplasia.

Conclusion.—Agenesis, aplasia, and hypoplasia of the ICA are rare findings. The primary collateral pathways included the circle of Willis, persistence of embryonic vessels, and transcranial collaterals via the ECA. These anomalies can have important implications for patients undergoing carotid endarterectomy.

▶ Anatomic variations are always of interest to surgeons. About 100 cases of congenital absence of the ICA have been reported. It happens, for some reason, 3 times more often on the left than on the right. Some cases are bilateral. Multiple collateral pathways exist. There are 6 main ones described by Lie in a 1968 publication.[1]

G. L. Moneta, MD

Reference

1. Lie TA: Congenital anomalies of the carotid arteries. Amsterdam: *Excerpta Medica*, 1968, pp 35-51.

13 Grafts and Graft Complications

Benefits, Morbidity, and Mortality Associated With Long-term Administration of Oral Anticoagulant Therapy to Patients With Peripheral Arterial Bypass Procedures: A Prospective Randomized Study
Johnson WC, and Members of the Department of Veterans Affairs Cooperative Study #362 (Boston Univ; VA Maryland Health Care System, Perry Point; et al)
J Vasc Surg 35:413-421, 2002   13–1

Introduction.—The risk-to-benefit ratio of warfarin in patients with lower extremity revascularization is controversial. The effect of warfarin plus aspirin therapy (WASA) versus aspirin therapy alone (ASA) on patient mortality and bypass patency rates was examined in a multicenter, prospective, randomized, nonmasked clinical investigation.

Methods.—Patients with patent bypasses on postoperative day 1 were stratified by center and by bypass material (prosthetic vs autogenous vein bypass); prosthetic bypasses were further stratified to those with 8-mm diameters versus 6-mm diameters. A total of 831 patients were randomly assigned in a long-term treatment program to either WASA (target international normalized ratio, 1.4-2.8; 325 mg/d) or ASA (325 mg/d). Warfarin therapy was usually 5 mg/d and was initiated as soon as the patient's condition allowed oral fluids. The main end point was bypass patency, and the secondary end points were mortality and morbidity.

Results.—There were 133 and 95 deaths, respectively, in the WASA and ASA groups (31.8% vs 23.0%; risk ratio, 1.41; 95% CI, 1.09-1.84; P = .0001). Major hemorrhagic events were more common in the WASA group (WASA, 35; ASA, 15; P = .02). For the prosthetic bypass group, no significant difference was found in the patency rate in the 8-mm bypass subgroup; a significant difference was found in the 6-mm bypass subgroup (femoral–popliteal; 71.4% WASA vs 57.9% ASA; P = .02). The patency rate in the vein bypass group was unaffected (75.3% WASA vs 74.9% ASA) (Fig 2).

Conclusion.—Long-term administration of WASA has only a few selected indications for improvement of bypass patency and is correlated with an increased risk of both morbidity and mortality.

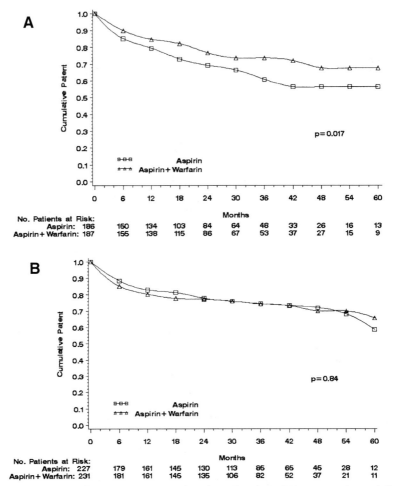

FIGURE 2.—Assisted primary patency rates of prosthetic (**A**) and vein (**B**) lower extremity arterial by-passes. (Reprinted by permission of the publisher from Johnson WC, and members of the Department of Veterans Affairs Cooperative Study #362: Benefits, morbidity, and mortality associated with long-term administration of oral anticoagulant therapy to patients with peripheral arterial bypass procedures: A prospective randomized study. *J Vasc Surg* 35:413-421, 2002. Copyright 2002 by Elsevier.)

▶ There are now 2 large randomized studies of the efficacy of warfarin and aspirin versus aspirin alone in preventing infrainguinal bypass graft occlusion. Both this study (VA cooperative 362) and the Dutch bypass oral anticoagulants or aspirin study (BOA) found a slight benefit of the combination of warfarin and aspirin in improving patency of prosthetic bypasses but at the expense of increased hemorrhagic events. (The benefit was primarily for above-knee prosthetic femoral-popliteal bypasses in VA 362.) BOA, however, found a benefit of warfarin also in vein bypass grafts that was not shown in VA 362. BOA, however, had a targeted international normalized ratio of 3.0 to 4.5 as opposed to 1.4 to 2.8 in VA 362. Overall, except possibly for very high risk distal vein grafts, warfarin doesn't appear to be an effective means to prevent vein graft occlusion. Like many others, we have used warfarin in some patients with infrainguinal vein grafts. However, given this study and the Dutch study, I think it is now time to say there really is no place for warfarin to prevent infrainguinal vein graft occlusion in patients who do not have a documented hypercoagulable state.

G. L. Moneta, MD

The Effect of Anticoagulation Therapy and Graft Selection on the Ischemic Consequences of Femoropopliteal Bypass Graft Occlusion: Results From a Multicenter Randomized Clinical Trial
Jackson MR, Johnson WC, Williford WO, et al (Dallas Veteran's Affairs Med Ctr; Univ of Texas, Dallas; Boston Veteran's Affairs Med Ctr; et al)
J Vasc Surg 35:292-298, 2002   13–2

Background.—Autogenous saphenous vein is the preferred graft material for infrainguinal bypass. Several studies have suggested acceptable patency for polytetrafluoroethylene (PTFE) for above-knee femoropopliteal bypass. A recent retrospective study, however, showed the ischemic consequences of femoropopliteal bypass graft occlusion were more severe with PTFE than with autologous saphenous vein. To confirm the conclusions of this study and to determine whether oral anticoagulation therapy may reduce the degree of ischemia after occlusion of PTFE and vein femoropopliteal bypass grafts, a prospective study was done.

Methods.—The study included 402 patients who underwent femoropopliteal bypass grafting (PTFE, 233; vein, 169) who were assigned randomly to a postoperative regimen of either warfarin and aspirin therapy or therapy with aspirin alone. The Society of Vascular Surgery recommended reporting standards (grade I, viable; grade II, threatened) were used to assess the grade of acute ischemia at the time of graft occlusion. Early graft occlusions were excluded.

Results.—During a mean follow-up of 36 months for the PTFE group and 39 months for the vein group, 100 graft occlusions occurred: 67 in the PTFE group and 33 in the vein group. One hundred patients were randomly assigned to either warfarin plus aspirin therapy (n = 48) or to aspirin only therapy (n = 52). The patients were well matched for age, atherosclerotic risk factors, operative indication, and preoperative ankle-brachial index. A greater percentage of the PTFE occlusions (48%) caused grade II ischemia compared with vein graft occlusions (18%). The ankle-brachial index at the time of graft occlusion was significantly lower in the PTFE grafts than in the vein grafts (0.28 vs 0.45). Patients who were taking warfarin and aspirin therapy at the time of graft occlusion had less grade II ischemia (28%) than did patients who were undergoing aspirin only therapy (55%). However, the incidence of severe ischemia after graft occlusion remained greater with PTFE grafts and warfarin plus aspirin therapy compared with all vein grafts (28% vs 18%). The incidence of grade II ischemia after vein graft occlusions was similar for warfarin plus aspirin therapy (20%) and aspirin only therapy (17%).

Conclusion.—The ischemic consequences of femoropopliteal bypass graft occlusion are worse with PTFE than with vein grafts. The use of warfarin plus aspirin therapy reduces the severity of acute ischemia after occlusion of a PTFE graft, as compared with that of aspirin only therapy, although not to the degree obtained with vein graft occlusion. Occlusion of femoropopliteal vein grafts seldom is accompanied by severe ischemia, and warfarin plus aspirin therapy does not improve this condition.

▶ My bias has always been that one of the best ways to put a patient on the pathway to critical limb ischemia is to perform a prosthetic infrainguinal bypass for claudication. This report provides some evidence for that bias.

G. L. Moneta, MD

Choice of Autogenous Conduit for Lower Extremity Vein Graft Revisions
Landry GJ, Moneta GL, Taylor LM Jr, et al (Oregon Health & Science Univ, Portland)
J Vasc Surg 36:238-244, 2002   13–3

Background.—Surgical revision for repair of stenosis is necessary in about 20% of LEVGs. Identifying a suitable autogenous conduit for revision of a lower extremity vein graft (LEVG) is often challenging. Options include contralateral or residual ipsilateral greater saphenous vein, lesser saphenous vein, or arm vein, either cephalic and basilic vein. Each of these conduit choices has advantages and disadvantages. Basilic vein harvesting requires deep exposure in proximity to major nerves. Yet it typically is a large vein that is unaffected by prior IV lines. It would therefore seem ideal for revisions in which relatively short venous segment is needed for an interposition within the graft or for extension to a more proximal inflow or distal outflow site. An experience with basilic veins compared with other sources of autogenous conduit for LEVG revisions is presented.

Methods.—All patients who underwent LEVGs were enrolled in a duplex scan surveillance program, and LEVGs that developed a focal area of increased velocity or uniformly low velocities throughout the graft, with appropriate lesions confirmed by angiography, were candidates for revision. This report includes all patients at the authors' institution who underwent LEVG revision with basilic vein segments from January 1, 1990, to September 1, 2001. These revisions were compared with LEVG revisions in which cephalic and saphenous veins were used.

Results.—A total of 130 basilic veins were used to revise 122 LEVGs. The mean follow-up period after revision was 28 ± 27 months. Patency was maintained in 93 grafts (71%) without further revision, and 37 grafts (29%) either needed additional revisions (22 grafts) or were occluded (15 grafts). However, only 4 (11%) of these adverse events were directly attributed to the basilic vein segment. Ten of 43 grafts revised with cephalic vein (23%)

were either revised or occluded, with 3 related to the cephalic vein segment. Twenty-four of 81 grafts revised with saphenous vein (30%) were either revised or occluded, of which 11 adverse events could be attributed to the saphenous vein segment. Two patients (1.5%) had complications from basilic vein harvesting, but no neurologic complications occurred from harvesting of the basilic veins.

Conclusions.—The basilic vein seems to be a reliable and durable conduit for segmental revision of LEVGs. Stenoses rarely occur within interposed basilic vein segments, and excellent freedom from a subsequent revision or occlusion can be obtained.

▶ The reason the basilic vein makes an excellent conduit for vein graft revision is that it is not subject to repeated venipunctures and is of relatively large caliber. It is a bit difficult to harvest, some of the branches are short and wide, the vein is thin, and important nerves are nearby. (Since the publication of this paper we have had 1 case of neuropraxia secondary to a basilic vein harvest.) Overall, however, this conduit should be kept in mind when a short piece of vein is needed. We use it in preference to harvesting residual saphenous veins.

G. L. Moneta, MD

Prospective Analysis of Endoscopic Vein Harvesting
Patel AN, Hebeler RF, Hamman BL, et al (Baylor Univ, Dallas)
Am J Surg 182:716-719, 2001   13–4

Background.—The use of continuous linear incisions for saphenous vein graft (SVG) harvesting results in 5% to 20% patient morbidity. Studies of bridging SVG harvest (BVH), noncontinuous parallel incisions, have shown a moderately improved patient morbidity rate. In contrast, studies of endoscopic SVG harvesting (EVH) have reported morbidity of just 2% to 5%. EVH was compared with BVH to determine whether EVH can significantly reduce the morbidity associated with SVG harvesting.

Methods.—A prospective database of 200 matched patients undergoing EVH and BVH was compared. All patients underwent coronary artery bypass grafting over a period of 4 months, from April to August 2000. None of the patients had a history of prior vein harvesting. Patients in the 2 groups were demographically similar.

Results.—The patients in the EVH group had significantly fewer wound complications, fewer mean days to ambulation, and a shorter total length of hospitalization. There was no difference between the groups in harvest time or vein injuries.

Conclusion.—EVH is associated with significantly fewer wound complications, fewer days to ambulation, and a shorter total length of hospitalization. EVH is superior to BVH for patients undergoing coronary artery bypass grafting.

▶ In this study, EVH did not result in an increased incidence of vein injury, although the actual number of vein injuries in each group was not reported. With this technique, most patients still receive an incisional harvest of their vein when the length of conduit required necessitates use of the below-knee saphenous vein. Wound complications were less with EVH, but no preoperative vein mapping was used. It is our bias that the use of vein mapping preoperatively may decrease wound complications associated with the open harvesting technique. I think the advantages of EVH are not as dramatic as suggested in this study.

G. L. Moneta, MD

Simvastatin Inhibits Human Saphenous Vein Neointima Formation Via Inhibition of Smooth Muscle Cell Proliferation and Migration
Porter KE, Naik J, Turner NA, et al (Univ of Leeds, England; Univ of Leicester, England)
J Vasc Surg 36:150-157, 2002   13–5

Background.—In vitro and in vivo studies have suggested the involvement of basement membrane–degrading matrix metalloproteinases (MMPs) and growth factors in mediating smooth muscle cell migration and proliferation. Statins are widely used in the treatment of atherosclerosis and are said to have other effects besides the reduction of cholesterol levels. The effects of simvastatin on the proliferation and migration of cultured human saphenous vein smooth muscle cells and the effects of simvastatin on neointimal formation and MMP activity in human saphenous vein organ cultures were investigated. The effects of marimastat, a specific MMP inhibitor, were also studied to provide clarification of the mode of action of simvastatin.

Methods.—Human saphenous vein specimens were obtained from patients who underwent coronary artery bypass grafting. The specimens were cultured for 14 days in the presence of 3 different concentrations of simvastatin and then processed for measurement of MMP activity and neointimal thickness measurements. Cultured saphenous vein smooth muscle cells were then used to develop growth curves in the presence of 10% fetal calf serum or 10% fetal calf serum supplemented with simvastatin or marimastat. Modified Boyden chambers were used to quantify migration through a Matrigel basement-membrane matrix.

Results.—Neointimal formation was reduced by simvastatin in a dose-dependent manner and in association with reduced MMP-9 activity (Fig 1). Simvastatin also inhibited smooth muscle cell proliferation and invasion. Marimastat also had a dose-dependent inhibitory effect on smooth muscle cell invasion; however, it had no effect on proliferation of smooth muscle cells.

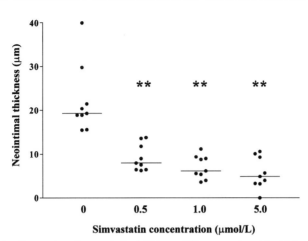

FIGURE 1.—Simvastatin reduces neointimal thickness. Veins were cultured for 14 days in a medium alone (control) or in presence of indicated concentrations of simvastatin before measuring neointimal thickness. *Horizontal bars* represent median values. **P < .01, compared with control. (Reprinted by permission of the publisher from Porter KE, Naik J, Turner NA, et al: Simvastatin inhibits saphenous vein neointima formation via inhibition of smooth muscle cell proliferation and migration. *J Vasc Surg* 36:150-157, 2002. Copyright 2002 by Elsevier.)

Conclusions.—Effective control of neointimal development in vivo requires a pharmacologic strategy that inhibits both the migration and proliferation of smooth muscle cells. These findings suggest that simvastatin may offer a promising therapeutic approach to the prevention of stenosis in saphenous vein grafts.

▶ Statins are turning out to be much more than cholesterol-lowering medications. They appear to have considerable anti-inflammatory effects, at least as far as inflammation is related to atherosclerosis. They also now appear to effect intimal hyperplasia through a variety of mechanisms. I wonder if everyone with clinical atherosclerosis should not be on a statin regardless of their cholesterol level?

G. L. Moneta, MD

Femoropopliteal Arteries: Immediate and Long-term Results With a Dacron-Covered Stent-Graft
Ahmadi R, Schillinger M, Maca T, et al (Univ of Vienna)
Radiology 223:345-350, 2002   13–6

Introduction.—One of many promising new techniques developed to potentially help improve the outcome of endovascular interventions in femoropopliteal arteries is the use of polyethylene terephthalate (Dacron)-covered vascular stent-grafts. The immediate and long-term outcomes after femoropopliteal implantation of a polyethylene terephthalate–covered stent-graft were prospectively examined in 30 consecutive patients with peripheral arterial disease with recurrent stenosis after percutaneous transluminal angioplasty.

Methods.—Patients took 100 gm of acetylsalicylic acid before and after placement of the polyethylene terephthalate–covered stent-graft. During the intervention, patients received 5000 IU of heparin intra-arterially after insertion of the introducer sheath. After implantation, IV heparin was continuously administered immediately after removal of the arterial sheath. Oral anticoagulation was continued for 6 months postoperatively (therapeutic level; international normalized ratio, 2.0-3.0).

Results.—Initial technical success was achieved in all 30 patients. A significant improvement in ankle-brachial index was observed from a preintervention mean of 0.5 to a postoperative mean of 0.8 ($P < .001$). Twelve patients (405) experienced postimplantation noninfectious fevers and elevation in both leukocyte and C-reactive protein levels. Seventeen patients reported persistent pain at the site of implantation for a mean of 5 days (range, 2-28 days). Early recurrent occlusion occurred within the first 24 hours in 5 patients (17%). At a mean follow-up of 60 months, 25 patients (83%) experienced restenosis. The primary patency rates at 6, 12, 36, and 72-month follow-up, respectively, were 27%, 23%, 17%, and 17%; secondary patency rates were 63%, 60%, 34%, and 34%, respectively.

Conclusion.—Implantation of polyethylene terephthalate–covered stent-grafts for the treatment of femoropopliteal lesions was associated with high early and late restenosis rates and a considerable incidence of complications, including fever and pain. These problems make the polyethylene terephthalate–covered stent-graft unacceptable for treatment of femoropopliteal arterial occlusive disease.

▶ It is rare to see people with sufficient courage to report the results of a second bad idea to treat the results of a first bad idea.

G. L. Moneta, MD

The Effectiveness of Muscle Flaps for the Treatment of Prosthetic Graft Sepsis

Graham RG, Omotoso PO, Hudson DA (Univ of Cape Town, South Africa)
Plast Reconstr Surg 109:108-113, 2002   13–7

Background.—The efficacy of muscle flaps for the treatment of prosthetic graft sepsis was examined in a retrospective analysis.

Study Design.—The results of all 21 patients treated with 27 muscle flaps for the management of prosthetic graft infections at Groote Schuur Hospital between January 1991 and July 2000 were reviewed. The most common site of infection was the groin. The patients underwent surgery with debridement, and cultures were obtained. The graft was left in situ, and the wound was closed with local muscle flaps. All patients received parenteral antibiotics until sepsis was clinically resolved. End points evaluated included flap survival, the limb salvage rate, and the mortality rate.

Findings.—The mortality rate was 0. Limb salvage was achieved in 71%, and sepsis did not recur in 36 months of follow-up. Of the 27 muscle flaps, 18 were sartorius flaps in the groin. The graft survival rate for these flaps was 94%, and the limb salvage rate was 71%.

Conclusions.—This report describes a series of 27 muscle flaps used for the treatment of prosthetic graft sepsis. This approach was successful in 71% of the patients: wounds healed, sepsis cleared, and limbs were salvage. These results further suggest that the sartorius muscle is a good choice for prosthetic graft infections of the groin.

▶ It is important to keep in mind the infected grafts treated with muscle flaps in this study were those where infection was *clearly* localized. Under such circumstances, I believe muscle flap coverage of exposed infected grafts can be effective. The authors use sartorius flaps with good results. We prefer rectus femoris flaps because of their more reliable blood supply.

G. L. Moneta, MD

Limitations in the Use of Rifampicin-Gelatin Grafts Against Virulent Organisms

Koshiko S, Sasajima T, Muraki S, et al (Asahikawa Med Univ, Japan)
J Vasc Surg 35:779-785, 2002   13–8

Background.—The efficacy and duration of antibacterial activity of rifampicin-gelatin grafts against methicillin-resistant *Staphylococcus aureus* (MRSA) was assessed in an animal model.

Methods.—Twenty-four rifampicin-gelatin grafts and 4 plain Gelseal grafts were placed in canine abdominal aorta inoculated with *Staphylococcus epidermis*, *Escherichia coli*, or MRSA. Grafts were retrieved 1 to 4 weeks later.

Findings.—On in vitro testing, the initial inhibition zones of rifampicin-gelatin grafts were 40 mm, 36 mm, and 11.8 mm against *S epidermidis*, MRSA, and *E coli*, respectively. After implantation, *S epidermidis*-inoculated rifampicin-gelatin grafts showed no graft infection. No colony growth was seen on plates streaked with perigraft fluids. Initial inhibition zones of *S epidermidis*-inoculated rifampicin-gelatin grafts were 20.1 mm at 1 week and 7.6 mm at 2 weeks. In *E coli*-inoculated and MRSA-inoculated rifampicin-gelatin grafts, perigraft abscess was observed in all 8 animals. Blood culture results indicated septicemia in 5 animals with patent grafts at death. Inhibition zones against *E coli* and MRSA were not apparent on plates streaked with the same organism. Initial inhibition zones of *E coli*- and MRSA-inoculated rifampicin-gelatin grafts on *S epidermidis*-streaked plates were 8 mm and 18.5 mm, respectively. Recolonization of high minimal inhibitory concentration strains in the MRSA group developed in the inhibition zones as early as 24 hours.

Conclusions.—Rifampicin-gelatin grafts appear to be a valid approach for *S epidermidis* infection. These grafts, however, were ineffective against

MRSA and *E coli* infections. Early development of high minimal inhibitory concentration MRSA strains or poor susceptibility could explain this latter observation.

▶ Rifampicin has antibacterial activity against *E coli* and MRSA and can be bound to the gelatin in gelatin-impregnated grafts by soaking the graft in a rifampicin solution. Unfortunately, in this case, 1 + 1 is actually less than 2 as rifampicin-treated grafts do not appear effective against preventing *E coli* and MRSA graft infections. Such grafts therefore cannot be recommended for in situ graft replacement of *E coli* or MRSA graft infections.

G. L. Moneta, MD

Abdominal Aortic Reconstruction in Infected Fields: Early Results of the United States Cryopreserved Aortic Allograft Registry

Noel AA, and Members of the United States Cryopreserved Aortic Allograft Registry (Mayo Clinic, Rochester, Minn; et al)
J Vasc Surg 35:847-852, 2002   13–9

Introduction.—Cryopreserved allografts have a number of potential advantages in the treatment of aortic and aortic graft infection. These include easy availability, avoidance of deep vein excision, maintenance of pelvic blood flow with in situ replacement, and a theoretical reduction in rates of reinfection. The results of aortic replacement with cryopreserved aortic allograft (CAA) in infected fields were assessed by review of data from various centers.

Methods.—The United States Cryopreserved Aortic Allograft Registry collects clinical data on patients who have undergone placement of a CAA in the United States after March 4, 1999. Thirty-one institutions submitted data for 56 patients (43 men and 13 women). Indications for CAA placement included primary graft infection (PGI), mycotic aneurysm (MA), aortoenteric erosion/fistula (AEE), and aortic reconstruction with concomitant bowel resection.

Results.—The mean patient age was 66 years. Indications were PGI (77%), MA (14%), AEE (7%), and elective aortic reconstruction with concomitant bowel resection (4%). Infectious organisms were identified in 33 (59%) patients; the most common was *Staphylococcus aureus*, present in 17 (52%) cases. Thirty-one patients (55%) needed an additional cryopreserved segment for reconstruction. One patient died in the operating room, another 6 died within 30 days, 3 died in hospital after 30 days, and 4 died during subsequent follow-up (the median follow-up was 2 months). Thus, the overall mortality rate was 25% (14 patients). Hemorrhage from the CAA and persistent infection were the cause of graft-related mortality in 2 (4%) patients. Graft-related complications were common and included persistent infection with perianastomotic hemorrhage (9%), graft limb occlusion (9%), and pseudoaneurysm (2%). Amputation was necessary in 3 (5%) patients.

Conclusion.—Cryopreserved aortic allografts are an option for replacement of infected aortic grafts. Early results indicate that graft-related mortality rates are low, but morbidity is high. Reinfection has not been reported as yet, but CAA is not currently recommended as preferred therapy for PGI, MA, or AEE. Two patients who underwent aortic reconstruction with concomitant bowel resection did well without complications.

▶ Do not for one moment be fooled by the results presented here. Cryopreserved grafts are not the "Holy Grail" for aortic graft infection. With only a mean follow-up of 5.3 months, 15% of the patients have had graft-related complications of hemorrhage, infection, or limb occlusion. This was a registry format and is likely to underestimate complications. In addition, we are still waiting for the late complications of graft limb stenosis. These grafts are very expensive and many are not long enough to complete the operation. To recommend these highly costly devices there has to be more convincing evidence of their increased efficacy over existing techniques of managing aortic graft infections.

G. L. Moneta, MD

The Use of Cryopreserved Femoral Vein Grafts for Hemodialysis Access in Patients at High Risk for Infection: A Word of Caution
Bolton WD, Cull DL, Taylor SM, et al (Greenville Hosp System, SC)
J Vasc Surg 36:464-468, 2002   13–10

Background.—The rise in the use of arteriovenous (AV) grafts has been associated with an increase in the number of graft infections. Infections of AV grafts occur at a rate of approximately 16% overall and between 18% and 35% in the thigh position. Several studies have reported success with the use of venous homografts for arteriovenous access and bypass in infected fields. The outcomes of arteriovenous graft placement with cryopreserved femoral veins in patients at high risk of graft infections are reported.

Methods.—From October 1999 to July 2001, about 3100 dialysis access operations were performed at a single center, and among these procedures, 20 patients underwent arteriovenous access grafting with cryopreserved femoral veins. All patients were determined to be at high risk of infection of the access because of active infections at the time of graft implantation, the location of the graft in the thigh, or a history of multiple access infections. The grafts were placed in the thigh (14 patients), upper extremity (3 patients), and chest wall (3 patients).

Results.—No early operative deaths or graft thromboses were seen. Three late deaths occurred: 2 from cardiac disease and 1 from a graft-related complication. Thirteen major graft-related complications (65%) occurred in 20 patients from 1 to 14 months after transplantation, including in 11 of these patients 3 generalized graft infections (15%) and 8 localized graft infections (40%) at dialysis needle access sites. Six graft infections were associated with graft rupture and hemorrhage, which resulted in the death of 1 patient from exsanguination. Two grafts thrombosed (10%), of which 1 was salvaged after a thrombectomy and revision. At a mean follow-up of 13 months, only 5 of 20 patients have a functioning arteriovenous graft that came from a cryopreserved femoral vein.

Conclusions.—The use of cryopreserved vein grafts for hemodialysis access in patients at high risk for infection is associated with a high incidence of infection and rupturing of the graft. The in situ replacement of infected polytetrafluoroethylene arteriovenous grafts with cryopreserved veins should only be considered if no suitable alternative sites can be found for access placement.

▶ Replacing one infected prosthetic graft with what amounts to another prosthetic graft has never seemed like a good idea to me. Everyone gets away with it once in a while, but bad ideas have a way of proving themselves as time goes by and experience accumulates. I am particularly concerned by the predilection of these grafts to rupture in the face of recurrent infection.

G. L. Moneta, MD

14 Vascular Trauma

An Analysis of Outcomes of Reconstruction or Amputation of Leg-Threatening Injuries
Bosse MJ, MacKenzie EJ, Kellam JF, et al (Carolinas Med Ctr, Charlotte, NC; Johns Hopkins Univ, Baltimore, Md; Univ of Maryland, Baltimore; et al)
N Engl J Med 347:1924-1931, 2002   14–1

Introduction.—Medical and surgical advances have improved the ability to reconstruct severely injured limbs. However, some reports indicate that functional outcome is often poorer after successful limb reconstruction than after treatment with early amputation and a good prosthesis. The functional outcomes of 569 patients with severe leg injuries who underwent reconstruction or amputation were compared.

Methods.—In this multicenter (8 level I trauma centers), prospective, observational trial, functional outcome measures included the Sickness Impact Profile, a multidimensional evaluation of self-reported health status (scores range from 0 to 100; scores for the general population average 2-3; scores >10 represent severe disability). Secondary outcomes included limb status and the presence or absence of major complications requiring a second hospitalization.

Results.—At 2-year follow-up, there were no significant differences in scores for the Sickness Impact Profile between the amputation and reconstruction groups (12.6 vs 11.8; $P = .53$). After adjusting for the characteristics of patients and their injuries, patients in the amputation group had functional outcomes that were similar to patients in the reconstruction group. The predictors of a poorer score for the Sickness Impact Profile were rehospitalization for a major complication, low educational level, nonwhite race, poverty, lack of private health insurance, poor social support network, low self-efficacy (the patient's confidence in being able to resume life activities), smoking, and involvement in disability compensation litigation. Patients who underwent reconstruction were more likely to be rehospitalized than those who underwent amputation (47.6% vs 33.9%; $P = .002$). Similar proportions of patients in the amputation group and in the reconstruction group had returned to work by 2 years (53.0% and 49.4%, respectively).

Conclusion.—Outcomes were similar for patients who underwent reconstruction and amputation. Patients with limb injuries at risk for amputation can be advised that reconstruction typically results in 2-year outcomes equivalent to those of amputation. However, patients who undergo reconstruction are at higher risk for complications, additional surgeries, and re-hospitalization.

▶ This is a very difficult study to analyze. Patients were not randomly assigned to reconstruction versus amputation. Patients undergoing amputation had more severe injuries than those undergoing reconstruction. While an attempt was made in the multivariant analysis to adjust for the different severity of injuries in the 2 groups, the complexity of the patients and their injuries makes it unlikely all confounding variables could possibly be considered. What is clear is that regardless of whether amputation or reconstruction is employed, the outcome of severe lower extremity injuries is greatly dependent on social factors such as economic status, support systems, race, and the presence or absence of private health insurance. Clearly, case managers and social workers must play a prominent role in the management of these types of patients.

G. L. Moneta, MD

A Quantitative Approach to Lower Extremity Vein Repair
Kuralay E, Demirkiliç U, Özal E, et al (Gülhane Military Med Academy, Ankara, Turkey)
J Vasc Surg 36:1213-1218, 2002   14–2

Background.—There is ongoing debate over the indications for complex reconstructions of the lower extremity veins. Patency rates after lower extremity venous repair were investigated in a quantitative fashion.

Methods.—A total of 130 patients underwent surgery to repair vascular injuries of the lower extremities over a 10-year period. There were 110 direct venous injuries in 97 patients. They involved the popliteal vein in 46 patients; the posterior tibial, anterior tibial, or peroneal veins in 45; the superficial femoral vein in 9; the common femoral vein in 7; and the deep femoral vein in 3. Most patients had associated fractures, nerve injuries, or other injuries. Patency rates and blood flow velocities were assessed with the use of duplex color US, performed in the early postoperative period and at late follow-up (mean, 6.2 years).

Results.—The severity of reperfusion injury, as indicated by extremity circumference, had a significant effect on venous blood flow velocity. After popliteal vein repair, mean flow velocity was 15 cm/sec in severe reperfusion injuries, with extremity diameters more than twice normal; versus 8.4 cm/sec in moderate injuries, with diameters of 1.5 to 2 times normal. Infrapopliteal vein repairs had flow velocities of less than 5 cm/sec and usually became occluded on the first day after surgery. Eleven patients, most with tibial fractures and extensive tissue loss, required amputation.

The 1-year patency rate was 100% for common femoral vein repairs and 89% for superficial femoral vein repairs; the 6-year patency rates were 100% and 78%, respectively. For popliteal vein repairs, the patency rate decreased from 86% at 1 year to 60% at 6 years. The patency rate was 100%

for popliteal veins undergoing thrombectomy without direct injury. Of all techniques used, patch angioplasty had the highest 6-year patency rate: 75%, compared with 58% for lateral repair, 43% for end-to-end anastomosis, and 36% for saphenous vein graft interposition.

Conclusions.—Quantitative outcome assessment shows good patency rates for femoral and popliteal venous repairs. However, infrapopliteal venous repairs are associated with low flow velocities and poor patency rates.

▶ This study cannot be used to determine if one technique of venous repair is superior to another. Obviously, one does not wish to narrow the lumen as a result of the repair. Therefore, in most cases, lateral repair of a venous injury is probably inadequate. However, the poor patency of the more complex techniques for repair of venous injuries likely reflects the nature and extent of the injury as much, or more, than the type of reconstruction employed. The good news is, most repairs proximal to the popliteal vein remain patent long term, and even if the repair does thrombose, pulmonary emboli were not noted in this series.

G. L. Moneta, MD

War Injuries of Major Extremity Arteries
Nanobashvili J, Kopadze T, Tvaladze M, et al (Tbilisi 1st Hosp, Georgia; Univ of Vienna)
World J Surg 27:134-139, 2003   14–3

Background.—Combat conditions are associated with significantly different types of wounds and constraints on medical and surgical treatment compared with peacetime. An experience with wartime injuries to the extremity arteries is reported.

Patients.—The 3-year experience included 99 combat-related injuries to the major blood vessels of the extremities treated at a Russian hospital. Forty percent of the patients were injured by mine fragments, 35% by high-velocity projectiles, and 25% by shotgun pellets. Fifty-seven percent of the injuries were to the upper limb and 43% to the lower limb. The median time to hospital admission was 8 hours after injury, at which time 39% of the patients were in severe hemorrhagic shock. Preoperative angiography was usually not needed to diagnose the arterial injury. Distal ischemia requiring arterial reconstruction was needed in 51% of the patients; there were no primary amputations.

Findings.—Axillary and popliteal artery injuries always required reconstruction, whereas injuries to the superficial femoral or brachial arteries did not. Reconstruction by end-to-end anastomosis was possible in only 38% of the cases; 56% required autologous venous bypass. In 22% of the patients uncontrolled wound infection developed, with complications including hemorrhage requiring arterial ligature in 8% of the cases and thrombosis in 65%. There was a 10% rate of secondary amputation after reconstruction. Sixty-eight percent of the major vessel injuries were accompanied by fractures, nerve damage, or venous injuries. Arterial damage in the forearm, popliteal region, and crural region was usually accompanied by venous injury as well. Venous damage in the upper extremity was usually managed with ligation, whereas repair was usually performed in the lower extremity.

Conclusions.—The experience highlights the complexity and treatment difficulties of combat injuries to the major blood vessels. Management priorities are aggressive debridement, drainage, immobilization, and prevention of infection. Because of the danger of infection, autologous vein bypass is the favored technique of reconstruction.

▶ Vascular surgeons tend to focus on the vascular repair after penetrating injury. An interesting point of this study is that wound complications are frequently the undoing of a good arterial repair. Once the arterial repair is complete, aggressive management of the wound both intraoperatively and postoperatively is required to prevent infection and disruption of the vascular repair.

G. L. Moneta, MD

Traumatic Rupture of the Aorta: Immediate or Delayed Repair?
Symbas PN, Sherman AJ, Silver JM, et al (Emory Univ, Atlanta, Ga; Grady Mem Hosp, Atlanta, Ga)
Ann Surg 235:796-802, 2002   14–4

Background.—Acute traumatic rupture of the thoracic aorta has traditionally been managed by repair of the injury as soon as possible. The primary basis for this is the premise that as many as 90% of patients will die within the first 24 hours after their injury. However, immediate repair of the transected aorta has also been associated with a surgical death rate of 0% to 54.2%. Delayed repair of the acute aortic tear, which allows the patient to recover from other major injuries, has been reported with increasing frequency in the literature. Whether delaying repair of the ruptured thoracic aorta in patients with other major injuries is safe and can positively affect survival was determined.

Methods.—A retrospective review was conducted of 30 consecutive patients with rupture of the thoracic aorta from blunt trauma treated from 1995 to 2001. Two patients died shortly after admission and were excluded from further consideration. The remaining 28 patients were grouped according to the time of repair of the rupture. Patients in group 1 underwent repair immediately after diagnosis, whereas patients in group 2, who had associated injuries that were likely to increase the risk of surgical death, had either repair more than 48 hours after injury or had no repair. Patients in group 2 had their mean arterial pressure maintained with medication at less than 70 mm Hg to eliminate shear stress on the aortic tear while under observation.

Results.—The patients had an average age of 36 years at the time of rupture. Of the 14 patients in group 1, 5 died during surgery or in the early postoperative period. In group 2, 2 of 9 patients with repair more than 48 hours after injury and 3 of 5 patients with no repair died of associated injury or illness. There were no cases of rupture of the traumatic pseudoaneurysm of the thoracic aorta in any of the patients who had associated injuries likely to increase the risk of surgical death.

Conclusion.—Delayed repair of acute traumatic aortic rupture is safe with appropriate treatment and should be considered in some patients.

▶ The ability to delay operation in patients with traumatic rupture of the thoracic aorta makes possible planning an endovascular procedure for these severely injured patients. (See also Abstract 14–5.)

G. L. Moneta, MD

Natural History of Traumatic Rupture of the Thoracic Aorta Managed Nonoperatively: A Longitudinal Analysis
Holmes JH IV, Bloch RD, Hall RA, et al (Univ of Washington, Seattle)
Ann Thorac Surg 73:1149-1154, 2002   14–5

Background.—Traumatic rupture of the thoracic aorta (TRA) is a surgical emergency. However, nonoperative management may be appropriate in a small subgroup of affected patients. The outcome of nonoperative management of TRA was investigated.

Methods.—One hundred forty-five patients admitted for TRA during a 16-year period were reviewed. Thirty of these patients underwent a period of nonoperative management. In this subgroup, the mean patient age was 44 years and 80% were male. The mean Injury Severity Score (ISS) was 34. In 15 patients, surgery was delayed to more than 24 hours (median, 3 days) after injury and diagnosis. The remaining 15 patients never underwent surgical repair.

Findings.—In the delayed surgery group, 3 patients had TRA progression within 5 days of injury. Two of these patients died. The 3 deaths in the delayed surgery group resulted from rupture in 1 case and intraoperative arrest in 2. Compared with the patients in the delayed surgery group, the patients who had no surgery were significantly older, had a higher ISS, and had more premorbid risk factors. Five of these patients died, all from severe injuries. The 10 survivors were alive at a median 2.5 years later, with no progression of injury or need for surgery. Complete radiographic resolution was documented in 5 of the 10 survivors, and the remaining 5 had asymptomatic, radiographically stable pseudoaneurysms.

Conclusions.—In selected patients with multiple severe associated injuries or high-risk premorbid conditions, TRA surgery may be delayed temporarily or even indefinitely. However, rapid TRA progression is still possible, necessitating serial radiographic assessments in the first week after injury and diagnosis.

▶ This study provides more evidence that immediate operation for traumatic thoracic aortic dissection is not necessary in many patients. (See also Abstract 14–4.)

G. L. Moneta, MD

15 Venous Thrombosis and Pulmonary Embolism

Incidence of Venous Thromboembolism in Hospitalized Patients vs Community Residents
Heit JA, Melton LJ III, Lohse CM, et al (Mayo Clinic, Rochester, Minn)
Mayo Clin Proc 76:1102-1110, 2001   15–1

Introduction.—Hospitalization may be among the most important factors affecting the risk of venous thromboembolism. The incidence of venous thromboembolism among hospitalized patients has never been determined because of an inability to define the actual population at risk. The incidence rates of deep venous thrombosis (DVT) and pulmonary embolism (PE) were assessed in hospitalized patients and compared with incidence rates in community residents.

Methods.—A retrospective review of completed medical records was examined in a population-based inception cohort of patients who resided in Olmsted County, Minnesota and had an incident DVT or PE between 1980 and 1990.

Results.—A total of 911 residents in Olmsted County experienced an initial lifetime event of definite, probable, or possible venous thromboembolism. Within this group, 253 had been hospitalized for a reason other than a diagnosis of DVT or PE (in-hospital cases) and 658 were not hospitalized at onset of an event (community residents). The average annual age- and gender-adjusted incidence of in-hospital venous thromboembolism was 960.5 (95% confidence interval, 795.1-1125.9) per 10,000 person-years and was over 100 times greater than the incidence among community residents at 7.1 per 10,000 person-years (95% confidence interval, 6.5-7.6).

The rate of venous thromboembolism increased substantially with advancing age for both groups; PE accounted for most of the age-related increase in the in-hospital group. Incidence rates changed little over time in the 2 groups, despite a decrease in the average length of hospital stay between 1980 and 1990.

299

Conclusion.—Venous thromboembolism is an important national health problem, particularly among elderly hospitalized patients. This finding underscores the need for accurate identification of hospitalized patients at risk for venous thromboembolism and a better understanding of the mechanism involved so that safe and effective prophylaxis can be used.

▶ There is an awful lot of DVT out there. The prevalence of the problem is why this is one of the largest sections of the YEAR BOOK.

G. L. Moneta, MD

Oral Contraceptives and Venous Thromboembolism: A Five-Year National Case-Control Study
Lidegaard Ø, Edström B, Kreiner S (Herlev Univ, Denmark)
Contraception 65:187-196, 2002   15–2

Background.—Many studies have investigated the influence of oral contraceptives (OCs) on the risk of venous thromboembolism (VTE). Apparently, the risk of VTE is increased by OCs, but differences in risk between OCs with second-generation progestins and those with third-generation progestins are unknown. The influence of different types of OCs on the risk of developing VTE was investigated in a 5-year case-control study conducted in Denmark.

Methods.—The study included all Danish women, aged 15 to 44 years, who experienced a first deep venous thrombosis or a first pulmonary embolism from 1994 through 1998. Control subjects were selected each year: 600 per year were selected in 1994 and 1995, and 1200 per year were selected from 1996 through 1998. Women who were pregnant or who had a history of thrombotic disease were excluded, thus leaving 987 cases and 4054 control participants for analysis. In multivariate analysis, adjustment was made for age, year, body mass index, length of OC use, family history of VTE, cerebral thrombosis or myocardial infarction, coagulopathies, diabetes, years of schooling, and previous birth. Current users of OCs were categorized according to estrogen dose, progestin type, duration of use, and first-, second-, or third-generation OC use.

Results.—Slightly more than half (52.5%) of the women with VTE were current users of OCs, and 32.6% were former users; 50.0% of control subjects were users, and 29.8% were former users. Compared with the risk of VTE among nonusers of OCs, the risk of VTE among current users was primarily influenced by duration of use. Risk was greatest during the first year of use (odds ratio, 7.0), then lessened with a longer duration of OC use (odds ratio, 3.6 for 1 to 5 years and 3.1 for >5 years). After adjustment for progestin types and length of use, the risk of VTE decreased significantly with a decreasing estrogen dose. The risk of VTE was also increased by smoking more than 10 cigarettes per day, a family history of VTE, body mass index of more than 30, and coagulation disturbances.

Conclusion.—The use of OCs was significantly related to the risk of VTE, particularly during the first years of use. Among current users of OCs, VTE risk was influenced by length of use, estrogen dose, and progestin type. The difference in risk between users of third- and second-generation OCs was 33% (after correction for estrogen dose and duration of use).

▶ This is about as close as one is going to get concerning a definitive epidemiologic study of the effects of OCs on the risk of deep venous thrombosis. The only problem is the study group is basically all Danish women aged 15 to 44 years. Generalization to other populations is perhaps inappropriate. Nevertheless, the main points are that the risk of deep venous thrombosis associated with OCs decreases over time. Obesity, smoking more than 10 cigarettes per day, hypercoagulable states, and a family history of venous thromboembolism all also increase the risk of venous thromboembolism in female patients.

G. L. Moneta, MD

Four Missense Mutations Identified in the Protein S Gene of Thrombosis Patients With Protein S Deficiency: Effects on Secretion and Anticoagulant Activity of Protein S

Tsuda H, Urata M, Tsuda T, et al (Kyushu Univ, Fukuoka, Japan)
Thromb Res 105:233–239, 2002   15–3

Background.—Congenital protein S (PS) deficiency is associated with an increased risk of thromboembolic disease and is classified as one of 3 types. Type I deficiency is characterized by low levels of both total and free PS; type II deficiency is characterized by a decreased PS activity level associated with normal levels of both total and free PS; and type III deficiency is characterized by a low free PS level with a normal level of total PS. A systematic hemostatic investigation found a high incidence of PS deficiency in Japanese patients with thrombosis. Four missense mutations, G54R, T589I, K155E, and Y595C, were identified in these patients. Whether these 4 missense genes have a causative role in PS deficiency was clarified.

Methods.—The 4 PS mutants and wild-type PS were stably expressed in human embryo kidney (HEK) 293 cells. Included in the analysis were hemostatic tests and gene analyses, mutagenesis, construction of expression vectors, expression of recombinant PS, Western blotting analysis, pulse-chase analysis, and measurement of activated protein C cofactor activity of recombinant PS.

Results.—Pulse-chase experiments showed intracellular degradation and decreased secretion of the Y595C mutant. The activated protein C cofactor activity of the G54R, K155E, and T589I mutants were inhibited by C4b-binding protein in a dose-dependent manner similar to that of wild-type PS.

Conclusions.—These findings indicate that the Y595C and K155E mutations are responsible for a secretion defect and decreased anticoagulant activity, respectively, in PS. However, the other 2 mutations investigated in this study, G54R and T589I, had no definitive association with an abnormality that resulted in a low level of plasma PS activity.

▶ PS deficiency turns out to be more complex than most readers of the YEAR BOOK would have realized. The PS gene has been identified and fully sequenced. It is affected by a number of mutations, not all of which produce clinical disease. This is about all most surgeons will get from this article, unless of course they understand cell culture techniques, polyclonal and antimonoclonal antibodies, mechanisms of mutagenesis, polymerase chain reactions, oligonucleotides, gene transfection, etc. I guess a second message is that if you want to do high-level basic science and do it well, you'd better be prepared to spend some serious time learning with experts.

G. L. Moneta, MD

"Long Haul" Flight and Deep Vein Thrombosis: A Model to Help Investigate the Benefit of Aspirin and Below-Knee Compression Stockings
Hollingsworth SJ, Dialysis M, Barker SGE (Royal Free and Univ College, London)
Eur J Vasc Endovasc Surg 22:456-462, 2001   15–4

Background.—Deaths of seemingly healthy young persons on "long haul" airline flights have raised awareness and prompted investigation of the true physiologic basis of this problem. The incidence of airline flight–associated deep vein thrombosis (DVT), progressing to the development of a pulmonary embolus and potentially death, has been difficult to assess. This report presented a potential model for simulating factors involved in long haul (more than 6 hours) flights that may contribute to the development of DVT.

Methods.—A total of 30 volunteers (19 men, 20 women) sat for 6 hours in a warm (more than 25°C), dry environment with restricted movement while consuming alcohol (40 mL of 40% alcohol/hr) and salted foods (300 g). Half of the volunteers received 150 mg aspirin and wore specially designed below-knee, compression stockings (class 1 profile). The other half of the volunteers functioned as the control group. Changes in full blood counts were recorded. Plasma was analyzed for D-dimer as an indication of DVT formation. Limb swelling was assessed from leg measurements.

Results.—In the control group, there were significant increases in platelet packing, total platelet numbers, and total numbers of white blood cells after 6 hours. In the group that received aspirin plus stockings, there were similar increases in total platelet numbers and total white blood cells. There were significant increases in both groups in all white blood cell types except basophils. The wearing of compression stockings by the intervention group prevented the calf swelling seen in the control group after 6 hours. None of the volunteers had DVT develop or a change in levels of D-dimer.

Conclusion.—Changes in the cellular components of blood, particularly white blood cells, combined with vasocompression and reduced blood flow, could predispose persons on long flights to development of deep vein thrombosis. The ability of aspirin and compression stockings to modify these potential risk factors for travel-related DVT could not be demonstrated.

▶ "Economy class syndrome" is resulting in more papers, lectures, and seminars than clinically significant DVT. The authors' data did not in any way prove aspirin and compression stockings are useful in preventing travel-related DVT. On the other hand, I bet every one of my residents would have volunteered for this study. Getting paid for sitting around for 6 hours drinking beer and eating chips has some appeal.

G. L. Moneta, MD

Duration of Prophylaxis Against Venous Thromboembolism With Enoxaparin After Surgery for Cancer
Bergqvist D, for the ENOXACAN II Investigators (Academic Hosp, Uppsala, Sweden; et al)
N Engl J Med 346:975-980, 2002   15–5

Introduction.—Venous thromboembolism is an important cause of death among patients with cancer, particularly those who undergo abdominal surgery. For these patients, the optimal duration of postoperative thromboprophylaxis has not been determined. The ENOXACAN (enoxaparin and cancer) II trial was a double-blind multicenter trial that compared the efficacy and safety of a 4-week regimen of enoxaparin prophylaxis with those of a 1-week regimen in patients undergoing elective surgery for abdominal or pelvic cancer.

Methods.—Patients undergoing planned curative open surgery for abdominal or pelvic cancer received enoxaparin (40 mg subcutaneously) daily for 6 to 10 days and were then randomly assigned to either enoxaparin or placebo for an additional 21 days. Patients underwent bilateral venography between days 25 and 31 or sooner if symptoms of thromboembolism occurred. The main endpoint was the incidence of venous thromboembolism between 25 and 31 days. The main safety endpoint was bleeding during the 3-week postrandomization period. Follow-up was 3 months.

Results.—The study included 322 patients in the intent-to-treat analysis. The rates of venous thromboembolism at completion of the double-blind phase for the placebo and enoxaparin groups were 12.0% and 4.8%, respectively ($P = .02$). This significant difference continued at 3 months (13.8% vs 5.5%; $P = .01$). Three patients in the enoxaparin group and 6 in the placebo group died within 3 months postoperatively. No significant between-group differences were noted in the incidence of bleeding or other complications during the double-blind or follow-up periods.

Conclusion.—Enoxaparin prophylaxis for 4 weeks after surgery for abdominal or pelvic cancer is safe and significantly diminishes the rate of venographically demonstrated thrombosis compared with the rate achieved by the use of enoxaparin prophylaxis for 1 week.

▶ It is now well appreciated that prophylaxis for deep venous thrombosis for 1 month after orthopedic surgery decreases the overall frequency of deep venous thrombosis compared with giving low molecular weight heparins for only the first postoperative week. The same conclusion appears to apply to patients undergoing surgery for abdominal or pelvic cancer. This decrease in deep venous thrombosis is achieved without increased risk of bleeding or other complications. This is a very well done and important study. Clinicians and insurance companies need to consider this information very carefully. It ought to change practice.

G. L. Moneta, MD

Endothelial Nitric Oxide Production During In Vitro Simulation of External Limb Compression

Dai G, Tsukurov O, Chen M, et al (Massachusetts Inst of Technology, Cambridge; Harvard Med School, Boston)
Am J Physiol 282:H2066-H2075, 2002   15–6

Background.—External pneumatic compression (EPC) is an effective prophylactic technique for deep vein thrombosis. There have been many studies aimed at optimizing or improving EPC performance from a hemodynamic perspective, but the biological correlates of various hemodynamic factors have not been clearly elucidated. The effects of EPC on nitric oxide (NO)—which is a critical mediator in the regulation of vasomotor and platelet function—were investigated.

Methods.—An in vitro cell culture system was developed to simulate blood flow and vessel collapse under conditions simulating EPC. Human umbilical vein endothelial cells were cultured and subjected to tube compression, pulsatile flow, or a combination of compression and flow. NO production and expression of endothelial NO synthetase (eNOS) messenger RNA (mRNA) expression were measured.

Results.—There was a rapid release of NO in the tube compression and pulsatile flow groups, followed by a sustained increase in NO release. The levels of NO production in these 2 groups were nearly identical, while the combined compression and pulsatile flow group produced the same low amount of NO as the control group. Conditions of pulsatile flow and tube compression also upregulate eNOS mRNA expression by a factor of 2.08 ± 0.25 and 2.11 ± 0.21, respectively, at 6 hours. Additional experiments with different modes of EPC demonstrated that NO production and eNOS mRNA expression respond to different time cycles of compression.

Conclusion.—These findings implicate the enhanced release of NO as a potentially significant factor in the prevention of deep vein thrombosis.

▶ It has been postulated that EPC reduces deep venous thrombosis by increasing velocity of venous flow and eliminating stasis. There may also be undetermined biochemical systemic effects as well. This study introduces NO production as a possible factor in reduction of deep venous thrombosis with EPC. Of all the studies evaluating the biochemistry of pneumatic compression, I think this one demonstrates the best science. However, the mechanical effects of external pneumatic compression are still likely the most important mechanism in achieving deep venous thrombosis reduction with this mode of prophylaxis.

G. L. Moneta, MD

Low Rate of Venous Thromboembolism After Craniotomy for Brain Tumor Using Multimodality Prophylaxis
Goldhaber SZ, Dunn K, Gerhard-Herman M, et al (Harvard Med School, Boston)
Chest 122:1933-1937, 2002   15–7

Background.—The most frequent complication of craniotomy for brain tumors is venous thromboembolism (VTE), so strategies that minimize this adverse postsurgical event are critically important. In a study conducted at an institution in which VTE after craniotomy for brain tumor is the leading cause of deep vein thrombosis (DVT) and pulmonary embolism (PE) among patients hospitalized for conditions other than VTE, an effort was made to minimize the development of VTE among patients undergoing craniotomy for brain tumor.

Methods.—This randomized, prospective, double-blind clinical trial included 150 patients undergoing craniotomy for brain tumor. The patients were randomly assigned to either enoxaparin, 40 mg/d, or heparin, 5000 U twice daily. All of the patients received graduated compression stockings and intermittent pneumatic compression.

Results.—None of these patients had symptomatic DVT or PE develop. The overall rate of asymptomatic VTE was 9.3%, and there was no significant difference in the rates between the 2 prophylaxis groups. Of the 14 patients determined to have VTE, 10 had thrombus limited to the deep veins of the calf.

Conclusions.—In this series of 150 consecutive patients undergoing craniotomy for brain tumor, the use of enoxaparin, 40 mg/d, or unfractionated heparin, 5000 U twice daily, in conjunction with graduated compression stockings, intermittent pneumatic compression, and predischarge surveillance venous US of the legs resulted in no symptomatic VTE in any patient. The low frequency of asymptomatic VTE (9.3%) consisted primarily of isolated calf DVT. It would appear from these findings that this comprehensive, multimodality therapy is a safe and effective approach to VTE prophylaxis in patients undergoing craniotomy for brain tumor.

▶ VTE after surgery for brain tumors is relatively common and fairly resistant to prophylactic measures. The authors achieved amazing results in preventing this complication. Their system of multimodality prophylaxis should be strongly considered for patients undergoing craniotomy for brain tumors.

G. L. Moneta, MD

Ability of Recombinant Factor VIIa to Reverse the Anticoagulant Effect of the Pentasaccharide Fondaparinux in Healthy Volunteers
Bijsterveld NR, Moons AH, Boekholdt SM, et al (Univ of Amsterdam; N V Organon, Oss, The Netherlands)
Circulation 106:2550-2554, 2002   15–8

Background.—Fondaparinux, a synthetic selective factor Xa inhibitor, has been found to be safe and effective for the postoperative prevention of venous thrombosis. However, as with any anticoagulant therapy, there is a risk of bleeding complications with fondaparinux, and a method to reverse these anticoagulant effects is needed. A study was undertaken to determine whether recombinant factor VIIa (rFVIIa) can neutralize the anticoagulant effects of subcutaneously administered fondaparinux.

Methods.—This randomized placebo-controlled study enrolled 16 healthy male subjects between the ages of 18 and 45 years, with a body mass index between 18 and 30 kg/m² and a maximum weight of 100 kg. None of the subjects had a personal or family history of thrombosis or bleeding disorders. The subjects received either a single subcutaneous dose of fondaparinux (10 mg) and a single intravenous bolus of (rFVIIa) (90 (g/kg), fondaparinux and placebo, or placebo and rFVIIa. Fondaparinux or placebo was administered 2 hours before rFVIIa (or placebo).

Results.—The injection of rFVIIa after fondaparinux normalized the prolonged activated partial thromboplastin and prothrombin times and reversed the decline in prothrombin activation fragments $1 + 2$ (F_{1+2}) observed with administration of fondaparinux alone. Thrombin-generation time and endogenous thrombin potential were inhibited by fondaparinux injection and normalized up to 6 hours after rFVIIa injection.

Conclusions.—These findings indicate that rFVIIa can normalize coagulation times and thrombin generation during fondaparinux treatment, with a duration of treatment effect ranging from 2 to 6 hours after rFVIIa injection. Thus, rFVIIa may be useful for the reversal of fondaparinux's anticoagulant effect in cases of serious bleeding complications or a need for acute surgery during treatment with fondaparinux.

▶ Fondaparinux is a synthetic direct inhibitor of factor Xa. It is highly effective in preventing venous thromboembolism in patients undergoing hip surgery and total knee arthroplasty. Up to now, no specific reversal agent had been identified. Recombinant factor VIIa increases thrombin generation and appears to overcome the effects of fondaparinux. The administration of factor VIIa has, however, been associated with thrombotic complications. In a clinical setting, it should probably be used only for extensive bleeding associated with fondaparinux therapy.

G. L. Moneta, MD

Long-term, Low-Intensity Warfarin Therapy for the Prevention of Recurrent Venous Thromboembolism
Ridker PM, for the PREVENT Investigators (Harvard Med School, Boston; et al)
N Engl J Med 348:1425-1434, 2003   15–9

Background.—Recurrent venous thromboembolism is a major clinical problem after cessation of anticoagulation therapy, with an estimated incidence of 6% to 9% each year. No therapeutic agent has been shown to provide an acceptable benefit-to-risk ratio for the long-term management of venous thromboembolism. The Prevention of Recurrent Venous Thromboembolism (PREVENT) trial was conducted to test the hypothesis that long-term, low-intensity warfarin therapy could safely and effectively reduce the risk of recurrent venous thromboembolism in patients with a previous idiopathic venous thrombosis.

Methods.—The study enrolled patients with idiopathic venous thromboembolism who had received full-dose anticoagulation therapy for a median of 6.5 months. The patients were randomly assigned to placebo or low-intensity warfarin with a target international normalized ratio of 1.5 to 2.0. Participants were followed up for recurrent venous thromboembolism, major hemorrhage, and death.

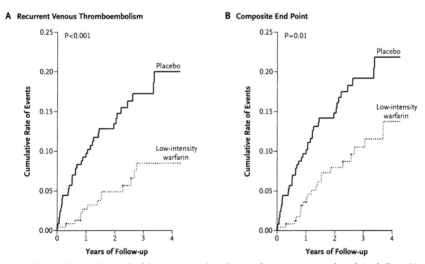

FIGURE 2.—Cumulative risk of the primary study end point of recurrent venous thromboembolism (**A**) and of the composite study end point of recurrent venous thromboembolism, major hemorrhage, or death from any cause (**B**). (Reprinted by permission of *The New England Journal of Medicine* from Ridker PM, for the PREVENT Investigators: Long-term, low-intensity warfarin therapy for the prevention of recurrent venous thromboembolism. *N Engl J Med* 348:1425-1434, 2003. Copyright 2003, Massachusetts Medical Society. All rights reserved.)

Results.—The intention was to enroll 750 patients, but the study was terminated early after randomization of 508 patients, who were followed up for up to 4.3 years. Of the 253 patients assigned to placebo, 37 had recurrent venous thromboembolism (7.2/100 person-years), as compared with 14 of 255 patients assigned to low-intensity warfarin (2.6/100 person-years). This represented a risk reduction of 64%. The risk reductions were similar for all subgroups, including patients with and without an identified inherited thrombophilia. Major hemorrhage occurred in 2 patients assigned to placebo and 5 patients assigned to low-intensity warfarin. There were twice as many deaths in the placebo group (8 patients) as in the low-intensity warfarin group (4 patients). Low-intensity warfarin was associated with a 48% reduction in the composite end point of recurrent venous thromboembolism, major hemorrhage, or death and a reduction of 76% to 81% in the risk of recurrent venous thromboembolism on per-protocol and as-treated analyses (Fig 2).

Conclusion.—Long-term, low-intensity warfarin therapy is highly effective for the prevention of recurrent venous thromboembolism.

▶ This is the most important article in this section of the YEAR BOOK. Note the data apply to patients with idiopathic venous thrombosis only.

G. L. Moneta, MD

An Association Between Atherosclerosis and Venous Thrombosis

Prandoni P, Bilora F, Marchiori A, et al (Univ of Padua, Italy; Univ of Amsterdam; Univ of Maastricht, The Netherlands)
N Engl J Med 348:1435-1441, 2003   15–10

Background.—The pathogenesis of venous thromboembolism has not been fully elucidated. Classic risk factors include cancer, surgery, immobilization, fractures, paralysis, pregnancy, childbirth, and use of estrogens. However, the cause of venous thromboembolism remains unexplained in about one third of patients. Atherosclerosis is associated with activation of both platelets and blood coagulation and an increase in fibrin turnover, all of which may predispose to blood coagulation. Whether atherosclerosis is associated with an increased risk of venous thrombosis was determined.

Methods.—US of the carotid arteries was performed in 299 unselected patients with deep venous thrombosis of the legs without symptomatic atherosclerosis and in 150 control subjects. The patient group included those with spontaneous thrombosis and those with secondary thrombosis from acquired risk factors. Both patients and controls were assessed for the presence of plaques.

Results.—At least one carotid plaque was identified in 72 of 153 patients with spontaneous thrombosis (47.1%), in 40 of 146 patients with secondary thrombosis (27.4%), and 48 of 150 control subjects (32%). The odds ratios for carotid plaques in patients with spontaneous thrombosis, compared with patients with secondary thrombosis and controls, were 2.3 and 1.8, respectively. The strength of this association did not change on multivariate analysis that adjusted for risk factors for atherosclerosis.

Conclusions.—An association was found between atherosclerotic disease and spontaneous venous thrombosis. Atherosclerosis may induce venous thrombosis, or the 2 conditions may have common risk factors.

▶ The association between atherosclerosis and venous thromboembolism found in this report applies only to patients with idiopathic venous thromboembolism. While this association is interesting, at this point it is not much more than an observation. Of immediate practical importance is increasing recognition that idiopathic venous thrombosis is really a different disease than venous thrombosis associated with obvious risk factors. (See Abstract 15–9.)

G. L. Moneta, MD

Initial Experience in Humans With a New Retrievable Inferior Vena Cava Filter
Asch MR (Mount Sinai Hosp/Univ Health Network, Toronto)
Radiology 225:835-844, 2002   15–11

Background.—For patients with venous thromboembolic disease who have contraindications to anticoagulant therapy, placement of inferior vena cava (IVC) filters has provided an effective treatment alternative. Late complications develop in 2% to 19% of patients, often after filter placement, leading to the suggestion that permanent filters not be used, particularly in young patients. In general, retrievable filters should be removed within 10 to 14 days of placement to avoid endothelialization. The efficacy of a new retrievable filter, the Recovery nitinol filter (RNF), was evaluated along with its safety of retrieval.

Methods.—The 16 men and 16 women evaluated were aged 18 to 83 years (mean, 53 years) and had RNF devices successfully placed for recent pulmonary embolism, recent deep venous thrombosis, or prophylaxis. Twenty were placed through the left femoral vein and 12 through the right femoral vein. Measures included efficacy of the filter and ability to remove it when the patient could safely resume full and uninterrupted anticoagulant therapy.

Results.—Two types of problems developed in insertion. Difficulty in 17 cases with releasing the filter legs from the splines of the stabilizer arm was overcome by moving the introducer sheath with a gentle twisting movement. This led to a change in the manufacturing process and no further release problems. None of the patients experienced either substantial puncture-site hematomas or other complications related to insertion or removal. The mean implantation period was 53 days (range, 5-134 days). Seven patients (22%) had thrombus in the filter when it was removed. In one patient with a large trapped thrombus, the filter had migrated 4 cm cephalad. Three deaths occurred while the filter was in place for 15 to 59 days (average, 38 days). All filter removals were successful and required less than 2 minutes to accomplish. During the 4- to 522-day period of follow-up for 22 patients, 1 patient had clinical symptoms of pulmonary embolism not substantiated on repeat CT angiography. None of the patients had clinical symptoms or imaging findings suggestive of caval abnormalities.

Conclusions.—The RNF was easily delivered via a femoral vein and readily removed percutaneously up to 134 days after insertion. None of the complications that developed were significant.

▶ Retrievable vena cava filters seem like a good idea. We have also been evaluating them at our institution. In some cases, the intended temporary filter has become permanent. Significant thrombus has been trapped within the filter, precluding its safe removal. There is a relatively narrow window for filter removal. It is recommended they be removed within 10 to 14 days of placement. Beyond that, endothelialization may make retrieval difficult.

G. L. Moneta, MD

Prevention of Deep-Vein Thrombosis in Ambulatory Arthroscopic Knee Surgery: A Randomized Trial of Prophylaxis With Low–Molecular Weight Heparin

Michot M, Conen D, Holtz D, et al (Kantonsspital Aarau, Switzerland)
Arthroscopy 18:257-263, 2002   15–12

Introduction.—Heparin prophylaxis is effective in decreasing the incidence of perioperative thromboembolic complications. In patients undergoing hip or knee replacement, there is a decrease in delayed deep vein thrombosis (DVT) and pulmonary embolism if prophylaxis with oral anticoagulation or low molecular weight heparin (LMWH) is continued after hospital discharge. The risk of DVT in patients undergoing arthroscopic knee surgery, however, is not well known and was assessed in a prospective, single-blind, randomized clinical trial.

Methods.—The incidence of DVT and the efficacy and safety of perioperative and postoperative prophylaxis against thromboembolism was examined in 218 consecutive outpatients scheduled for ambulatory arthroscopic knee surgery. Of 130 patients who were randomly assigned, 66 were treated with LMWH (dalteparin: 2500 IU if ≤70 kg and 5000 IU if >70 kg, initiated perioperatively and administered once daily for 4 weeks). Sixty-four patients were placed in a control group with no prophylaxis. All patients underwent bilateral compression US before surgery and 12 and 31 days postoperatively.

Results.—Thromboembolism was significantly lower in the treatment versus control group (1.5% vs 15.6%; 95% CI, 7.8%-26.8%; $P = .004$). Eighty percent of DVT was observed within the first 14 postoperative days. No severe side effects occurred with LMWH therapy. Five percent of patients refused continued subcutaneous LMWH injections.

Conclusion.—The risk of DVT is high among patients undergoing ambulatory arthroscopic knee surgery without antithrombotic prophylaxis. Perioperative and postoperative prophylaxis with dalteparin is effective and safe in decreasing this risk.

▶ DVT was reduced by LMWH in patients undergoing arthroscopic knee surgery. All DVT in this study was confined to the calf veins. Only US was used to evaluate DVT. Compared with venography, US is less accurate in detecting asymptomatic calf DVT. The true incidence of DVT in both patient groups may therefore be higher than observed.

G. L. Moneta, MD

Extended Outpatient Therapy With Low Molecular Weight Heparin for the Treatment of Recurrent Venous Thromboembolism Despite Warfarin Therapy
Luk C, Wells PS, Anderson D, et al (Univ of Western Ontario, London, Canada; Ottawa Civic Hosp, Ontario, Canada; Queen Elizabeth II Health Sciences Centre, Halifax, Nova Scotia, Canada; et al)
Am J Med 111:270-273, 2001   15–13

Introduction.—Low molecular weight heparin is among several different approaches advocated for patients who have symptomatic recurrent venous thromboembolism while receiving oral anticoagulants. An experience with extended low molecular weight heparin therapy for patients who had recurrent venous thromboembolism while receiving warfarin is presented.

Patients.—This retrospective analysis included data on 827 patients enrolled in prospective databases of 3 tertiary care hospitals. Of these, 32 patients had symptomatic, objectively documented episodes of thromboembolism while receiving warfarin therapy. Sixty-three percent of patients who had a recurrence while receiving warfarin had cancer. Treatment consisted of 200 U/kg/d low molecular weight heparin (dalteparin).

Outcomes.—Three patients (9%) had an additional symptomatic recurrence while taking dalteparin. Overall, 19 patients (59%) died during dalteparin therapy. However, all but 1 of these deaths were caused by cancer; none was attributable to a pulmonary embolism or hemorrhage.

Conclusions.—Cancer is associated with recurrent venous thromboembolism during warfarin therapy. The recurrences during warfarin therapy may be successfully managed with extended low molecular weight heparin therapy. Further study of this treatment, including randomized trials, is needed.

▶ Think cancer if a compliant patient with venous thromboembolism has a recurrent venous thromboembolism while on warfarin therapy.

G. L. Moneta, MD

Randomized Prospective Study Comparing Routine Versus Selective Use of Sonography of the Complete Calf in Patients With Suspected Deep Venous Thrombosis

Gottlieb RH, Voci SL, Syed L, et al (Univ of Rochester, NY)
AJR 180:241-245, 2003   15–14

Background.—Most pulmonary emboli arise from lower extremity veins, but there is controversy as to whether emboli originate only from the thigh or from both the thigh and the calf. Some reports suggest that calf sonography can be safely omitted in patients with suspected deep vein thrombosis, unless they have evidence of calf thrombi. A randomized trial of routine versus clinically indicated calf examination for patients with suspected deep vein thrombosis is reported.

Methods.—Over 2 years, patients with suspected deep venous thrombosis were randomly assigned to "complete calf" or "incomplete calf" protocols. In the complete calf group (235 patients), all deep calf veins were evaluated by ultrasonography: in the incomplete calf group (261 patients), the calf was evaluated only when symptoms or physical signs were present. In the latter group, 57.5% of the patients underwent at least focal examination of the calf because of signs or symptoms. Three-month outcomes were compared between groups.

Results.—No adverse outcomes occurred in patients in the complete calf group. In the incomplete calf group, there was 1 case each of thigh deep venous thrombosis and pulmonary embolism, for an adverse outcome rate of 0.8%. This difference was nonsignificant. A total of 7 isolated thrombi in the deep calf veins were detected, 3 in the complete calf group and 4 in the incomplete calf group (Table 3).

Conclusions.—For patients with suspected deep venous thrombosis, routine evaluation of the deep veins of the calf, compared with calf vein evaluation for signs and symptoms only does not result in an increase in adverse

TABLE 3.—Patient Outcomes

Results	Complete Calf Protocol Group*		Incomplete Calf Protocol Group†	
	No.	%	No.	%
Thigh deep venous thrombosis	0	0.0	1	0.4
Pulmonary embolism	0	0.0	1	0.4
Death‡	7	3.0	7	2.7

*Patients randomly assigned to protocol that routinely evaluated the calf.
†Patients randomly assigned to protocol evaluating only the calf for signs and symptoms.
‡All deaths that occurred within 3 months of baseline sonography were due to factors other than pulmonary embolus.
(Courtesy of Gottlieb RH, Voci SL, Syed L, et al: Randomized prospective study comparing routine versus selective use of sonography of the complete calf in patients with suspected deep vein thrombosis. *AJR* 180:241-245, 2003. Reprinted with permission from the *American Journal of Roentgenology*.)

outcomes. Routine examination of the calf does not identify additional cases of clinically significant calf thrombi.

▶ For some reason, many people agonize about evaluating the calf veins to rule out lower extremity deep venous thrombosis. I realize the calf veins can at times be difficult to evaluate, but it rarely adds more than 10 minutes to a deep venous thrombosis examination, so why not "just do it" and stop creating a giant controversy of a nonproblem?

G. L. Moneta, MD

Prospective Study of Color Duplex Ultrasonography Compared With Contrast Venography in Patients Suspected of Having Deep Venous Thrombosis of the Upper Extremities
Baarslag H-J, van Beek EJR, Koopman MMW, et al (Academic Med Ctr, Amsterdam; Royal Hallamshire Hosp, Sheffield, England)
Ann Intern Med 136:865-872, 2002   15–15

Background.—Only a few small prospective studies have been done to determine the role of US in the diagnosis of deep venous thrombosis (DVT) of the upper extremities. Both US and compression US are difficult to perform in the upper extremity because of the region's anatomical features, the overlying bony structures, and the inability to visualize the central intrathoracic venous system. The diagnostic accuracy of color duplex US was assessed in comparison with contrast venography for diagnosis of upper extremity DVT.

Methods.—At a Dutch teaching hospital, 126 consecutive inpatients and outpatients with suspected DVT of the upper extremities underwent contrast venography after duplex US. A 3-step protocol involving compression US, color US, and color Doppler US was used to determine the accuracy of

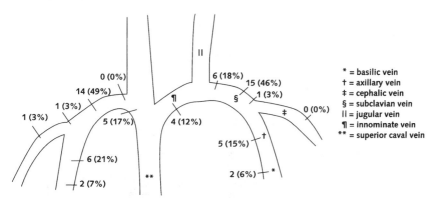

FIGURE 2.—Distribution of 29 thrombi in the right upper-extremity veins and 33 thrombi in the left upper-extremity veins on digital subtraction angiography. (Courtesy of Baarslag H-J, van Beek EJR, Koopman MMW, et al: Prospective study of color duplex ultrasonography compared with contrast venography in patients suspected of having deep venous thrombosis of the upper extremities. *Ann Intern Med* 136:865-872, 2002.)

duplex US. The sensitivity, specificity, and likelihood ratios for US as a whole were calculated, and the independent value of each step was assessed.

Results.—Venography was not feasible in 23 of 126 patients (18%), and US was not feasible in 1 of 126 patients (0.8%). The results of US were inconclusive in 3 patients. Venography showed thrombosis in 44 of 99 patients (44%). In 36 patients (36%), the thrombosis was related to IV catheters or malignant disease (Fig 2). The sensitivity and specificity of duplex US were 82% and 82%, respectively. Venous incompressibility correlated well with thrombosis, but only 50% of isolated flow abnormalities proved to be related to thrombosis.

Conclusions.—These results suggest that duplex US may be the preferred method for the initial diagnosis of patients with suspected thrombosis of the upper extremities. However, contrast venography should be used in patients with isolated flow abnormalities.

▶ When performing upper extremity venous duplex examinations to rule out DVT, my vascular laboratory technicians are fond of pointing out absence of phasic flow without detectable thrombosis. The implication is these patients may have central thrombosis not detected by US. Well, it turns out about half of these patients will have central DVT. If you are going to consider treating central upper extremity DVT with anticoagulation, a venogram should be obtained when there is absence of phasic flow and no visible thrombus. Enough patients will have central DVT to warrant the study.

G. L. Moneta, MD

Venous Thrombosis Associated With Peripherally Inserted Central Catheters: A Retrospective Analysis of the Cleveland Clinic Experience
Chemaly RF, de Parres JB, Rehm SJ, et al (Cleveland Clinic Found, Ohio; Univ Hosps of Cleveland, Ohio)
Clin Infect Dis 34:1179-1183, 2002   15–16

Introduction.—Peripherally inserted central catheters (PICCs) are generally safe, yet their use can be associated with infection, venous thrombosis (VT), pulmonary embolism, phlebitis, catheter malpositioning, and catheter fractures. The incidence and risk factors for VT associated with PICC lines was determined with retrospectively reviewed data collected over a period of 34 months.

Methods.—All upper extremity ultrasonograms and venograms with positive findings for VT between January 1, 1994, and October 31, 1996, were reviewed. Patient medical records were reviewed for data concerning the diagnosis that led to the administration of outpatient parenteral antibiotic therapy (OPAT), antibiotics used during OPAT, discharge information, clinical manifestations of and therapy for any thrombotic complication, and evidence of pulmonary embolism diagnosed either by ventilation-perfusion scanning or pulmonary angiography. Also evaluated were 107 control subjects in whom PICCs were placed during the same time period. Predisposing conditions were documented for both groups, including a history of deep venous thrombosis (DVT) and pulmonary embolism, malignancy, hypercoagulable states, neuromuscular disease, and the presence of AIDS.

Results.—Fifty-one (2.4%) of 2063 patients who had PICCs placed during the evaluation period had 51 known PICC-associated VTs. Two patients diagnosed with pulmonary embolism as a complication of the PICC. Risk factors for VT were younger age, a history of VT, discharge to a skilled-nursing facility, and therapy with amphotericin B.

Conclusion.—VT is an important complication of PICC placement. It may be more common than previously recognized and may be complicated by pulmonary embolism. Clinicians need to maintain a high index of suspicion, particularly for high-risk patients.

▶ The authors found only a 2.5% incidence of upper extremity VT after ipsilateral PICC line placement. They, however, did not look very hard as patients were evaluated at the discretion of attending physicians. Other studies surveying all patients have found evidence of thrombosis in up to 56% of patients. I think PICC lines should be avoided if an upper extremity vein may be needed as an arterial substitute or for dialysis access.

G. L. Moneta, MD

Appropriate Indications for Venous Duplex Scanning Based on D-dimer Assay
Shitrit D, Levi H, Huerta M, et al (Shaare Zedek Med Ctr, Jerusalem)
Ann Vasc Surg 16:304-308, 2002   15–17

Background.—The current gold standard for diagnosis of deep venous thrombosis (DVT) is duplex US. Duplex US is, however, frequently ordered without regard for objective clinical findings or appropriateness of the test. Wide, and perhaps inappropriate, use of this test strains the budgets and personnel resources of vascular laboratories. As a result, the rapid D-dimer assay has recently been used as a predictor of the absence of DVT. The rapid D-dimer assay was evaluated for its capability to exclude DVT in subgroups of patients with specific risk factors of malignancy, poor postoperative status, and cellulitis.

Methods.—A total of 126 consecutive patients with suspected DVT underwent clinical assessment, D-dimer testing with quantitative Miniquant D-dimer assay, and duplex scanning according to standard criteria for the diagnosis of DVT. The sensitivity, specificity, negative predictive value (NPV), and positive predictive value (PPV) were calculated for the D-dimer assay versus duplex scanning for the various risk factors.

Results.—The overall sensitivity, specificity, NPV, and PPV for the D-dimer assay were 94%, 57%, 54%, and 46%, respectively. Among the various subgroups, the highest values were found among the cellulitis subgroup: the sensitivity, specificity, NPV, and PPV were 100%, 97%, 97%, and 50%, respectively.

Conclusions.—These findings indicate that the Miniquant D-dimer assay is a useful screening procedure in select groups of patients with DVT, including patients with cellulitis and those without malignancy or poor postoperative status. The use of this D-dimer assay could provide cost savings and reduce costs by reducing the number of negative duplex venous examinations for DVT.

▶ Something has to be done about all of the venous duplex studies performed off-hours for marginal indications. Based on articles such as this, it seems reasonable to perform D-dimer testing on patients with very low probabilities of having a DVT and who do not have a clinical condition associated with elevated D-dimer. The problem will be educating physicians regarding whom to initially screen with D-dimer testing. It took years for emergency room doctors and internists to recognize the futility of trying to exclude DVT on history and physical alone. Getting them to understand the subtleties of D-dimer testing when confronted with mild bilateral leg swelling or cellulitis at 2 AM may be too much to ask.

G. L. Moneta, MD

Validity of D-dimer Tests in the Diagnosis of Deep Vein Thrombosis: A Prospective Comparative Study of Three Quantitative Assays
Larsen TB, Stoffersen E, Christensen CS, et al (Aalborg Hosp, Denmark)
J Intern Med 252:36-40, 2002   15–18

Background.—The diagnostic reliability of 3 quantitative D-dimer assays, compared with US, in the diagnosis of deep venous thrombosis (DVT) was determined.

Methods.—One hundred thirteen outpatients suspected of having DVT were included in the prospective study. The assays tested were 2 new quantitative D-dimer assays—VIDAS New and Auto Dimer—and an established quick test—the Nycocard D-dimer assay. The Auto Dimer assay was assessed on 3 different coagulation analyzers.

Findings.—Forty-three percent of the patients were confirmed to have DVT. The VIDAS New and Auto Dimer assays had sensitivities of 90% and 88%, respectively, with specificities of 42% and 44%. The negative predictive values of these assays were 85% and 83%, respectively. The Nycocard D-dimer assay had a 63% sensitivity, a 67% specificity, and a 71% negative predictive value.

Conclusion.—The VIDAS New and Auto Dimer D-dimer assays were nearly identical in diagnostic performance. However, neither appears to be suitable as the only screening method for DVT when there is a high pretest probability of DVT. A differential strategy is needed to distinguish between patients with low and high clinical probability using a D-dimer test or US.

▶ Not all D-dimer tests are the same. Know the results of the test you wish to include in your algorithm to rule out DVT.

G. L. Moneta, MD

Clinical Prediction of Deep Venous Thrombosis Using Two Risk Assessment Methods in Combination With Rapid Quantitative D-Dimer Testing
Cornuz J, Ghali WA, Hayoz D, et al (Univ of Lausanne, Switzerland; Univ of Calgary, Alberta, Canada)
Am J Med 112:198-203, 2002   15–19

Background.—The probability of deep venous thrombosis (DVT) can be assessed on the basis of a physician's clinical assessment or a prediction rule (the Wells score) that considers an amalgamation of signs, symptoms, and the presence or absence of an alternative diagnosis. A comparison of the 2 methods, in isolation and in combination, was undertaken to evaluate the pretest probability of DVT.

Methods.—The 278 patients (mean age, 60 years) had been referred with suspected DVT and were placed in low, moderate, and high risk groupings based on their clinical assessments and Wells scores. Rapid quantitative D-dimer testing was carried out (cutoff, 500 µg/mL), as were US examinations and follow-up evaluations for the presence of DVT.

Results.—Twenty-nine percent of the patients had a final diagnosis of DVT. Eighty patients were given diagnoses at the initial visit, and 2 were given diagnoses during the 3-month follow-up; 60% had proximal DVT. Five patients died, but none of the deaths were directly attributable to venous thromboembolism. For 80% of the patients, the physician's estimate and the Wells score agreed on their classification into the moderate or low probability groups. Physicians may have included clinical features other than those considered in the Wells score because agreement was only fair between the 2 methods. However, the overall accuracy for the 2 methods was similar (area under the receiver operating characteristic curve, 0.72), and higher accuracy values were seen when the analysis was restricted to patients with proximal DVT (0.78 for physicians and 0.77 for the Wells score). The D-dimer measurement had an overall negative predictive value of 96%. Not performing a duplex US in patients who had a low pretest probability on Wells scoring and a D-dimer level of 500 µg/mL or less would have omitted 28 US examinations (10% of the 278 patients); thus, a negative D-dimer test was helpful in cases of low clinical probability, but a positive test was not. Similar results were obtained when the analysis was restricted to patients with proximal DVT and to outpatients.

Conclusions.—The prediction of DVT in these patients was similar whether the Wells score or the physician's implicit clinical assessment was used. Even though the agreement between the physicians' estimates and the Wells score was only fair, pretest probabilities derived from either method showed similar accuracy when combined with rapid D-dimer measurement for all types of DVT or for proximal DVT only.

▶ The authors contend that patients with low clinical probability of DVT and a negative D-dimer assay have a 100% negative predictive value to exclude DVT. For those who want to use D-dimer testing to decrease the number of negative venous duplex examinations, this is good news. The bad news is it requires physicians to learn the Wells screening system. This system requires higher math (the ability to both add and subtract are required). I doubt this algorithm will pass "the ease of use test" in clinical practice.

G. L. Moneta, MD

Usefulness of a Semiquantitative D-dimer Test for the Exclusion of Deep Venous Thrombosis in Outpatients
Schutgens REG, Esseboom EU, Haas FJLM, et al (St Antonius Hosp, Nieuwegein, The Netherlands; Univ Hosp, Utrecht, The Netherlands)
Am J Med 112:617-621, 2002   15–20

Introduction.—The diagnosis of deep vein thrombosis (DVT) is usually made from US of the lower extremity veins. Plasma D-dimer levels, which measure the degradation products of cross-linked fibrin, may be valuable in the exclusion of DVT. Several clinical and laboratory variables that may compromise the accuracy of a semiquantitative D-dimer test were examined retrospectively in 704 patients with suspected DVT.

Methods.—All patients underwent a semiquantitative D-dimer test and US. The performance of the D-dimer test was assessed in 61 patients receiving anticoagulants, in 127 with previous thrombosis, in 47 with malignancy, and in 39 patients with more than one of these characteristics. The remaining 508 patients acted as a reference group.

Results.—There were 254 patients (36%) with evidence of DVT. For the reference group, the D-dimer test had a sensitivity of 99% (174 of 176; 95% CI, 96%-100%) and a negative predictive value of 98% (98 of 100; 95% CI, 93%-100%). Compared with the sensitivity found for the reference group, the sensitivity of the D-dimer test in patients receiving oral anticoagulants was 75% (6 of 8; 95% CI, 35%-97%; P = .01). For patients with prior thrombosis, the sensitivity was 96% (51 of 53; 95% CI, 87%-100%); it was 100% (29 of 29; 95% CI, 88%-100%) in patients with cancer. D-dimer test results were abnormal in 553 patients (79%), including 43 patients (91%) with cancer.

Conclusion.—The semiquantitative D-dimer test had a high sensitivity and negative predictive value for excluding DVT, except, possibly, for patients receiving oral anticoagulants. The test may not be worthwhile in patients with cancer and in patients older than 70 years because the test results are usually positive in this cohort.

▶ Bottom line: (1) Previous DVT/no longer anticoagulated: D-dimer over US; (2) Previous DVT/anticoagulated: US over D-dimer; (3) No previous DVT/anticoagulated:US over D-dimer

G. L. Moneta, MD

The Use of a D-Dimer Assay in Patients Undergoing CT Pulmonary Angiography for Suspected Pulmonary Embolus
Burkill GJC, Bell JRG, Chinn RJS, et al (Chelsea and Westminster Hosp, London)
Clin Radiol 57:41-46, 2002   15–21

Introduction.—D-dimer is a specific fibrin degradation product that is increased in venous thrombotic disease and several other clinical states. The Accuclot D-dimer (Sigma Diagnostics, St Louis, Mo) test is a rapid latex agglutination assay. Its diagnostic efficacy was compared with that of pulmonary angiography in patients with suspected acute pulmonary embolism (PE).

Methods.—All patients referred to the CT unit for evaluation of suspected acute PE underwent measurements of pulse oximetry, respiratory rate, heart rate, and blood sampling for D-dimer immediately before undergoing CT. A high-resolution CT pulmonary angiogram was performed. Images were independently interpreted at a work station with cine-paging and z-dimension (2D) reformation by 3 consultant radiologists blinded to both clinical and laboratory data. If a PE was detected, the level of the most proximal embolus was noted. Discordant imaging findings were re-read collectively and a consensus was achieved.

Results.—Of 101 patients evaluated, 28 (28%) had positive CT pulmonary angiogram for PE and 65 (65%) were positive for D-dimer. Twenty-six patients were positive both by CT and D-dimer. Thirty-four patients had negative CT and negative D-dimer results. The negative predictive value of the Accuclot D-dimer test for excluding a PE on spiral CT was 0.94; when the D-dimer test was combined with pulse oximetry, the negative predictive value improved to 0.97.

Conclusion.—A negative Accuclot D-dimer assay was highly predictive for a negative CT pulmonary angiogram in suspected PE. If the D-dimer assay were included in the diagnostic algorithm, a negative D-dimer can be useful in avoiding further investigation when the clinical likelihood of a PE is considered low. When the pretest probability of a PE is high—on the basis of the patient's history, physical examination, and respiratory measurements—a negative D-dimer result should not exclude further investigation (Fig 1).

▶ D-dimer may also be useful in minimizing CT pulmonary angiography (CTA) to detect PE. However, note 2 patients in this study had a positive CTA and a negative D-dimer. In both of these patients the PE detected by CTA was at the segmental level, but that doesn't ensure, if untreated, that the next PE won't

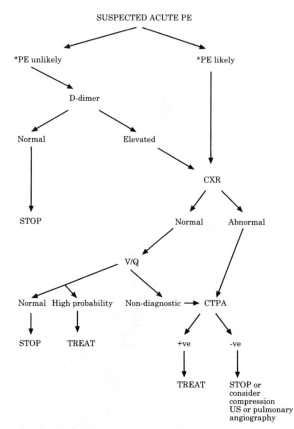

SUSPECTED ACUTE PE

*PE unlikely   *PE likely

D-dimer

Normal   Elevated

CXR

STOP   Normal   Abnormal

V/Q

Normal   High probability   Non-diagnostic → CTPA

STOP   TREAT   +ve   -ve

TREAT   STOP or
consider
compression
US or pulmonary
angiography

FIGURE 1.—Algorithm for the diagnosis of pulmonary embolism. *Based on scoring system by Wells PS, Anderson DR, Rodger M, et al: Derivation of a simple clinical model to categorize patient probability of pulmonary embolism: Increasing the model's utility with the SimpliRED D-dimer. *Thromb Haemost* 83:416-420, 2000. (Courtesy of Burkill GJC, Bell JRG, Chinn RJS, et al: The use of a D-dimer assay in patients undergoing CT pulmonary angiography for suspected pulmonary embolus. *Clin Radiol* 57:41-46, 2002.)

be a saddle embolus. We need more data to give serious consideration to using D-dimer testing to rule out PE in patients with clinically suspected PE.

G. L. Moneta, MD

Placement of Vena Cava Filters: Factors Affecting Technical Success and Immediate Complications

Savin MA, Panicker HK, Sadiq S, et al (St Joseph Mercy-Oakland, Pontiac, Mich; William Beaumont Hosp, Royal Oak, Mich; Wayne State Univ, Detroit; et al)
AJR 179:597-602, 2002   15–22

Introduction.—No trials have addressed the safety and effectiveness of vena cava filters as a function of technique and operator specialty. Factors influencing the technical success and immediate complications of placement of vena cava filters were retrospectively examined.

Methods.—The medical records of 148 consecutive patients who underwent filter placement between December 1995 and February 1999 were examined for cavography, technical success, complications, and operator specialty.

Results.—The records were complete for 143 filter placements in 142 patients. Cavography was performed before filter placement in 120 patients, including 3 misplacements (2.5%). Ten other misplacements (43%) were not preceded by cavography. Radiologists and surgeons performed 114 and 29 filter placements, respectively. Cavography was performed before 98% and 28% of placements by radiologists and surgeons, respectively ($P <$ .0001). Of 13 filter misplacements, 12 were placed by surgeons and 1 was placed by a radiologist ($P <$ .0001). Major complications occurred in 3 placements by surgeons and in none by radiologists (10% vs 0%; $P <$ .01).

Conclusion.—Vena cava filters were placed with higher technical success and less complications when preceded by cavography. The greater success and fewer complications for radiologists versus surgeons may reflect more education and experience with imaging-guided procedures and greater adherence to cavography protocol on the part of the former.

▶ This study likely developed out of a local turf war. It is not going to be popular among the surgeons at the authors' institution. Training is important. I wonder if the radiologists remaining at this institution (3 of the 5 authors are gone) are now helping train the individuals who actually take care of the patients before and after the procedure.

G. L. Moneta, MD

Prophylactic and Therapeutic Inferior Vena Cava Filters to Prevent Pulmonary Emboli in Trauma Patients
Carlin AM, Tyburski JG, Wilson RF, et al (Wayne State Univ, Detroit)
Arch Surg 137:521-527, 2002   15–23

Background.—Inserting inferior vena cava filters (IVCFs) may serve as effective prophylaxis to decrease pulmonary embolism (PE) in patients with trauma. The experience with the use of prophylactic and therapeutic IVCFs at one level 1 trauma center during a 10-year period was analyzed.

Methods.—Two hundred patients with blunt trauma undergoing IVCF placement were included in the retrospective review. Insertion of the IVCF was considered therapeutic in 122 patients diagnosed as having DVT and/or PE. Seventy-eight patients had no evidence of DVT or PE, but were considered at high risk for PR. In these patients, IVCF insertion was considered prophylactic.

Findings.—The number of IVCFs inserted for prophylaxis increased significantly from 4% of all filters between 1991 and 1996 to 57% between 1997 and 2001. The mean age was older in the therapeutic IVCF group, but mean Injury Severity Scores were comparable between groups. The mortality rate was 11% in patients during the period of therapeutic IVCF insertion and only 3% during the period of prophylactic IVCF insertion. Mortality from PE was unchanged, however. No PE developed in any of the patients with prophylactic IVCF insertion. The incidence of PE declined in all patients with blunt trauma, from 0.29% before 1997 to 0.15% after 1997, when 57% of the IVCF placements were prophylactic.

Conclusions.—Clinicians should consider prophylactic IVCF insertion in trauma victims at high risk for PE and with obvious contraindications to anticoagulation and sequential compression devices. Patients with major pelvic fractures combined with lower extremity long-bone fractures and those with bilateral lower extremity long-bone fractures should undergo prophylactic IVCF placement within 48 hours after injury.

▶ I try to include articles in the YEAR BOOK that are important and may improve practice. Sometimes it is important to point out that a study published in a major journal is not worth the tree that died for its publication. The authors' conclusions in this paper are not substantiated by their data. There was no consistent method of diagnosis. Deaths from PE were not reduced by placing prophylactic filters. Historic controls were used. I wonder if this is number 569? (See Abstract 15–22.)

G. L. Moneta, MD

Medical Literature and Vena Cava Filters: So Far So Weak

Girard P, Stern J-B, Parent F (Institut Mutualiste Montsouris, Paris; Hôpital Antoine Béclère, Clamart, France)
Chest 122:963-967, 2002
15–24

Background.—Vena cava interruption is incomplete treatment for venous thromboembolic disease. Anticoagulant therapy effectively prevents a pulmonary embolism in the very large majority of patients with deep venous thrombosis, so only absolute contraindications to and documented failures of anticoagulant therapy in patients with acute venous thromboembolism are widely accepted indications for interruption of the inferior vena cava. A systematic literature review was performed to clarify the indications for filter placement.

Methods.—The MEDLINE database was searched for relevant articles on vena cava filters for the years 1975 through 2000.

Results.—A total of 568 articles were identified. Each reference was analyzed according to predetermined criteria. Almost two thirds (65%) of the articles were retrospective studies (33.3%) or case reports (31.7%); 12.9% were animal or in vitro studies, 7.4% were prospective studies, 6.7% were reviews, and 8.1% reported on miscellaneous related topics. Among the prospective studies, only 16 studies included 100 patients or more. There was only 1 randomized controlled trial, and heterogeneity among series precluded any relevant comparison. A similar search for articles involving hep-

TABLE 3.—Categorical Indications for Filter Placement

Indications
Contraindication to anticoagulation (absolute or relative)
Complication of anticoagulation
Failure: objectively documented extension of existing DVT or new DVT or PE while therapeutically anticoagulated
Hemorrhage: major or minor
Thrombocytopenia
Skin necrosis
Drug reaction
Evidence/probability of poor compliance
Prophylaxis: no thromboembolic disease
Prophylaxis with thromboembolism in addition to anticoagulation
Failure of previous device to prevent PE; central extension of thrombus through an existing filter or recurrent PE
In association with another procedure: thrombectomy, embolectomy, or lytic therapy

*Reporting standards as recommended by the Vena Cava Filter Consensus Conference.
Abbreviations: DVT, Deep venous thrombosis; PE, pulmonary embolism.
(Courtesy of Girard P, Stern J-B, Parent F: Medical literature and vena cava filters: So far so weak. *Chest* 122:963-967, 2002.)

arin and venous thromboembolism showed that 47.4% of the 531 references identified were randomized controlled trials.

Conclusions.—Until more relevant data become available, literature reviews of vena cava filters will continue to be narrative, and many, if not most, indications for filter placement will be a matter of opinion (Table 3).

▶ After 25 years and 568 references, I am sad to say I have to agree with the authors' conclusions. Perhaps the "Camel Dung Award" should be revived and given to a whole field of medical investigation.

G. L. Moneta, MD

Early Results of Thrombolysis vs Anticoagulation in Iliofemoral Venous Thrombosis: A Randomised Clinical Trial

Elsharawy M, Elzayat E (Ismailia, Egypt; Suez Canal Univ, Ismailia, Egypt)
Eur J Vasc Endovasc Surg 24:209-214, 2002   15–25

Introduction.—Systemic anticoagulation is standard treatment for deep vein thrombosis (DVT). Some suggest catheter-directed thrombolysis for iliofemoral DVT will preserve valve function and diminish the incidence of postphlebitic syndrome. Local thrombolysis and anticoagulation were compared with anticoagulation alone in patients with iliofemoral DVT.

Methods.—Thirty-five consecutive eligible patients were randomly assigned to treatment with either catheter-directed thrombolysis followed by anticoagulation or to anticoagulation alone. Clot lysis and deep venous reflux were examined via duplex US and plethysmography at a 6-month follow-up.

Results.—Complete data were available for all patients. At a 6-month follow-up, the patency rate was better in patients treated with thrombolysis than in those treated with anticoagulation alone (13/18, 72% vs 2/17, 12%; $P < .001$). Venous reflux was higher in patients in the anticoagulation alone group than in those in the thrombolysis group (7 patients, 41% vs 2 patients, 11%; $P = .04$).

Conclusion.—Patients treated with catheter-directed thrombolysis and anticoagulation had better patency and competence than those treated with standard anticoagulation alone.

▶ I am not yet an advocate for thrombolytic therapy for acute DVT. I am an advocate for science, and this seems like a reasonably well-done study. I wonder why these guys in Egypt were able to do a pretty good trial of thrombolytic therapy for DVT while in the United States we have not done squat to objectively evaluate this therapy. (This is a thinly veiled nudge.)

G. L. Moneta, MD

16 Chronic Venous and Lymphatic Disease

Chronic Venous Insufficiency: Clinical and Duplex Correlations. The Edinburgh Vein Study of Venous Disorders in the General Population
Ruckley CV, Evans CJ, Allan PL, et al (Royal Infirmary of Edinburgh, Scotland; Univ of Edinburgh, Scotland)
J Vasc Surg 36:520-525, 2002   16–1

Background.—The prevalence of chronic venous insufficiency, chronic pathologic changes in the skin and subcutaneous tissue of the lower leg, in the general population was determined, and its clinical features were correlated with those of sonographically proven venous reflux.

Methods.—In this cross-sectional survey of the general population, ambulatory men and women ages 18 to 64 years were randomly selected from 12 general practices. The 1566 study participants were then examined for chronic venous insufficiency. Eight segments of the deep and superficial veins were assessed for reflux by means of duplex scanning.

Results.—The mean age of the 867 women selected was 44.8 years; the 699 men chosen for participation in the study had a mean age of 45.8 years. Of the 1566 participants screened, 124 received a diagnosis of chronic venous insufficiency, with 95 persons with grade I, 19 persons with grade II, and 10 persons with grade III disease. The age-adjusted prevalence for the whole population was 9.4% in men and 6.6% in women. The prevalence of chronic venous insufficiency was closely correlated with age and sex and was 21.2% in men older than 50 years of age and 12% in women older than 50 years of age (Table 1). Heaviness; tension; and a sense of swelling, aching, and itching were significantly associated with worsening grade of chronic venous insufficiency, and chronic venous insufficiency was associated with reflux in all deep and superficial segments. The frequency of reflux in both superficial and deep segments increased with increasing severity of disease. In 30.8% of the study participants with chronic venous insufficiency in the left leg, the reflux was limited to the superficial system.

Conclusions.—These findings revealed a steep increase in the prevalence of chronic venous insufficiency with increasing age. A strong correlation was noted between venous symptoms and the presence and severity of chronic venous insufficiency. In approximately one third of the study participants,

TABLE 1.—Prevalence of CVI, in Either Leg or Both Legs, According to Age and Sex

Age (y)	Men	Women	Within Age Group P Value Between Sexes*
18-33	—	1.0 (2)	NS
34-49	3.3 (9)	4.0 (13)	NS
>50	21.2 (60)	12.0 (40)	.002
Within sex P value	.001	.001	

Data are n (%) unless indicated otherwise.
The values represent percentages of subjects with CVI within that age band.
*P > .05 is not significant (NS).
Abbreviation: CVI, Chronic venous insufficiency.
(Reprinted by permission of the publisher from Ruckley CV, Evans CJ, Allan PL, et al: Chronic venous insufficiency: clinical and duplex correlations. The Edinburgh Vein Study of venous disorders in the general population. *J Vasc Surg* 36:520-525, 2002. Copyright 2002 by Elsevier.)

chronic venous insufficiency was associated with incompetence limited to the superficial system. The severity of clinical features is significantly correlated with the prevalence of valvular reflux in the deep and superficial systems.

▶ The authors sought to assess the prevalence of chronic venous insufficiency in a cross-section of the general population. Their finding that chronic venous insufficiency increases with age is expected. Only 10 out of 1553 patients, however, had a history of or a current venous ulcer. This seems low and may be explained by the relatively young age of the patients studied. Their finding that chronic venous insufficiency is more prevalent in men than women is unexpected and unexplained.

G. L. Moneta, MD

The Mechanism of Venous Valve Closure in Normal Physiologic Conditions

Lurie F, Kistner RL, Eklof B (Univ of Hawaii, Honolulu)
J Vasc Surg 35:713-717, 2002   16–2

Background.—The mechanism of venous valve closure in physiologic conditions was investigated in situ to clarify the role of reversed flow through the valve in closure of valve cusps. The temporal relations between movements of valve cusps, changes in geometry of the venous sinus, and blood flow were also studied.

Methods.—Duplex US scanning was performed in 12 healthy volunteers. On the basis of real-time US scan records of the saphenofemoral junction, the time relationship between flow and venous valve movements was determined. A planimeter was used to measure the size and shape of the common femoral vein and proximal greater saphenous vein.

Findings.—Only 1 participant had reverse flow below the valve. In this subject, the maximum peak velocity of the reverse flow was 0.8 cm/s, and the duration was 0.2 seconds. Reverse flow was documented just before and just after valve closure. The average duration of the outflow wave below the valve was 816 ms, which did not differ significantly from the time of the valve cycle. Valve closure coincided with reduction in flow velocities. The first detectable movement of the valve cusps was noted a mean 108 ms after flow deceleration began. The mean time from the first cusp movement to complete valve closure was 139 ms. During the valve cycle, both the size and shape of the sinus changed, the size of the sinus increasing as much as 127% over the baseline value. The sinus also became more spheric. These changes coincided with the movements of the valve cusps, the first detectable change in size occurring at a mean 80 ms after the first detectable movement of the cusps toward closure.

Conclusions.—Venous valve closure does not rely on reverse flow through the valve. Venous valve closure coincides with the reduction in flow velocities and in the ballooning of the sinus.

▶ This is an interesting physiologic study that challenges the concept that a short period of reverse flow is necessary for venous valve closure.

G. L. Moneta, MD

Primary Varicose Veins: The Sapheno-femoral Junction, Distribution of Varicosities and Patterns of Incompetence

Cooper DG, Hillman-Cooper CS, Barker SGE, et al (Royal Free and Univ College London)
Eur J Vasc Endovasc Surg 25:53-59, 2003   16–3

Background.—Primary varicose veins (VVs) can occur with an intact, functional saphenofemoral junction (SFJ), with initial pathologic chances occurring in more distal valves. Patterns of varicose disease and underlying venous incompetence were studied with the use of venous duplex scans in a large series of patients with primary VVs.

Methods.—The retrospective study included 706 limbs of 481 patients referred for evaluation of primary VVs. There were 475 women and 231 men, with a median age of 50 years. For each limb, the color flow duplex scan findings were analyzed in detail, focusing on SFJ competence, perforating vein competence, and locations of VVs.

Results.—The SFJ was competent in 46% of the limbs scanned. Of these limbs, nearly two thirds had no incompetent perforating vessels. Overall, VVs were more frequent in limbs without any incompetent perforating vessels. When incompetent perforators were present, VVs were found mainly below the knee. Sixty-two percent of the limbs had incompetent segments both above and below the knee. For both women and men, incompetence was more commonly limited to above-knee segments than to below-knee segments (Fig 2).

Conclusions.—This study suggests primary VVs can develop in isolated segments of the superficial venous system, either at the site of underlying

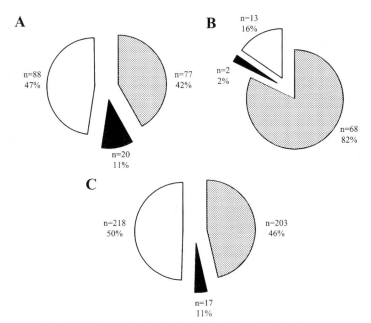

FIGURE 2.—Correlation between the distribution of varicosities and that of an incompetent segment of the long saphenous system (**A**) above-knee only, (**B**) below-knee only, and (**C**) combined above- and below-knee. Sites of varicosities: striped segments, calf only; filled segments, thigh only; open segments, calf and thigh. Numbers are total numbers per group of incompetent segment with percentage (of total group) in parenthesis. (Reprinted from Cooper DG, Hillman-Cooper CS, Barker SGE, et al: Primary varicose veins: The sapheno-femoral junction, distribution of varicosities and patterns of incompetence. *Eur J Vasc Endovasc Surg* 25:53-59, 2003. Copyright 2003 by permission of the publisher.)

main trunk incompetence or distal to it. The findings question the theory that VVs result from valve dysfunction or in a descending pattern. Rather, the observed patterns support a pattern of spreading incompetence, with an initial abnormality giving rise to varicosities mainly in tributaries.

▶ The authors found no consistent pattern of superficial or perforator incompetence in patients with VVs. Since this is a retrospective study, it may be that the authors' routine clinical evaluation is not sufficiently detailed to pick up all sites of incompetence. I am, however, intrigued by the notion that VVs develop from a primary wall abnormality (the "egg") with associated incompetence secondary to the wall abnormality (the "chicken"). Of interest is that deep venous incompetence had virtually no association with development of VVs. Therefore, I don't think that the presence of deep venous insufficiency should preclude treatment of VVs and may not increase recurrence of VVs after their treatment.

G. L. Moneta, MD

The Prevalence of Thrombophilia in Patients With Chronic Venous Leg Ulceration

MacKenzie RK, Ludlam CA, Ruckley CV, et al (Royal Infirmary, Edinburgh, Scotland; Heartlands Hosp, Birmingham, England)

J Vasc Surg 35:718-722, 2002   16–4

Background.—Thrombophilia is a risk factor for deep venous thrombosis (DVT), and DVT is a major risk factor for chronic venous ulceration (CVU). However, the relationship between thrombophilia and CVU is unclear. The prevalence of thrombophilia in patients with CVU and its possible association with a history of or duplex scan evidence of DVT were investigated in the current study.

Methods and Findings.—Eighty-eight patients with CVU were enrolled in the prospective study. Fifty-three were women (median age, 76 years) and 35 were men (median age, 61 years). Thirty-six percent had a history of, or duplex scan evidence of, previous DVT. Coagulation abnormalities included 4 cases of antithrombin, 5 of protein C, and 6 of protein S deficiency; 14 cases of activated protein C resistance—11 cases of factor V Leiden mutation, 3 cases of prothrombin 20210A mutation—8 cases of lupus anticoagulant, and 12 cases of anticardiolipin antibodies. Thrombophilia did not correlate significantly with previous DVT, deep reflux, or disease severity.

Conclusions.—In these patients with CVU, the prevalence rate of thrombophilia was 41%, which is 2 to 30 times greater than that in the general population and comparable to that in pateints with previous DVT. Thrombophilia appears to be unassociated with a history of DVT, pattern of reflux, and disease severity in patients with CVU.

▶ This study documented an astounding prevalence of thrombophilia (41%) in patients with venous leg ulcers. The exact importance of this is unclear as the presence of thrombophilia did not relate to a history of DVT or duplex evidence of a previous DVT. I, however, tend to think the thrombophilia is important and that we know DVT can be asymptomatic and can be cleared by endogenous fibrinolysis, leaving little evidence of residual DVT. I don't think we are quite ready to recommend thrombophilia testing in all patients with venous leg ulcers. If the thrombophilia does not relate to evidence of DVT or other symptoms, why bother to treat the thrombophilia indefinitely with a difficult to manage and somewhat dangerous anticoagulant?

G. L. Moneta, MD

The Influence of Obesity on Chronic Venous Disease

Danielsson G, Eklof B, Grandinetti A, et al (Univ of Hawaii, Honolulu; Straub Clinic and Hosp, Honolulu, Hawaii)

Vasc Endovasc Surg 36:271-276, 2002   16–5

Introduction.—There is evidence of an association between obesity and varicose veins, especially in women, but not all studies have confirmed a relationship between obesity and the more severe stages of chronic venous disease (CVD). Patients with CVD who underwent duplex US scanning were evaluated for the impact of body mass index (BMI) on the clinical severity of their disease.

Methods.—The study group consisted of 272 patients (173 women and 99 men) with a mean age of 60 years. Patients were classified according to the clinical, etiologic, anatomical, and pathophysiologic (CEAP) system and BMI. Reflux time was measured in seconds, with reflux time greater than a half second defined as pathologic. Peak reverse flow velocity was measured in centimeters per second. A multisegment reflux score (total score) was calculated for both reflux duration and peak reverse flow velocity.

Results.—The total number of limbs studied was 401. The mean BMI of the group was 28.9, and 61% of patients were overweight (BMI, 25 kg/m² or more). A significant association was found between BMI and clinical severity, and this association persisted after adjustment for total peak reverse flow velocity and total reflux score. Patients who were overweight were more likely than those of normal weight to have skin changes and ulcers, even when total reflux time and total peak reverse flow velocity were similar.

Among patients with varicose veins, obesity was present in 15%. Among those with open venous ulcer, however, 58% were obese. Pacific Islanders had the highest average BMI and the highest prevalence of skin changes (56.8%), but ethnicity was not significantly related to skin changes in analyses controlled for age, gender, and BMI.

Conclusion.—Obesity may be an independent risk factor for skin changes and disease progression in patients with CVD. Weight reduction should be emphasized in patients with venous disease.

▶ This is one of the clearest demonstrations of the adverse impact of obesity on venous disease that I am aware of. I think we all recognize the high prevalence of obesity in our patients with difficult-to-manage venous insufficiency. I'd always assumed the obesity adversely affected the venous disease itself. However, in this study no correlation with values of venous reflux was found. The authors suggest obesity may act through a separate mechanism to influence skin changes associated with chronic venous insufficiency. Certainly this may be true, but it has always been difficult to correlate measures of reflux with severity of skin changes. We need to consider that our tests of venous reflux may not be as specific as we would hope.

G. L. Moneta, MD

Lower Limb Venous Insufficiency and Tobacco Smoking: A Case-Control Study

Gourgou S, Dedieu F, Sancho-Garnier H (CRLC Val d'Aurelle—Paul Lamarque, Montpellier, France; Laboratoires Knoll France, Rungis)
Am J Epidemiol 155:1007-1015, 2002   16–6

Introduction.—The role of tobacco smoking in venous insufficiency has not been clearly demonstrated, but smoking is a major factor in oxidative stress, hypoxia, and endothelial damage. The possible association between tobacco smoking and lower extremity venous insufficiency was examined in a case-control study.

Methods.—A total of 460 general practitioners in France each collected data on 4 cases and 4 matched controls. Patients enrolled by each physician were 1 woman younger than 45, 2 women older than 45, and 1 man. Each control was the next eligible matched patient seen after the case patient. A questionnaire administered by physicians collected data on participants' medical history, smoking habits, alcohol consumption, physical activity, and known risk factors for lower limb venous insufficiency.

Results.—The statistical analysis included 1806 case patients and 1806 control subjects. Both groups had an average age of 48 years. Clinical symptoms of venous disorders differed significantly between men and women. Disease onset was earlier in women, symptoms were more often bilateral, pain was more likely to be severe, and edema and varicosities were more often present. Case patients had a mean body mass index significantly greater than that of control subjects. Compared with control subjects, a higher proportion of case patients reported prolonged standing on the job. The latter group were less likely to engage in sports activities and were more likely to show clinical signs of alcohol abuse. Smoking was present in more case patients than in control subjects. Compared with control subjects who smoked, case patients were more likely to smoke dark tobacco, unfiltered cigarettes, and more than 19 cigarettes a day and to have started smoking at a younger age.

Conclusion.—Patients with lower limb venous insufficiency showed known risk factors associated with the disorder. The strongest risk factors included family history (odds ratio [OR], 7.7), regular prolonged standing at work (OR, 2.7), heat exposure (OR, 2.0), and more than 4 pregnancies (OR, 3.4). Multivariate analysis adjusted for other risk factors confirmed a significant association between tobacco smoking and lower limb venous insufficiency, with an OR of 2.4 for 20 or more cigarettes per day.

▶ Smoking is also bad for veins.

G. L. Moneta, MD

Plasma Matrix Metalloproteinase-9 as a Marker of Blood Stasis in Varicose Veins

Jacob M-P, Cazaubon M, Scemama A, et al (CHU Xavier Bichat, Paris)
Circulation 106:535-538, 2002   16–7

Background.—The pathophysiologic process of varicose veins has not been well-explored. Suggestions have been made regarding the involvement of polymorphonuclear (PMN) leukocyte adhesion to endothelial cells. Previous clinical investigations have demonstrated the involvement of leukocyte activation in chronic venous ulcers. Intermediate biological markers of these interactions induced by stasis in varicose veins were further evaluated in this study.

Methods.—Blood was sampled from 22 patients in the supine position at rest and after a 30-minute period of dependency both in the varicose vein (limbs hanging down) and in the brachial vein (arm hanging down) as a paired control. Oxygen partial pressure (PVO_2) and 12 biological markers were measured with the use of enzyme-linked immunosorbent assay kits. Angiotensin-converting enzyme activity was determined by means of a specific substrate. Matrix metalloproteinases (MMPs) 9 and 2 were evaluated with the use of gelatin zymography.

Results.—No markers were significantly changed in the brachial vein after 30 minutes of arm dependency. However, a decrease was seen in varicose vein PVO_2 after 30 minutes of lower extremity dependency. Thrombomodulin, von Willebrand factor, vascular endothelial growth factor, and MMP-2 were not modified in these conditions, but several markers in varicose veins were altered after 20 minutes of lower extremity dependency. These markers included the proteins released by proteolysis from the endothelial membrane intercellular adhesion molecule-1, vascular cell adhesion molecule-1, and angiotensin-converting enzyme. Varicose vein, leukocyte markers lactoferrin, myeloperoxidase, and interleukin-8 were not modified, but L-selectin shed from the leukocytes increased. In addition, a major increase in pro-MMP-9, which is released from tertiary granules during PMN activation, was observed.

Conclusions.—The significant increase in plasma pro-MMP-9 activity presents evidence of PMN activation and granule release in the varicose vein in response to postural blood tests. The detection of membrane proteins shed from the endothelium or leukocytes in the plasma provides evidence of pericellular proteolysis.

▶ This study provides very convincing evidence to support the hypothesis that venous stasis stimulates an increase in metalloproteinase-9 within the venous effluent of lower extremity veins consistent with specific activation of neutrophils. The investigators hypothesize that this metalloproteinase release is accompanied by a transient increase in L-selectin release also consistent with leukocyte activation. The clinical stage of venous disease was documented in all patients, and anatomic evidence of venous reflux was confirmed with duplex US. However, each patient's arm served as the internal control

comparison. These authors discount the possibility that there may be both local and systemic activation of neutrophils in patients with venous ulcers. No
patients without venous disease were studied for these experiments. Thus,
the changes reported by these investigators may represent a gross underestimation of an important physiologic response. Since there are no adequate
animal models for venous stasis disease, clinical studies with human beings
must be designed to get the most bang for the buck—that is, appropriate controls whenever possible.

M. T. Watkins, MD

Synthesis of Collagen Is Dysregulated in Cultured Fibroblasts Derived From Skin of Subjects With Varicose Veins as It Is in Venous Smooth Muscle Cells
Sansilvestri-Morel P, Rupin A, Jaisson S, et al (Servier Research Inst, Suresnes, France; European Hosp Georges Pompidou, Paris)
Circulation 106:479-483, 2002   16–8

Background.—Alterations in tissue remodeling occur in varicose veins, and evidence exists that the content of elastin, laminin, fibronectin, and collagen are modified. In previous studies, it has been shown that cultured smooth muscle cells derived from human varicose veins retain at least some of the dysregulation of the synthesis of extracellular matrix proteins. Several studies have indicated that, in some hereditary conditions, the loss of integrity of matrix proteins in the skin reflects similar changes in major blood vessels such as the aorta. This study determined whether the phenotypic modulations observed in the venous smooth muscle cells of patients with varicose veins are also present in their dermal fibroblasts.

Methods.—Twelve control skin biopsy specimens were obtained from patients (mean age, 71.9 years) undergoing endarterectomy or coronary bypass surgery with and without varicose veins. Collagen type I, type III, and type V were compared in dermal fibroblasts.

Results.—The synthesis of collagen type I, the release of its metabolites, and the expression of its messenger RNA (mRNA) were increased in fibroblasts from patients with varicose veins. The synthesis of collagen type III was decreased, but this decrease was not correlated with a decrease in either mRNA expression or metabolite release. Matrix metalloproteinases (MMP)-2, -7, -8, -9, and -13 and their inhibitors (TIMP-1 and -2) were quantified in both cell types; however, only the production of proMMP-2 was increased in cells derived from patients with varicose veins.

Conclusions.—The synthesis of collagen types I and III may be dysregulated in dermal fibroblasts of patients with varicose veins. Comparable findings were reported in smooth muscle cells derived from varicose veins, which suggests that a systemic alteration of tissue remodeling is present in patients with varicose veins.

▶ This study purports to provide in vitro data to suggest that dermal fibro-blasts grown from limbs of patients with varicose veins have dysregulated col-lagen synthesis. I cannot endorse these results since the control fibroblasts were derived from the neck and chest, not the leg. Parts are not parts, and ap-propriate source of control fibroblasts for these studies should come from the limb, not the neck or the chest.

M. T. Watkins, MD

Varicose Veins Possess Greater Quantities of MMP-1 Than Normal Veins and Demonstrate Regional Variation in MMP-1 and MMP-13
Gillespie DL, Patel A, Fileta B, et al (Uniformed Services Univ, Bethesda, Md; Walter Reed Army Med Ctr, Washington, DC)
J Surg Res 106:233-238, 2002   16–9

Background.—Previous studies have found a decrease in elastin and col-lagen in varicose veins compared with normal veins. In this study, whether the changes seen in the composition of the varicose vein wall may be related to alterations in extracellular matrix remodeling proteins, such as matrix metalloproteases and serine proteases, was investigated. Regional variation of the expression of these enzymes within the leg was also investigated.

Methods.—One-cm segments of proximal and distal greater saphenous vein (GSV) were obtained from 15 patients with venous insufficiency under-going GSV ligation and stripping. Samples were also obtained from 7 pa-tients undergoing GSV harvesting for coronary artery bypass grafting. All patients with venous insufficiency had incompetence of the greater saphe-nous vein by color flow duplex scans. Vein specimens were examined for ma-trix metalloproteinases MMP-1, MMP-3, MMP-13, and for tryptase, and reduced glyceraldehyde-phosphate dehydrogenase (GAPDH) messenger RNA (mRNA) by means of semiquantitative reverse transcriptase-poly-merase chain reaction analysis or Western blot analysis as appropriate. Western blots were analyzed with the use of scanning densitometry and stan-dardized to normal control veins and values expressed as the median densi-tometric index. Nonparametric statistical methods were used for analysis.

Results.—MMP-1, MMP-13, and tryptase mRNA were amplified from both proximal and distal segments of all greater saphenous veins studied. However, MMP-3 mRNA was not found in either segment of any of the veins examined. Semiquantitative analysis of reverse transcriptase-poly-merase chain reaction products comparing the ratio of MMP-1, MMP-13, or tryptase mRNA to GAPDH mRNA showed no difference between case patients and control subjects and no differences between proximal and distal vein segments. Western blot analysis showed larger quantities of MMP-1 in varicose veins than in nondiseased veins from patients undergoing coronary artery bypass grafting. An investigation of the regional variation in proteases revealed lower amounts of MMP-1 in distal than in proximal vein segments, and significantly less MMP-13 in distal segments of varicose veins than in proximal vein segments.

Conclusions.—Veins of the lower leg have significantly reduced amounts of proteolytic enzymes in comparison with veins of the upper thigh. MMP-1 is increased in varicose veins in comparison with control veins, even though no difference in mRNA expression was observed. This study also identified regional variation of MMP-1 and MMP-13 in diseased varicose veins. The differences observed in MMP-1 and MMP-13 quantities between normal and varicose veins may be the result of posttranscriptional regulatory controls.

▶ This well-designed study compares the molecular and biosynthetic profile of a number of MMPs in normal patients and those with documented venous insufficiency. The data are convincing and are presented with precision in a comprehensive manner. The findings regarding posttranscriptional changes may implicate decreased turnover of the MMPs in the walls of varicose veins. This is an excellent article with potential for numerous follow-up studies!

M. T. Watkins, MD

Effect of Venous Ulcer Exudates on Angiogenesis In Vitro
Drinkwater SL, Smith A, Sawyer BM, et al (St Thomas' Hosp, London)
Br J Surg 89:709-713, 2002   16–10

Background.—Some venous ulcers never heal, despite intensive treatment. Angiogenesis is a part of normal wound healing; thus, angiogenesis may have an important part of the mechanism of healing of venous ulcers. Whether venous leg ulcer wound exudates stimulate or inhibit angiogenesis was determined.

Methods.—Fluid exudate was obtained from 16 patients with venous ulcers over 4 hours. Five of these ulcers had not healed after more than 1 year of compression bandaging, and 5 were rapidly healing ulcers. In addition, fluids from acute wounds were collected from subcutaneous drains in 7 patients as a control. Vascular endothelial growth factor (VEGF) at 2 ng/mL acted as a positive control. The extent of angiogenesis was expressed as the ratio of the mean tubule length in the test wells over that in blank control wells.

Results.—Angiogenesis was significantly inhibited by venous ulcer exudates compared with fluids from acute wounds and VEGF. Exudates from the 5 nonhealing venous ulcers inhibited angiogenesis to a significantly greater degree than did exudates from the 5 rapidly healing venous ulcers.

Conclusions.—This study of experimental angiogenesis found that angiogenesis was inhibited by fluid exudate from venous ulcers, particularly from slow-healing ulcers.

▶ It has been suggested by others that impaired angiogenesis may be a factor in nonhealing of recalcitrant venous ulcers. This study suggests inhibition of VEGF may play a role in nonhealing venous ulcers. Other biochemical abnormalities are also undoubtedly present (see Abstract 16–11).

G. L. Moneta, MD

A Reduction in Serum Cytokine Levels Parallels Healing of Venous Ulcers in Patients Undergoing Compression Therapy
Murphy MA, Joyce WP, Condron C, et al (Royal College of Surgeons, Dublin; Cavan Gen Hosp, Ireland)
Eur J Vasc Endovasc Surg 23:349-352, 2002   16–11

Background.—Chronic venous disease is the most common and least understood cause of lower leg ulceration. Ambulatory venous hypertension appears to act through largely unknown mechanisms to promote the tissue damage of chronic venous disease. This may be modified by compression therapy. Recent studies have also implicated vascular endothelial growth factor (VEGF) and tumor necrosis factor-α (TNFα) in the tissue damage associated with chronic venous disease. Production of both factors is known to be upregulated in vessel wall cells subject to hypertension. Local venous levels of VEGF and TNFα were determined in limbs with venous ulcers before and after treatment with graduated compression.

Methods.—The study group included 8 patients with venous ulcers and 8 patients with varicose veins only. For the patients with ulcers, serum samples were obtained from the superficial veins in the lower limbs, and additional samples were obtained after 4 weeks of treatment with 4-layered graduated compression. Serum from the arms of these patients served as a control. Sandwich enzyme-linked immunosorbent assay was used to determine the concentrations of VEGF and TNFα proteins.

Results.—VEGF and TNFα levels were elevated in both groups of patients. In the patients with venous ulcers, compression treatment resulted in reductions in the levels of both cytokines to below control values. These changes correlated with healing of the ulcers, as determined by reduction in the ulcer size.

Conclusions.—These findings are the first to suggest a central role for both TNFα and VEGF in the pathogenesis of venous ulceration, which may constitute a causative link between venous hypertension and the cutaneous changes of chronic venous disease.

▶ The findings of Drinkwater et al suggest VEGF is good for venous ulcers in that it may stimulate angiogenesis (see Abstract 16–10). In this study, however, healing of venous ulcers correlated with a decrease in VEGF, a finding seemingly contradictory to Drinkwater et al. Arguing with these authors (the senior author is Kevin Burnand) is not for the faint of heart. Perhaps it is possible that cytokines other than VEGF have a more deleterious effect on venous ulcers than VEGF has benefit. In such a scenario, a decrease in the bad cytokine may be more important than an increase in a good cytokine.

G. L. Moneta, MD

Why Insurers Should Reimburse for Compression Stockings in Patients With Chronic Venous Stasis
Korn P, Patel ST, Heller JA, et al (Cornell Univ, New York; New York Hosp)
J Vasc Surg 35:950-957, 2002   16–12

Background.—Chronic venous stasis ulcers are associated with substantial morbidity and cost. Compression stockings (CSs) can decrease recurrence rates in patients with previous ulceration. However, Medicare and other insurers do not provide reimbursement for the costs of CSs and patient education. Using a Markov decision analysis model, the authors analyzed the cost efficacy of a strategy of reimbursement for CSs and patient education versus a strategy that does not provide these resources.

Methods.—The model was based on a hypothetical 55-year-old patient with previous venous stasis ulceration. Published data were used to estimate the mean time to ulcer recurrence, the mean time to ulcer healing, the probabilities of hospitalization and amputation after ulcer development, and quality-adjustment factors. Costs were calculated from the authors' hospital accounting system.

Findings.—The CSs and patient education strategy was associated with a savings of $5904 and 0.37 quality-adjusted life years compared with the strategy that did not provide these resources. When revenue loss related to missed work was included in the analysis, the cost savings increased to $17,080 during the patient's lifetime. In a sensitivity analysis, CSs and patient education was still cost effective if amputations and the cost of ulcer treatment were eliminated or if the cost of prophylaxis was increased to 600% of the base case. The mean time to recurrence would have to be reduced from 53 to 21.2 months before the CSs and patient education strategy was no longer cost effective.

Conclusion.—Even with the most conservative assumptions, prophylactic CSs and patient education for patients with previous venous stasis ulceration was a cost-saving strategy. Insurers should provide reimbursement for these interventions.

▶ In the sensitivity analysis of this study, the authors found that compliance with the use of elastic compression stockings to prevent recurrence of venous ulcers needed to be reduced to 52% before a program of prophylactic use of elastic compression stockings after healing of venous ulcers was no longer cost saving. Compliance needed to be reduced to 16% before the use of elastic compression stockings after healing of venous ulcers was no longer cost effective. I don't know precisely who reads these Markov decision analysis studies, but I hope the people from Medicare would at least read this one.

G. L. Moneta, MD

The Effect of Long Saphenous Vein Stripping on Quality of Life

MacKenzie RK, Paisley A, Allan PL, et al (Royal Infirmary of Edinburgh, Scotland; Univ of Edinburgh, Scotland; Heartlands Hosp, Birmingham, England)
J Vasc Surg 35:1197-1203, 2002   16–13

Background.—Stripping of the long saphenous vein (LSV) in the treatment of varicose veins may be effective in reducing the recurrence of varices. However, this practice may also increase morbidity rates. The effects of stripping on health-related quality of life (HRQOL) is unknown. The effects of long saphenous vein surgery, with and without successful stripping of the LSV, on HRQOL were evaluated in the United Kingdom.

Methods.—This prospective study included 102 consecutive patients who underwent varicose vein surgery with attempted stripping of the LSV to the knee. HRQOL was assessed preoperatively and at 4 weeks, 6 months, and 2 years after surgery with the Aberdeen varicose vein severity score (AVSS) and the Short-Form 36 (SF-36). The AVSS functioned as a disease-specific assessment, and the SF-36 was used as a generic assessment tool. Patients defined as stripped were those in whom complete stripping from the thigh to the knee was confirmed with postoperative duplex scanning at 2 years. Patients defined as incompletely stripped were those in whom any LSV remnant was

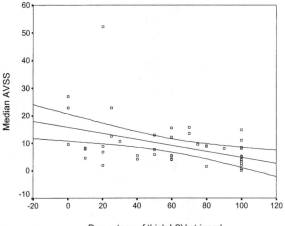

Percentage of thigh LSV stripped

FIGURE 2.—Scatterplot of median Aberdeen varicose vein severity score (AVSS) at 2 years after surgery versus percentage of long saphenous vein (LSV) stripped in thigh in patients without preoperative deep venous reflux. *Lines* represent mean linear regression prediction line with 95% CIs. Spearman rank correlation, –0.357. P = .003. (Reprinted by permission of the publisher from MacKenzie RK, Paisley A, Allan PL, et al: The effect of long saphenous vein stripping on quality of life. *J Vasc Surg* 35:1197-1203, 2002. Copyright 2002 by Elsevier.)

found in the thigh after surgery. Deep venous reflux (DVR) was defined as reflux of 0.5 seconds or more in at least the popliteal vein.

Results.—Complete HRQOL data at all 4 time points were obtained from 66 of 102 patients (65%). No significant differences were found at baseline between patients who were stripped (25 patients) and those who were incompletely stripped (41 patients) in terms of AVSS, SF-36, age, sex, DVR, or CEAP grade. However, significantly more patients in the incompletely stripped group underwent surgery for recurrent disease (71% vs 32%). Both groups obtained significant improvements in AVSS scores for as much as 2 years (Fig 2). When adjustment was made for recurrent disease, stripping provided additional benefits on the AVSS tool at 6 months and at 2 years, which was statistically significant in patients without preoperative DVR but which was not significant in patients with preoperative DVR. Scores on the SF-36 were not affected by stripping.

Conclusions.—Surgery of the LSV results in significant improvement in disease-specific HRQOL for as long as 2 years. Stripping to the knee confers an additional benefit to patients without DVR.

▶ Clumsy surgeons take note. This study couldn't have better results for you. Even patients who had basically botched operations on the greater saphenous vein benefited from LSV surgery.

G. L. Moneta, MD

Persistent Popliteal Fossa Reflux Following Saphenopopliteal Disconnection
Rashid HI, Ajeel A, Tyrrell MR (Kent and Sussex Hosp, Tunbridge Wells, England)
Br J Surg 89:748-751, 2002   16–14

Background.—Saphenopopliteal disconnection (SPD) has a higher recurrence rate of reflux than saphenofemoral disconnection. Flush ligation of the saphenopopliteal junction is necessary for a durable procedure, and failure to identify the saphenopopliteal junction is a common cause of recurrent short saphenous varices. This retrospective study reviewed the technical success of SPD in patients with short saphenous vein varices as judged by preoperative and postoperative color-coded duplex imaging.

Methods.—All patients scheduled for SPD over a period of 4 years underwent preoperative color-coded duplex imaging to localize the saphenopopliteal junction. The operations were performed with the patient under general anesthesia and in the prone position, with planned full popliteal fossa exposure. Patients underwent a follow-up imaging procedure 6 weeks after surgery.

Results.—From a total of 69 patients who underwent SPD during the study period, complete data were available for 59 patients with a median age of 55 years (range, 27-78 years). There were 8 staged bilateral procedures. Postoperative duplex scans identified 23 patients (39%) with the incompetent saphenopopliteal junction successfully disconnected (ideal result), 12 patients (20%) with incompetent saphenopopliteal junction disconnected successfully but with persisting venous reflux in superficial veins (satisfactory result), 8 duplex failures (14%), and 13 surgical failures (22%) (incompetent saphenopopliteal junction completely missed during surgery). Three patients (5%) suffered major postoperative complications consisting of 2 deep vein thromboses and 1 popliteal vein injury, and 1 patient suffered a sural nerve palsy.

Conclusion.—Despite preoperative duplex localization of the saphenopopliteal junction, SPD is an unreliable technique for the treatment of varicose veins.

▶ I doubt a truly disconnected saphenopopliteal junction grew back together. In the presence of varicosities in the region of the proximal lessor saphenous vein duplex, identification of the saphenopopliteal junction is difficult. I believe this examination can be improved by beginning proximal in the thigh and working toward the saphenopopliteal junction. Absolute identification of the saphenopopliteal junction through an adequate-sized incision is required to achieve success with this procedure. This is not a "keyhole" procedure.

G. L. Moneta, MD

Endovascular Obliteration of Saphenous Reflux: A Multicenter Study
Merchant RF, DePalma RG, Kabnick LS (Reno Vein Clinic, Nev; Univ of Nevada, Reno; Vein Ctr of New Jersey, Morristown)
J Vasc Surg 35:1190-1196, 2002   16–15

Background.—The clinical outcomes in patients treated with endovenous saphenous vein (SV) obliteration (closure technique) were assessed in terms of complete SV occlusion, near-complete SV occlusion, or SV recanalization.

Methods.—This prospective registry study had a follow-up period of 24 months. A total of 286 patients were enrolled from 30 clinical sites with saphenous vein reflux as determined by duplex scanning. A total of 319 limb treatments were performed. The intervention included endovenous catheter obliteration of insufficient saphenous veins with temperature-controlled radiofrequency heat, without high ligation of the saphenofemoral junction. The main outcome measures were the status of occlusion of the treated vein segments, the presence of varicose veins and reflux, clinical symptom scores, physician evaluation of the success of the procedure, and the patient's satisfaction with the procedure.

Results.—At 12 months' follow up, 83.6% of treated limbs were classified as having complete occlusion, 5.6% were categorized as having near complete occlusion, and 10.8% were recanalized. At 24 months, 85.2% of treated veins were classified as having complete occlusion, 3.5% were classified as having near complete occlusion, and 11.3% were recanalized. Varicose veins were present in 95% of limbs before treatment. The presence of varicose veins in limbs with complete occlusion was 10.5%, 7.3%, 5.7%,

TABLE 6.—Patient Satisfaction Assessment (By Patient)

	Follow-up Time Period					
	6 Months		12 Months		24 Months	
	n/N	% Satisfied	*n*/N	% Satisfied	*n*/N	% Satisfied
Complete occlusion	163/169	96.4	166/175	94.9	104/108	96.3
Near-complete occlusion	14/16	87.5	12/12	100	5/5	100
Recanalization	9/14	64.3	17/25	68.0	12/15	80.0

(Reprinted by permission of the publisher from Merchant RF, DePalma RG, Kabnick LS: Endovascular obliteration of saphenous reflux: A multicenter study. *J Vasc Surg* 35:1190-1196, 2002. Copyright 2002 by Elsevier.)

and 8.3% at 1 week, 6 months, 12 months, and 24 months, respectively, and a similar presence of varicose veins was found in limbs with near complete occlusion at each follow-up interval. Overall, 91.4% of 232 limbs followed up to 12 months and 90.1% of 142 limbs followed up to 24 months were free of saphenous vein reflux, regardless of the technical outcome. Paresthesia occurred in 3.9% of limbs at 1 year and in 5.6% of limbs at 2 years. The mean symptom severity scores declined from 2.0 preoperatively to 0.07, 0.0, and 0.50 for complete occlusion, near-complete occlusion, and recanalized limbs, respectively, at 6 months. The symptom severity scores continued to decline at 12 months but rose at 24 months to 0.10, 0.40, and 0.63 for complete occlusion, near-complete occlusion, and recanalized limbs, respectively. Patient satisfaction was obtained in 195 of 212 patients (92%) at 1 year and in 121 of 128 patients (94.5%) at 2 years (Table 6).

Conclusions.—Endovascular obliteration of saphenous reflux without high ligation reduces the presence of varicosities and reflux. Patient satisfaction is high at 2 years regardless of the technical outcome.

▶ Registry studies seem to be popular in venous disease. We have had registries for thrombolytic therapy, registries for SEPS, and now a registry for the VNUS closure device. I hope we don't see any more registries. A lot of effort is expended but the nonrandomized nature of the studies combined with minimal oversight and monitoring of data quality really only allow one to conclude whether a procedure is technically possible and basically safe. It is interesting that only about 60% of the patients in this registry had other adjunctive therapies such as surgical removal of branch varicosities and/or sclerotherapy. This suggests many of the patients had truly minimal venous disease and the indications for operation were somewhat aggressive.

G. L. Moneta, MD

Endovenous Treatment of the Greater Saphenous Vein With a 940-nm Diode Laser: Thrombotic Occlusion After Endoluminal Thermal Damage by Laser-Generated Steam Bubbles

Proebstle TM, Lehr HA, Kargl A, et al (Univ of Mainz, Germany; Dornier MedizinLaser GmbH, Germering, Germany)
J Vasc Surg 35:729-736, 2002

16–16

Introduction.—The efficacy, treatment-associated adverse effects, and putative mechanisms of action of endovenous laser treatment (EVLT) were determined in 26 patients with 31 limbs of clinical stages C_{2-6}, E_P, $A_{S,P}$, P_R. Incompetent greater saphenous veins (GSVs) were verified by duplex scanning in all patients.

Methods.—Twenty-one patients had unilateral incompetent GSVs, and 5 had bilateral incompetent GSVs. All patients were treated in an outpatient setting. A 600-µm fiber was introduced into the GSV with the use of an 18-gauge needle below the knee and was advanced to the saphenofemoral junction. After infiltration of tumescent local anesthesia, multiple laser pulses of energy of 15 J and a wavelength of 940 nm were administered along the vein with the use of a standardized technique. In 16 patients, D-dimers were identified in peripheral blood samples 30 minutes after completion of EVLT and on postoperative day 1 in 20 patients. One GSV that was surgically removed after EVLT underwent histopathologic examination. An experimental in vitro setup was constructed to investigate the mechanism of laser action within a blood-filled tube.

Results.—A median of 80 laser pulses (range, 22-116 laser pulses) were applied to the treated veins. On day 1, 7, and 28, all limbs except 1 (97%) demonstrated a thrombotically occluded GSV. In 1 patient, the vessel exhibited incomplete occlusion. The distance of the proximal end of the thrombus to the saphenofemoral junction was a median of 1.1 cm (range, 0.2-5.9). Adverse effects included ecchymoses and palpable induration along the thrombotically occluded GSV that lasted for 2 to 3 weeks. Two limbs (6%) had thrombophlebitis of a varicose tributary. The D-dimers in peripheral blood were normal in 14 of 16 patients tested at 30 minutes after completion of the procedure and elevated in 7 of 20 patients tested on day 1 after EVLT.

The 940-nm laser was demonstrated via in vitro experiments and the histopathologic examination of 1 explanted GSV to cause indirect heat damage to the inner vein wall. A threshold energy of 15 J is required to heat the surrounding blood until it reaches boiling temperature and produces steam bubbles. Steam bubbles are proposed to be the cause of injury to the vein wall (Fig 3).

Conclusion.—Endovascular laser treatment of the GSV with a 940-nm diode laser is effective in causing thrombotic vessel occlusion and is associated with minor adverse effects. Laser-induced or indirect local heat injury of the inner vein wall by steam bubbles originating from boiling blood may be the pathophysiologic mechanism of action in EVLT.

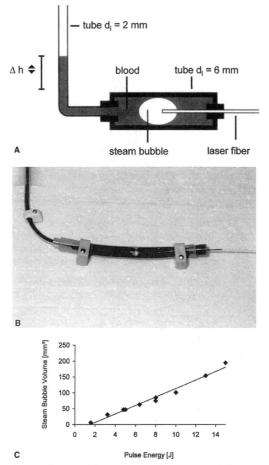

FIGURE 3.—**A**, Schematic drawing of the in vitro setup for examining the laser-generated steam bubble formation. The laser fiber was inserted into a silicone tube of 6-mm diameter filled with heparinized blood. During delivery of laser energy, heating and boiling of the blood finally lead to the formation of a steam bubble, pushing the corresponding blood volume out of the tube. Thus, the movement of the blood level in the smaller 2-mm diameter tube allowed the calculation of the volume of the steam bubble in reverse. **B**, Visible steam bubble formation during delivery of a laser pulse of 15 J. **C**, Dependency of the steam bubble volume for various amounts of energy delivered by the laser beam. (Reprinted by permission of the publisher from Proebstle TM, Lehr HA, Kargl A, et al: Endovenous treatment of the greater saphenous vein with a 940-nm diode laser: Thrombotic occlusion after endoluminal thermal damage by laser-generated steam bubbles. *J Vasc Surg* 35:729-736, 2002. Copyright 2002 by Elsevier.)

▶ This is another method of endovascular obliteration of the GSV (see also Abstract 16–15). The treated veins were quite small, all less than 1 cm in diameter at the saphenofemoral junction. Follow-up with this technique is even shorter than that of the VNUS system. All the points made with respect to Abstract 16–15 apply equally here.

G. L. Moneta, MD

Powered Phlebectomy (TriVex) in Treatment of Varicose Veins

Cheshire N, Elias SM, Keagy B, et al (St Mary's Hosp, London; Englewood Hosp, NJ; Univ of North Carolina, Chapel Hill; et al)
Ann Vasc Surg 16:488-494, 2002   16–17

Introduction.—Phlebectomy in patients with varicose veins is time-consuming, involves multiple scars, and may be associated with postoperative nerve damage, wound infections, and recurrence. The safety and efficacy of the powered varicose vein extractor for ablation of primary veins was evaluated in a prospective, noncomparative, multicenter, pilot investigation.

Methods.—One hundred fourteen patients (117 limbs) were recruited from 4 centers in Europe and 4 centers in the United States. The safety of the varicose vein extractor was assessed by recording the nature and severity of all adverse events and complications. The efficacy and performance were examined with the use of an 11-point box scale marked by each patient, an independent trial nurse, and the surgeon. Surgeries were performed with the patients under general, spinal, or epidural anesthesia. Tumescent anesthesia was added with infusions of dilute lidocaine with epinephrine. Transillumination was achieved with the use of a specially designed cannula. Vein extraction was performed with the use of a vein resector with a rotating tubular inner cannula encased in a stationary outer sheath dissector.

Results.—Eighty-four percent of limbs were clinical, etiologic, anatomical, pathophysiologic (CEAP) class 2, and 16% were class 3 or 4. Accompanying greater saphenous vein stripping was performed in 67% of limbs in the United States and in 88% of those in Europe. The median duration of the operative procedures was 45 minutes (range, 11-119 minutes); 94% of the procedures were completed with between 2 and 5 incisions. The duration of the powered phlebotomy portion of the procedure was 14 minutes (range, 3-75 minutes). One of 114 patients experienced deep venous thrombosis. There was 1 death of myocardial infarction at 29 days.

Conclusion.—Transilluminated powered phlebectomy used in varicose vein removal is quick and efficacious and conserves operating time. Results were satisfactory to both patients and physicians.

▶ Another gadget for veins. This one is for branch varicosities. It also accomplishes its goals reasonably well. There is, however, significant postoperative ecchymosis after this procedure and incisions are required to place the device. It is also concerning that 25% of the patients had parasthesia 6 weeks postoperatively. The primary potential advantage of this device appears to be in reducing operating times. No cost analysis is presented, but I am pretty sure the device and disposables cost more than a #11 scalpel blade and a small hemostat. As with other recent interventions in venous disease, I doubt that this device would stand the scrutiny of a randomized trial.

G. L. Moneta, MD

Intravascular Ultrasound Scan Evaluation of the Obstructed Vein

Neglén P, Raju S (River Oaks Hosp, Jackson, Miss)

J Vasc Surg 35:694-700, 2002   16–18

Background.—The extent and severity of obstructive venous lesions appear worse on intravascular US scan (IVUS) than on venography. Iliac vein intraluminal and mural morphologic observations with IVUS were analyzed and the degree of stenosis on venous IVUS studies was compared with that on single-plane transfemoral venography.

Methods.—Three hundred four consecutive limbs were analyzed by IVUS and standard single-plane transfemoral venography during balloon dilation and stenting of an obstructed iliac venous segment. In 173 limbs, stenotic areas were calculated by measures of diameters and with the IVUS software before and after dilation and stenting. In addition, preoperative measures of hand/foot differential pressure and dorsal foot venous pressure, and increases in intraoperative transfemoral hyperemia-induced pressure were obtained after intra-arterial injection of papaverine.

Findings.—Fine intraluminal and mural details were identified on IVUS that were not seen with venography, including trabeculation, frozen valves, mural thickness, and external compression. The median stenosis was 50% on venography and 80% on IVUS. With IVUS as the standard, the sensitivity and negative predictive value of venography were 45% and 49%, respectively, for the detection of a venous area stenosis of more than 70%. The actual stenotic area was more severe when determined directly with IVUS, probably because of the noncircular lumen geometry of the stenosis. None of the preoperative or intraoperative pressure measurements were associated with the degree of stenosis. Stenosis was more severe when collaterals were present and the actual stenotic area was greater and the rate of hyperemia-induced pressure gradient higher.

Conclusions.—Venous IVUS appears to be superior to single-plane venography for the diagnosis of iliac venous outflow obstruction. Apparently, no preoperative or intraoperative pressure test is currently available to sufficiently determine the hemodynamic significance of the stenosis.

▶ The important question is, what is a significant venous stenosis? If the "stenosis" does not result in collateral formation and has no pressure gradient, it may be that in the low-pressure distensible venous system our concept of what is a crucial stenosis needs to be modified. The idea that treatment of a lesion has no associated abnormal physiology doesn't make a lot of sense to me. One wonders if this is extrapolation of the "ocular-stenotic reflux" to the venous system.

G. L. Moneta, MD

Randomised Trial of Pre-operative Colour Duplex Marking in Primary Varicose Vein Surgery: Outcome Is Not Improved

Smith JJ, Brown L, Greenhalgh RM, et al (Imperial College of Science, Technology and Medicine, London)
Eur J Vasc Endovasc Surg 23:336-343, 2002   16–19

Background.—Recurrence rates for varicose vein surgery have been reported at 21% over 10 years. Several techniques for reducing the recurrence rates in varicose vein surgery have been suggested. One of the most important aspects of varicose vein surgery is correct preoperative assessment of patients. Clinical examination has been shown to be poor for the diagnosis of reflux in varicose veins, and even handheld Doppler has its limitations. The capability of color duplex US was investigated for accurate location and preoperative marking of incompetent venous sites in patients scheduled for varicose vein surgery.

Methods.—This prospective randomized controlled trial was conducted in the regional vascular service of one hospital in London. The study group consisted of 149 consecutive patients undergoing primary varicose vein surgery. One half of the patients (72 patients) were randomly assigned to receive duplex marking before surgery. All patients underwent color duplex scanning at 6 weeks and 12 months postoperatively to determine the accuracy of surgery and the presence of residual/recurrent varicose veins. In addition, all patients completed the Aberdeen Varicose Veins Questionnaire, the SF-36, and the EuroQol quality-of-life questionnaires. The main outcome measures were duplex evidence of venous incompetence and quality of life measures with the use of the SF-36 and the Aberdeen questionnaires.

Results.—The preoperative marking of primary varicose veins by skilled ultrasonographers did not result in any statistically significant improvement in accuracy or recurrence rates after surgery. The quality of life was significantly improved in both groups after surgery, but no difference was found between the groups in improved quality of life.

Conclusions.—This study found no additional benefit from preoperative color duplex marking over clinical and handheld marking in patients with primary varicose veins of the long saphenous system. However, the role of preoperative color duplex marking in the short saphenous system is less well elucidated.

▶ I do not use duplex US to mark individual sites of incompetence before most varicose vein operations. I think the combination of the obliterative nature of the operation and a good dissection of the saphenofemoral junction basically takes care of the problem in a large majority of cases. I do map the saphenous vein before stripping as I think it allows more precise placement of the incision over the saphenous vein below the knee.

G. L. Moneta, MD

17 Technical Notes

Totally Laparoscopic Aortobifemoral Bypass: A New and Simplified Approach
Coggia M, Bourriez A, Javerliat I, et al (Ambroise Paré Univ Hosp, Boulogne, France; René Descartes Univ, Paris)
Eur J Vasc Endovasc Surg 24:274-275, 2002   17–1

Introduction.—Two major technical problems are associated with laparoscopic infrarenal aortic surgery: exposure of the aorta and performance of the aortic anastomosis. Described is a simple laparoscopic approach to the infrarenal abdominal aorta that allows a totally laparoscopic aortic anastomosis.

Surgical Technique.—The patient is placed in right lateral and rotated decubitus, and the abdomen is rotated at 45° (Fig 1). The abdomen slope achieved with the maximal right rotation of the operating table reaches 65°. The video monitor is viewed distally on the left side of the patient, and the surgeon faces the patient's abdomen. The 0° endoscope is positioned through a 10 mm-trocar introduced on the anterior axillary line 3 cm under the costal margin. A left retrocolic dissection is performed in the line of the Tdd fascia, down to reach the level of the left renal vein. Because of this position, the small bowel and left mesocolon fall to the right. The infrarenal aorta is exposed up to the common iliac arteries. A complete dissection of the left and right sides of the aorta is performed. After dissection, the operating table is rotated to the left, which permits a conventional approach to the femoral arteries. The table is then positioned back to its maximal right rotation. The vascular prosthesis is introduced through 1 of the trocars. The right tunnel is started away from the groin, and the right limb of the prosthesis is brought to the groin incision with the use of an aortic clamp. The proximal and distal coelioscopic clamps are positioned through 10 mm-trocars, and aortic anastomosis is performed with the use of 2 polypropylene hemicircumferential running sutures, knotted on a prosthetic pledget earlier. The left prosthetic limb is brought to the groin incision. When the 2 graft limbs are positioned, the operating table is positioned on the left, which allow the femoral anastomoses to be performed.

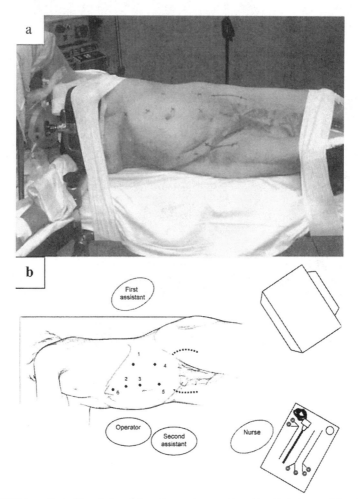

FIGURE 1.—a, Typical installation of the patient on the operating table with the bust and the pelvis rotated. b, Basic operating room setup after the maximal right rotation of the operating table and sites of trocar insertion. *1*, 10-mm trocar for laparoscope. *2 and 3*, 10-mm trocars for operator instruments. *4*, 5-mm trocar for suction/irrigation. *5 and 6*, 10-mm trocars for proximal and distal coelioscopic aortic clamps. (Reprinted from Coggia M, Bourriez A, Javerliat I, et al: Totally laparoscopic aortobifemoral bypass: A new and simplified approach. *Eur J Vasc Endovasc Surg* 24(3):274-275, 2002. Copyright 2002 by permission of the publisher W B Saunders Company Limited London.)

Conclusion.—This approach prevents the need for sophisticated techniques of retraction to pull the viscera aside and provides stable aortic exposure during performance of the laparoscopic aortic anastomosis.

▶ The French surgeons continue to push laparoscopic aortic surgery. Indeed, the approach detailed in this paper appears more user friendly than that previously described. Given the rapid advances of catheter-based techniques for aortic intervention, for the foreseeable future I doubt laparoscopic aortic surgery is going to be a major focus of investigation. I do think laparoscopic approach to the aorta may be of value for treating pesky type II endoleaks unresponsive to catheter-based interventions.

G. L. Moneta, MD

Novel Anastomotic Method Enables Aortofemoral Bypass for Patients With Porcelain Aorta

Sasajima T, Inaba M, Azuma N, et al (Asahikawa Med Univ, Japan)
J Vasc Surg 35:1016-1019, 2002   17–2

Background.—Patient high-risk factors and/or local anatomic factors may prevent the use of aortofemoral bypass in patients unsuited for a catheter-based procedure. One of these anatomic factors is porcelain aorta, a

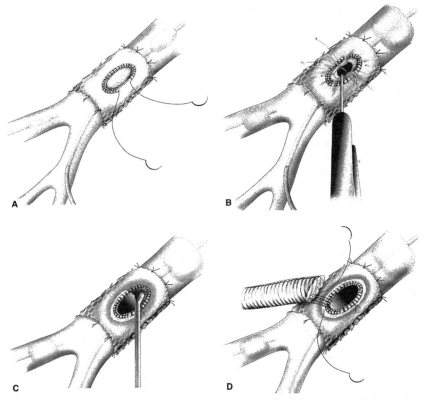

FIGURE 2.—Anastomotic techniques. **A,** Mesh wrapping of anastomotic site. Longitudinal suture line should be located at posterolateral aspect of aorta. Mesh is fixed with adventitia at suture line and proximal and distal margins. **B,** Exposed calcification is penetrated with airdrill. **C,** Opening is properly enlarged for anastomosis with laminectomy ronguer. **D,** Anastomotic suturing is performed between polyester graft and mesh-reinforced adventitia. (Reprinted by permission of the publisher from Sasajima T, Inaba M, Azuma N, et al: Novel anastomotic method enables aortofemoral bypass for patients with porcelain aorta. *J Vasc Surg* 35:1016-1019, 2002. Copyright 2002 by Elsevier.)

condition that can be found in patients who are diabetic or undergoing dialysis. A new method for obtaining aortofemoral bypass in patients with porcelain aorta was presented.

Methods.—This technique was performed in 9 patients between May 1995 and March 2001 (Fig 2). The portion of the distal aorta for anastomosis is wrapped with a double polytetrafluoroethylene mesh and fixed to the adventitia with continuous sutures. The adventitia of the anastomotic site is cut over the mesh until the calcified surface is revealed. Margins of the mesh and the peeled adventitia are then fixed along the anastomotic margin with continuous sutures. The aorta and distal arteries are occluded with balloon catheters, after which the anastomosis is performed between a graft and the mesh-reinforced adventitia with continuous sutures.

Results.—There were no anastomotic complications or operative deaths in the 9 patients, and satisfactory mid term results were obtained with follow-up from 3 to 62 months after surgery. There was 1 death from coronary heart disease 3 years after surgery without a graft-related complication.

Conclusion.—The anastomotic method is a safe and effective alternative to axillofemoral bypass in patients with porcelainized aorta.

▶ This seems a classic example of making something more difficult than it has to be. We have had good results with highly calcified vessels with a small handheld dental drill to facilitate passage of the needle through the aortic wall.

G. L. Moneta, MD

Treatment of Abdominal Aortic Anastomotic Pseudoaneurysm With Percutaneous Coil Embolization

Fann JI, Samuels S, Slonim S, et al (Stanford Univ, Calif; VA Palo Alto HCS, Stanford, Calif)
J Vasc Surg 35:811-814, 2002   17–3

Background.—Para-anastomotic pseudoaneurysm is a late complication of abdominal aortic reconstruction for occlusive or aneurysmal disease. These pseudoaneurysms and para-anastomotic true aortic aneurysms are associated with high morbidity and mortality rates. The case of a patient who underwent treatment with coil embolization of an intra-abdominal pseudoaneurysm at the distal anastomosis of a previously surgically repaired abdominal aortic aneurysm was described.

> *Case Report.*—Man, 76, was seen with chronic obstructive pulmonary disease with supplemental oxygen and steroid therapy, cor pulmonale, coronary artery disease with stable angina, hypothyroidism, and prostate carcinoma. He had had previous hormone and radiation therapy and had a history of right pneumonectomy for carcinoma. The patient had lower abdominal pain radiating to the back 4½ years earlier and had a CT-documented fusiform infrarenal abdominal aortic aneurysm. There was no evidence of rupture. This ini-

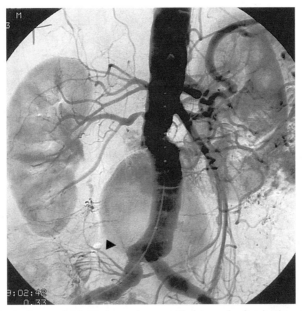

FIGURE 1.—Angiogram of abdominal aorta shows small leak (*arrowhead*) at distal anastomosis of aortic tube graft with enhancement of pseudoaneurysm. (Reprinted by permission of the publisher from Fann JI, Samuels S, Slonim S, et al: Treatment of abdominal aortic anastomotic pseudoaneurysm with percutaneous coil embolization. *J Vasc Surg* 35:811-814, 2002. Copyright 2002 by Elsevier.)

tial aneurysm was surgically repaired with a transperitoneal approach. The patient was then readmitted 13 months later with a 1-month history of mild abdominal pain and a pulsatile abdominal mass.

A pseudoaneurysm was diagnosed on angiography (Fig 1). Endovascular coil embolization was attempted because of the small size of the defect. Postprocedure angiographic results showed complete exclusion of the pseudoaneurysm (Fig 2). The patient's abdominal pain resolved 24 hours after embolization. Follow-up CT showed no flow and no contrast extravasation into the excluded pseudoaneurysm. At 3.5 years after coil embolization, an abdominal duplex US scan showed an excluded aneurysm sac measuring 5 cm with no flow into the sac.

▶ I cannot recommend coil embolization for treatment of anastomotic aneurysms. It seems to me a stent graft could have been easily placed to exclude the pseudoaneurysm.

G. L. Moneta, MD

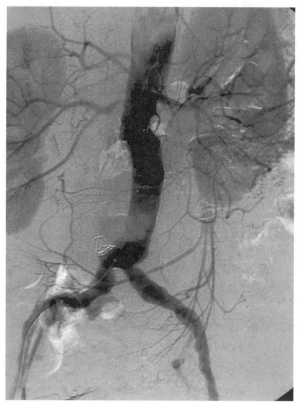

FIGURE 2.—Angiogram of abdominal aorta after coil embolization of site of leak at distal aortic anastomosis. Leak is no longer visualized. (Reprinted by permission of the publisher from Fann JI, Samuels S, Slonim S, et al: Treatment of abdominal aortic anastomotic pseudoaneurysm with percutaneous coil embolization. *J Vasc Surg* 35:811-814, 2002. Copyright 2002 by Elsevier.)

Retrograde Subintimal Angioplasty Via a Popliteal Artery Approach

Cutress ML, Blanshard K, Shaw M, et al (Leicester Gen Hosp, England)
Eur J Vasc Endovasc Surg 23:275-276, 2002   17–4

Background.—The use of percutaneous subintimal angioplasty for the treatment of long superficial femoral artery occlusions in patients with claudication or critical limb ischemia has been well described. However, failure of this procedure may result in therapeutic dilemmas. A technique involving popliteal artery puncture to recanalize these occlusions in a retrograde subintimal manner was described.

   Case Series.—Retrograde subintimal angioplasty via the popliteal artery was performed in 4 patients aged 71 to 77 years. Two patients had stable claudication, and 2 had critical ischemia caused by superficial femoral artery occlusions. In all of these patients, conventional antegrade subintimal angioplasty was unsuccessful. Entry into the subintimal space distal to the occlusion was obtained with a 0.035-inch-diameter angled guidewire in combination with a 5F catheter. The subintimal position of the guidewire was confirmed with injection of dilute contrast. The guidewire-catheter combination was then advanced to traverse the occlusion in a retrograde manner. The guidewire was then manipulated to enter the true lumen, and the catheter was replaced with a balloon catheter 5 to 6 mm in diameter and 8 cm long. Serial rapid inflations and deflations were performed throughout the length of the occluded segment and repeated once. This technique produced primary angioplasty success in all 4 patients, and there were no complications. Symptomatic and hemodynamic patencies were present in all patients 2 months after the procedures.

Conclusions.—Retrograde subintimal angioplasty may be an effective therapeutic technique for the treatment of patients not amenable to antegrade procedures. The need for reconstructive surgery in patients with claudication and critical ischemia can be avoided with this technique. Further evaluation of this technique is needed in studies of large numbers of patients with long-term follow-up to determine its durability and potential implications for clinical practice.

▶ The authors advocate this retrograde approach for subintimal angioplasty for patients who fail antegrade subintimal angioplasty or who are not technically suitable for antegrade subintimal angioplasty. There is currently a little flurry of interest in subintimal angioplasty. My prediction is that interest in both the antegrade and retrograde techniques will be a passing fad.

G. L. Moneta, MD

First Clinical Experience With an Anastomotic Device to Facilitate Aorto-mesenteric Saphenous Vein Bypass
Schmidli J, Heller G, Englberger L, et al (Univ Hosp, Berne, Switzerland)
J Vasc Surg 36:859-862, 2002   17–5

Background.—Manual suturing is the gold standard for construction of avascular anastomoses. However, the use of minimally invasive anastomotic devices in cardiac surgery has generated interest regarding whether this technique can be used with other vascular anastomoses. The first clinical experience with the aortic connector system during vascular surgery for a patient who needed aortomesenteric bypass with an autologous saphenous vein graft is described. One of the features of this system is its unique aortic cutter, a separate device with a rotating cutter blade, which is used to create a perfectly round hole in the aorta (Fig 5). After the cutter is removed with the core plug of aortic wall, bleeding from the circular defect in the aorta can be controlled with digital compression. The loaded aortic connector system is

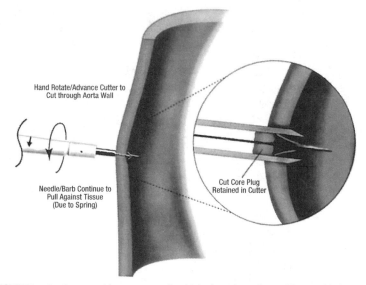

FIGURE 5.—Aortic cutter with puncture needle with barbs and round rotatable cutter blade creates hole through aorta. (Courtesy of St Jude Medical, Inc.) (Reprinted by permission of the publisher from Schmidli J, Heller G, Englberger L, et al: First clinical experience with an anastomotic device to facilitate aortomesenteric saphenous vein bypass. *J Vasc Surg* 36:859-862, 2002. Copyright 2002 by Elsevier.)

then inserted into the new aortic ostium (Fig 6). The connector is then released to construct the proximal anastomosis of the vein graft (Fig 7).

Case Report.—Woman, 53, had diffuse atherosclerosis and an end-to-side aortobifemoral bypass graft that eventually necessitated revision with a femorofemoral graft after one limb of the bifurcation graft became occluded. She also had recurrent episodes of abdominal pain, diarrhea, and weight loss. The patient had severe abdominal pain develop 2 weeks after the graft revision and had a blood leukocyte count of 30,000/mL. Critical mesenteric ischemia was believed to be the cause of the abdominal pain, so the patient was advised to

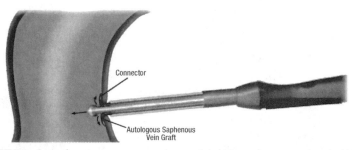

FIGURE 6.—Inserted aortic connector system into aortic hole. Internal struts are released with push of button at top of handle. (Reprinted by permission of the publisher from Schmidli J, Heller G, Englberger L, et al: First clinical experience with an anastomotic device to facilitate aortomesenteric saphenous vein bypass. *J Vasc Surg* 36:859-862, 2002. Copyright 2002 by Elsevier.)

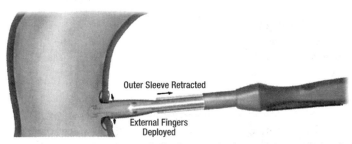

Outer Sleeve Retracted

External Fingers
Deployed

FIGURE 7.—Aortic connector system is pulled back. External and internal struts are deployed. (Courtesy of St Jude Medical, Inc.) (Reprinted by permission of the publisher from Schmidli J, Heller G, Englberger L, et al: First clinical experience with an anastomotic device to facilitate aortomesenteric saphenous vein bypass. *J Vasc Surg* 36:859-862, 2002. Copyright 2002 by Elsevier.)

undergo aortomesenteric revascularization. The procedure was performed with the sutureless aortic anastomosis of an aortosuperior mesenteric artery vein graft. The patient's postoperative course was uneventful. A postoperative arteriogram showed the aortomesenteric vein graft to be patent.

▶ I am worried the small anastomosis constructed with this device, combined with a 90° angle, might make the vein graft prone to kink when the mesentery returns to the anatomic position. The device seems better suited for aortorenal bypass, where there is less chance of kinking of the graft.

G. L. Moneta, MD

Endovascular Management of Iliac Limb Occlusion of Bifurcated Aortic Endografts
Bohannon WT, Hodgson KJ, Parra JR, et al (Southern Illinois Univ, Springfield)
J Vasc Surg 35:584-588, 2002   17–6

Background.—Iliac limb occlusion complicating aortic endografting is difficult to treat with surgical thrombectomy, as the graft may become dislodged or components may separate during thrombectomy. An endovascular approach to iliac limb occlusion in 3 patients with bifurcated aortic endografts is reported.

Patients and Outcomes.—The patients were 3 men, aged 61 to 75 years, who underwent placement of AneuRX bifurcated stent grafts for the treatment of abdominal aortic aneurysms. Two weeks to 5 months later, the patients had extremity pain and reduced ankle/brachial indices related to occlusion of the iliac limb of the endograft. All 3 cases were successfully managed with the use of the Angiojet thrombectomy catheter. In the first patient, who had a narrow aortic bifurcation with external compression of the endograft limb, a kissing balloon technique with bilateral brachial access was needed to dilate the bifurcation.

The other 2 patients had undergone treatment for common iliac artery aneurysms at the time of aortic endograft placement. In 1 of these, arterial access was via the ipsilateral common femoral artery. A left brachial approach was used in the third patient, who required an urgent open approach to the distal thromboembolus. However, the iliac limb was cleared by an endoluminal approach that avoided graft manipulation. All iliac limbs remained patent at 6 to 12 months' follow-up, with no evidence of endoleak or graft migration.

Conclusions.—For patients with acute occlusion of an iliac limb after bifurcated aortic endograft placement, an endovascular approach with the use of the Angiojet catheter can achieve successful recanalization. This technique avoids the risk of graft dislodgement associated with traditional thrombectomy approaches and minimizes reoperation in the ipsilateral groin. Distal thrombolysis or surgical thrombectomy may still be needed in patients with extensive thrombosis or emboli.

▶ Aortic endograft limb occlusions represent failure of the aortic endograft technique. Most such occlusions may be managed with endovascular techniques that involve some method of clot dissolution generally followed by placement of additional stents to treat the underlying lesions leading to the thrombosis. The authors employed a mechanical thrombectomy device for clot dissolution. Standard infusions of lytic agents probably work just as well.

G. L. Moneta, MD

Superior Mesenteric Artery-to-Renal Artery Bypass: A Rare but Useful Alternative for Renal Artery Revascularization

Jaroszewski DE, Fowl RJ, Stone WM (Mayo Clinic, Scottsdale, Ariz)
Ann Vasc Surg 16:235-238, 2002   17–7

Introduction.—The most frequently used inflow arteries for renal revascularization are the aorta, arteries of the celiac axis, and iliac arteries. When these arteries are diseased, the superior mesenteric artery (SMA) may be an alternative choice for renal artery graft inflow, although there is a theoretic risk of inducing mesenteric ischemia. A successful superior mesenterorenal artery bypass with the use of a normal caliber SMA was performed in a patient with left renal artery stenosis.

> *Case Report.*—Woman, 73, was seen for recent severe exacerbation of chronic hypertension that was poorly controlled despite 5 medications. A stent had previously been placed in a stenotic right renal artery, but a guidewire was not able to be placed across the 90% left renal artery stenosis. Angiography also showed a 60% to 70% celiac artery stenosis. The SMA was normal and had no signs of stenosis. Her aorta and iliac arteries were diffusely diseased, therefore the SMA was chosen as the inflow artery for a left renal artery graft. An end-to-side anastomosis between the SMA and a saphenous vein graft was accomplished with an end-to-end anastomosis to the left renal artery. A postoperative angiogram showed a widely

patent left superior mesenterorenal bypass graft. At 31 months' follow-up, the patient had no symptoms of mesenteric ischemia and her blood pressure was normal with only 3 medications.

Conclusion.—A normal diameter SMA may be used as an alternative inflow artery for renal artery revascularization without causing mesenteric ischemia.

▶ I don't see any reason why a normal SMA could not serve as an inflow source for renal revascularization. This falls into the category of something to keep in the back of your mind. It obviously is not anyone's first choice for inflow for a renal artery bypass.

G. L. Moneta, MD

Percutaneous Bedside Femorofemoral Bypass Grafting for Acute Limb Ischemia Caused by Intra-Aortic Balloon Pump

Lin PH, Bush RL, Conklin BS, et al (Baylor College of Medicine, Houston; Emory Univ, Atlanta, Ga)
J Vasc Surg 35:592-594, 2002   17–8

Background.—The complication rate associated with intra-aortic balloon pump (IABP) placement ranges from 8% to 18%, with complications including limb ischemia, pseudoaneurysm, ileofemoral artery dissection, thromboembolism, and localized wound infection, with acute lower limb is-

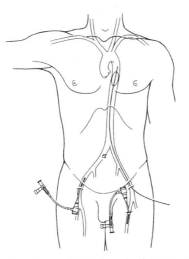

FIGURE 1.—With US scanning guidance, a 7F introducer sheath was inserted in an antegrade fashion in the superficial femoral artery just below the intra-aortic balloon pump catheter site. The contralateral common femoral artery was accessed percutaneously, and then a 9F introducer sheath was inserted in a retrograde fashion. (Reprinted by permission of the publisher from Lin PH, Bush RL, Conklin BS, et al: Percutaneous bedside femorofemoral bypass grafting for acute limb ischemia caused by intra-aortic balloon pump. *J Vasc Surg* 35:592-594, 2002. Copyright 2002 by Elsevier.)

chemia being the most common complication. When this complication occurs, a femorofemoral bypass graft is often necessary. This report presents a minimally invasive endovascular technique for creating a percutaneous temporary femorofemoral bypass graft at the bedside in patients with IABP-induced limb ischemia.

> *Technique.*—Before graft placement, it is necessary to ensure there is a palpable pulse in the donor (contralateral) common femoral artery. The superficial femoral artery in the ischemic limb is accessed with US scanning guidance, and the introducer sheath is inserted (Fig 1). Dilators are inserted into their respective introducer sheaths (Fig 3).
>
> A heparinized saline solution is connected and infused via the side port of the contralateral introducer sheath to maintain a partial thromboplastin time that is 1.5 times the baseline level. The IABP catheter is removed once the patient has been successfully weaned from it. The PTFE graft is test-clamped to ensure the ipsilateral foot remains adequately perfused before disconnection of the femoral graft and removal of the groin sheaths.

Results.—In patients with IABP-induced limb ischemia who were treated with percutaneous femorofemoral bypass grafting, there was no periprocedural morbidity or mortality. This approach was successful in resolving IABP-induced limb ischemia in all patients. At a mean follow-up of 7 ± 4.8

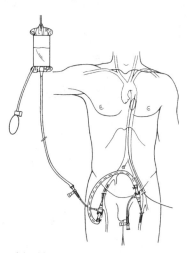

FIGURE 3.—The insertion of the dilator into the introducer sheath kept the 1-way valve open, which established a femorofemoral bypass graft from the contralateral common femoral artery to the ipsilateral ischemic superficial femoral artery. A heparinized saline solution was infused via the side port of the contralateral introducer sheath to maintain a prothrombin time 1.5 times the baseline level. (Reprinted by permission of the publisher from Lin PH, Bush RL, Conklin BS, et al: Percutaneous bedside femorofemoral bypass grafting for acute limb ischemia caused by intra-aortic balloon pump. *J Vasc Surg* 35:592-594, 2002. Copyright 2002 by Elsevier.)

months, there was no recurrent ischemia, limb loss, or groin-related infection.

Conclusion.—This report describes a percutaneous endovascular technique for creation of a temporary femorofemoral bypass graft to relieve acute leg ischemia caused by placement of an intra-aortic balloon pump. This temporary bypass grafting technique may eliminate the potential for graft infection or wound complications associated with a formal femoro-femoral bypass grafting.

▶ The authors utilize this technique in 4 patients and left the external femoral-femoral bypass in place for up to 5 days. Ideally the arteries in the donor groin are normal to minimize the chance of what we term an "ischemia transfer," that is, improving the bad leg at the expense of the good leg.

G. L. Moneta, MD

Initial Experience With Dorsal Venous Arch Arterialization for Limb Salvage

Rowe VL, Hood DB, Lipham J, et al (Univ of Southern California, Los Angeles)
Ann Vasc Surg 16:187-192, 2002   17–9

Background.—Unfortunately, conventional surgical options are not available for arterial reconstruction of lower extremity arterial disease when a distal arterial target is not available. The efficacy of a new technique for limb salvage, dorsal venous arch arterialization (DVAA), is discussed.

Methods.—Between February and October 2000, 6 patients (ages 27-64 years) with 7 affected limbs underwent DVAA. All had a lower extremity arteriogram and a tibia/plantar artery duplex scan showing unreconstructable arterial disease. The DVAA method was used for each patient and included the use of a retrograde balloon catheter, arterial dilator disruption, and a direct valvulectomy. Variables assessed to determine clinical outcomes were patency, limb salvage rate, and changes in toe pressure.

Results.—At a mean follow-up of 4.7 months, 71.5% of the grafts remained patent. The mean toe pressure measures increased by 211% from 21.3 mm Hg preoperatively to 45.4 postoperatively. The limb salvage rate was 86%. None of the patients died. Two early graft failures occurred, 1 at day 1 and the other at 1.5 months, both in patients with Buerger's disease.

Conclusions.—These preliminary findings suggest that DVAA may be a viable option for end-stage limb salvage.

▶ Arterialization of the venous system to treat limb ischemia continues to pop up once in a while in the vascular literature. It reflects both the human propensity for optimism over logic and the dangers of drawing big conclusions from small series. No conclusions regarding efficacy are possible from a series this size; the best one can hope is that "it doesn't hurt too much." If you are going to try this, it appears important to ensure lyses of the venous valves in the venous arch and to inform the patient that, at least initially, they will have a swollen, blue foot.

G. L. Moneta, MD

Microtibial Embolectomy

Mahmood A, Hardy R, Garnham A, et al (Univ Hosp Birmingham NHS Trust, England)
Eur J Vasc Endovasc Surg 25:35-39, 2003   17–10

Background.—The optimal management of acute arterial occlusion of the crural and pedal vessels has not been elucidated. Surgical thromboembolectomy, bypass reconstruction, and percutaneous intra-arterial thrombolysis are the most frequently performed procedures. However, surgery is the procedure of choice in patients with a severely ischemic limb in whom immediate revascularization is required or thrombolysis is contraindicated. Microtibial embolectomy is a useful technique in patients with limb-threatening acute arterial occlusion affecting native crural and pedal vessels, particularly when thrombolysis is contraindicated or ineffective. For example, thrombolysis may not be effective in the presence of old, well-organized clot or athero-emboli originating from ruptured vessel wall plaque ("trash"). An experience with microtibial embolectomy was reviewed.

Methods.—A retrospective case note review was conducted to evaluate the efficacy of microtibial embolectomy in a series of patients who were treated from 1990 to 1999. The data collected included the causes and degree of ischemia, additional procedures required, vessel patency, limb salvage, and complications.

Results.—Exploration of the crural/pedal vessels with ankle-level arteriotomies was conducted in 22 limbs in 12 patients under local anesthesia, in 9 patients under general anesthesia, and 1 patient under epidural anesthesia. The causes of ischemia were cardiac emboli in 8 patients, "trash foot" in 7 patients, emboli from aortic and popliteal aneurysms in 3 patients, and thrombotic occlusion of crural vessels in 4 patients. At up to 5 years of follow-up, the vessel patency rate was 69% and the limb salvage rate was 62%. Of the 7 patients with trash foot, 6 were salvaged. In the remaining patient, amputation was required at 3 months postoperatively. The 30-day mortality rate was 22%.

Conclusions.—Microtibial embolectomy is an effective treatment for acute occlusion of the crural/pedal arteries, including trash foot, and provides the potential for limb salvage to a large proportion of patients.

▶ The best patients for this procedure are those with acute embolism and intact pulses to the ankle. I suspect patients with chronic tibial and pedal artery disease would not do well. Apparently, none of the patients in this series had diabetes or chronic renal failure. Transverse arteriotomy with primary closure using interrupted 8-0 sutures worked as well as a longitudinal arteriotomy with patch closure.

G. L. Moneta, MD

Obturator Bypass: A Classic Approach for the Treatment of Contemporary Groin Infection
Patel A, Taylor SM, Langan EM III, et al (Greenville Hosp System, SC)
Am Surg 68:653-659, 2002   17–11

Introduction.—Infectious groin problems in vascular surgery often involve foreign prosthetic material or remnants of percutaneous femoral closure devices. The use of extra-anatomical bypass through the obturator foramen (obturator bypass) as an approach for treating limb ischemia after an arterial groin infection was evaluated.

Methods.—Between July 1992 and June 2001, 12 patients with severe vascular infections of the groin underwent obturator bypass surgery. Nine patients had isolated vascular graft infections, and 3 infections occurred after percutaneous interventional femoral access procedures. Six patients had systemic sepsis and draining sinuses, 2 had infected pseudoaneurysms, and 4 had bleeding. Treatment included debridement of the groin wound, sartorius muscle flap coverage of the femoral vessels, antibiotics, and synthetic obturator bypass with the use of the following: lower abdominal extraperitoneal incision from an aortobifemoral bypass graft limb to the superficial femoral artery in 6 patients, native iliac to femoral artery in 3 patients, iliac to popliteal artery in 2 patients, and aortobifemoral bypass limb to the popliteal artery in 1 patient. Graft patency and limb salvage were determined.

Results.—Two deaths occurred secondary to multisystem organ failure on postoperative days 6 and 9. There were 4 major complications that necessitated reoperation within the first 30 postoperative days. At a mean follow-up of 37 months, there were 10 survivors (83%) in whom groin wounds healed and were infection free. Graft patency at 60 months was 80%, and limb salvage was 60%. Late graft infections did not occur.

Conclusion.—The obturator bypass is effective and durable in revascularization of the septic groin.

▶ Vascular surgeons need to be aware of this technique in the management of arterial infection in the groin. I think, however, in modern practice all but the most extensive infections can be managed with arterial debridement and a femoral vein graft combined with muscle flap coverage.

G. L. Moneta, MD

Cutting Balloon Percutaneous Transluminal Angioplasty for Salvage of Lower Limb Arterial Bypass Grafts: Feasibility

Engelke C, Morgan RA, Belli A-M (St George's Hosp, London)
Radiology 223:106-114, 2002   17–12

Introduction.—Conventional percutaneous transluminal angioplasty (PTA) has poor durability when applied to neointimal hyperplastic lesions in peripheral arterial bypass grafts. Cutting-balloon PTA was evaluated as a new nonsurgical treatment option in this situation.

Methods.—Cutting-balloon PTA was used to treat a total of 16 anastomotic stenoses of infrainguinal bypass grafts in 15 patients (9 men, 6 women; mean age, 71 years). Seven patients had prosthetic grafts, 2 had prosthetic-vein composite grafts, 5 had venous grafts, and 1 had an ileofemoral stent-graft. After cutting-balloon PTA, conventional PTA was performed to increase the anastomotic diameter. In patients with stenotic vein grafts, cutting-balloon PTA was performed after conventional PTA had failed; in the rest, cutting-balloon PTA was performed as a primary procedure. The study definition of success was a greater than 50% improvement in the luminal diameter or a residual stenosis of no greater than 20%.

Results.—In 6 of 6 cases, attempts to perform conventional PTA before cutting-balloon PTA failed. The technical success rate of cutting-balloon PTA was 94%: just 1 failure occurred, with no clinical complications. At 5 to 7 months' follow-up, 2 cases of local restenosis and 1 of graft occlusion occurred. The 6-month primary graft patency rate was 84%, and the secondary patency rate was 92%. At 12 and 18 months, primary and secondary graft patency rates were 67% and 83%, respectively (Fig 3).

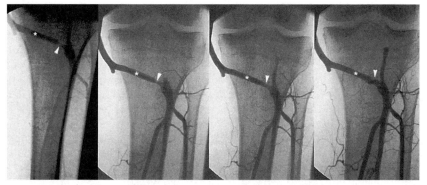

FIGURE 3.—Posterior unsubtracted angiograms show a femoropopliteal vein bypass graft (*) with distal anastomosis below the knee. **Far left,** Image shows a distal anastomotic stenosis (*arrowhead*). **Left middle,** Image shows the result of initial conventional PTA with 6-mm diameter balloon that failed to dilate the rigid stenosis (*arrowhead*) of neointimal hyperplasia. **Right middle,** Image shows the result after subsequent cutting-balloon PTA with 4.0-mm diameter balloon that achieved partial dilatation of the resistant stenosis (*arrowhead*). **Far right,** Image shows the final result after subsequent conventional PTA that achieved normal vessel diameter (*arrowhead*), which was maintained during a follow-up of 4 months. (Courtesy of Engelke C, Morgan RA, Belli A-M: Cutting balloon percutaneous transluminal angioplasty for salvage of lower limb arterial bypass grafts: Feasibility. *Radiology* 223:106-114, 2002. Radiological Society of North America.)

Conclusions.—This experience demonstrates the feasibility of cutting-balloon PTA for patients with neointimal hyperplasia causing stenosis of peripheral arterial bypass grafts. Cutting-balloon PTA may offer a higher technical success rate and a higher short-term patency rate than conventional PTA of infrainguinal bypass grafts. This technique could offer a new alternative to atherectomy and conventional PTA for salvage of infrainguinal bypass grafts.

▶ The authors exhibit either remarkable courage or remarkable stupidity in using this technique to treat stenoses occurring at a prosthetic graft to native artery anastomosis. It is generally believed the prevention of pseudoaneurysms at prosthetic graft native artery anastomoses requires an intact suture line. There are 3 possibilities for the authors' patients apparently not developing pseudoaneurysms: (1) the authors were lucky and didn't cut the suture; (2) the assumption that an intact suture line is required is incorrect; or (3) not enough time has gone by. At this time, I don't recommend this device for anastomoses involving prosthetic grafts.

G. L. Moneta, MD

Intraoperative Lidocaine Injection Into the Carotid Sinus During Endarterectomy
Maher CO, Wetjen NM, Friedman JA, et al (Mayo Clinic, Rochester, Minn)
J Neurosurg 97:80-83, 2002   17–13

Introduction.—Many surgeons inject the carotid sinus with a local anesthetic agent at the time of endarterectomy to alleviate intraoperative and postoperative hemodynamic instability. The influence of carotid sinus injection with lidocaine on perioperative hemodynamics and complications was prospectively examined in 92 consecutive patients who underwent carotid endarterectomies performed by a single surgeon.

Methods.—The mean age of 58 men and 42 women was 69.3 years (range, 45-78 years). Eight procedures were bilateral. Patients were randomly assigned to either injection of 0.5 mL of 1% lidocaine into the carotid sinus nerve or to no injection of lidocaine before arteriotomy. All patients were treated postoperatively with the use of a standard endarterectomy protocol.

Results.—No significant between-group differences were found in the incidence of hypertension, hypotension, or the use of vasoactive medications in the operating room after restoration of carotid artery (CA) blood flow, in the recovery room, or in the ICU.

Conclusion.—Injection of lidocaine into the carotid sinus at the time of an endarterectomy is not correlated with a significant improvement in any hemodynamic measures from the time of restoration of CA blood flow to post-operative day 1.

▶ The authors found that routine injection of the carotid sinus with lidocaine at the time of carotid endarterectomy is worthless in preventing hemodynamic instability associated with carotid endarterectomy. I agree and don't use this technique except for about once every 2 years to treat bradycardia arising during dissection of the artery.

G. L. Moneta, MD

Duplex Scan–Directed Placement of Inferior Vena Cava Filters: A Five-Year Institutional Experience

Conners MS III, Becker S, Guzman RJ, et al (Vanderbilt Univ, Nashville, Tenn)
J Vasc Surg 35:286-291, 2002   17–14

Introduction.—Placement of an inferior vena cava (IVC) filter at the bedside may have important advantages for critically ill patients. A large experience with bedside IVC filter placement under duplex scan guidance is reviewed.

Methods.—This 5-year experience included 284 patients undergoing duplex-directed IVC filter placement (Fig 2). In addition to chart review, the study included follow-up data collected by questionnaire and telephone interview.

Findings.—The patients were 203 men and 81 women (mean age, 41 years). Most patients had spinal cord injuries, closed head injuries, or multiple trauma. The review also identified 41 patients in whom duplex-directed IVC filter placement could not be carried out, for reasons such as poor visualization of the IVC, thrombosis, and unsuitable anatomy. In 83% of pa-

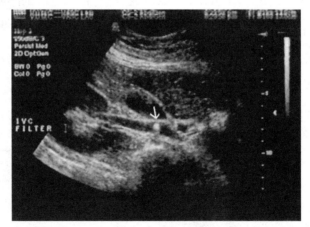

FIGURE 2.—Greenfield filter tip (*arrow*) at right renal vein–inferior vena cava junction. (Reprinted by permission of the publisher from Conners MS III, Becker S, Guzman RJ, et al: Duplex scan–directed placement of inferior vena cava filters: A five-year institutional experience. *J Vasc Surg* 35:286-291, 2002. Copyright 2002 by Elsevier.)

tients undergoing filter placement, the indication was venous prophylaxis without current thromboembolism. Another 12% had contraindications to anticoagulation, 7% had current thromboembolism, and 3% had complications of anticoagulant therapy.

None of the patients died of causes related to the procedure, and none had sepsis. A 4% rate of technical complications occurred, including filter misplacement, access thrombosis, filter migration, bleeding, and IVC occlusion. One patient with a misplaced filter subsequently had pulmonary emboli. Hospital charges for duplex-directed filter placement were significantly lower than those for fluoroscopic placement.

Conclusions.—This 5-year experience supports the use of duplex US-directed placement of IVC filters at the bedside. Complication rates are similar to those of fluoroscopic filter placement, and the procedure has the advantages of convenience, reduced radiation exposure, and avoidance of IV contrast.

▶ The authors have amassed a large experience with US guidance for placement of IVC filters, most of which were placed for the marginal indication of prophylaxis. A word of caution is needed. Since most of the patients did not have deep venous thrombosis, the likelihood of running into unexpected iliac vein thrombus is low. The authors used US to try and rule out iliac thrombus before placement but isolated iliac vein thrombus is unusual. I doubt they can reliably achieve excellent visualization with US of the iliac veins in critically ill ICU patients. The low complication rate may therefore reflect their patient population. In patients with known deep venous thrombosis, I think a pre-placement contrast study would be safer.

G. L. Moneta, MD

Retroperitoneoscopic Lumbar Sympathectomy
Beglaibter N, Berlatzky Y, Zamir O, et al (Hadassah Univ, Jerusalem)
J Vasc Surg 35:815-817, 2002   17–15

Background.—Lumbar sympathectomy is effective in relieving vasomotor tone, increasing blood flow through collateral vessels, and interrupting afferent pain pathways. This procedure is indicated in patients with nonreconstructable peripheral vascular disease as a means to slow or limit gangrene in thromboangiitis obliterans (Buerger's disease) and in vasospastic disorders (such as Raynaud's disease). Lumbar sympathectomy may also be indicated in patients with severe hyperhydrosis, frostbite, or reflex sympathetic dystrophy (RSD; causalgia). The application of the principles of balloon-assisted total preperitoneal groin hernia repair to the performance of retroperitoneoscopic lumbar sympathectomies is reported.

Methods.—A series of 27 consecutive unselected patients (21 men, 6 women; mean age, 45 years; range, 21-28 years) underwent 29 successful retroperitoneoscopic lumbar sympathectomies. Ischemia of the lower limb was present in 22 patients, and severe reflex sympathetic dystrophy was present in 5 patients. The retroperitoneal space was developed with a balloon trocar inserted through a small incision in the patient's flank. Additional trocars were used for endoscopic instruments. The sympathetic chain from second lumbar vertebrae to the fourth lumbar vertebrae was resected.

Results.—Retroperitoneoscopic lumbar sympathectomy was successfully performed in all 27 patients, with no operative or postoperative complications. The mean operative time was 136 minutes, and the mean duration of hospital stay was 1.4 days. All of the patients showed significant improvement in pain or dystrophic changes.

Conclusions.—Retroperitoneoscopic lumbar sympathectomy is a new technique that combines the advantages of minimally invasive surgery and the proved effectiveness of open sympathectomy.

▶ This innovative procedure is further testimony to the ingenuity and inventiveness of surgeons skilled in the use of the laparoscope. Although one cannot argue with the technical success of the described procedure, I would point out that the general length of time required to perform this procedure is long, compared with a standard, straightforward retroperitoneal lumbar sympathectomy. Moreover, I am somewhat surprised by the number of procedures performed, although the time interval is not reported. I question whether this procedure is truly preferable to percutaneous chemical sympathectomy, which in experienced hands has similar results and is less invasive than open or retroperitoneoscopic sympathectomy. Since the number of sympathectomies performed by any vascular surgeon is relatively small, it seems unlikely to me that this procedure will receive widespread acceptance. In my own practice, percutaneous, chemical sympathectomy will remain the procedure of choice.

F. B. Pomposelli, Jr, MD

Subject Index

A

Author Index